Mind-Body Practices in Healthcare

Edited by Marcelo Saad and Roberta de Medeiros

Published in London, United Kingdom

Mind-Body Practices in Healthcare
http://dx.doi.org/10.5772/intechopen.1006761
Edited by Marcelo Saad and Roberta de Medeiros

Contributors
Ananda Balayogi Bhavanani, Asaf Gitler, Brittany Heavens, Carmit Katz, Danica Anderson, Elena Borodulina, Engin Büyüköksüz, Ines Tchienga, Ingunn Hagen, Marcelo Saad, Monika Pathania, Nadine J. Pelling, Navdeep Ahuja, Olga Kozlova, Olga Maslova, Praag Bhardwaj, Priyanka Pathak, Proshanto Kr. Saha, Ratna Jyothi Kakumanu, Roberta de Medeiros, Shivani Patil, Simi Gogoi, Vasiliy Pyatin, Yori Gidron, Yosef Kula

First published in London, United Kingdom, 2025 by IntechOpen
IntechOpen is the global imprint of INTECHOPEN LIMITED, registered in England and Wales, registration number: 11086078, 167-169 Great Portland Street, London, W1W 5PF, United Kingdom

For EU product safety concerns: IN TECH d.o.o., Prolaz Marije Krucifikse Kozulić 3, 51000 Rijeka, Croatia, info@intechopen.com or visit our website at intechopen.com.

British Library Cataloguing-in-Publication Data
A catalogue record for this book is available from the British Library

Mind-Body Practices in Healthcare
Edited by Marcelo Saad and Roberta de Medeiros
p. cm.
Print ISBN 978-1-83635-073-6
Online ISBN 978-1-83635-072-9
eBook (PDF) ISBN 978-1-83635-074-3

Meet the editors

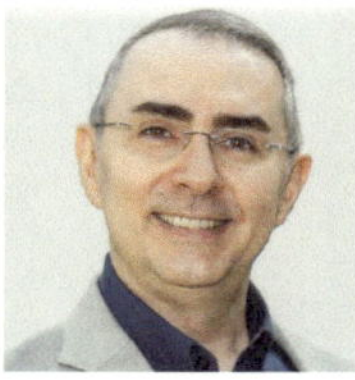

Marcelo Saad, MD, Ph.D., is a board-certified physician in Rehabilitation Medicine and Acupuncture. He earned his doctorate in Rehabilitation Sciences at the Federal University of S. Paulo (Brazil). He is the current director of the Spiritist-Medical Association of S. Paulo and coordinator of the Research Department at the Brazilian Spiritist-Medical Association. As an independent researcher, he is also engaged in event organization, scientific publication, editorial collaborations with journals and books, technical lectures, and scholarly tasks. His primary fields of interest are religiosity in healthcare, anomalous phenomena of consciousness, and complementary spiritual therapies.

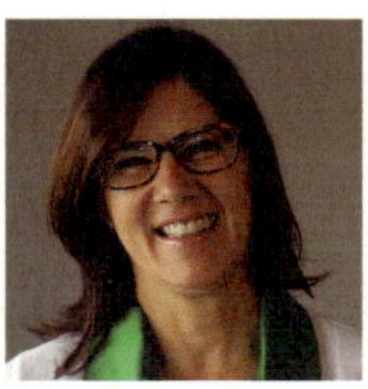

Roberta de Medeiros, Ph.D., is a biologist who holds a doctorate in Comparative Physiology from Universidade Estadual Paulista (Botucatu, Brazil). She has experience in teaching and research in Neurophysiology and Human Physiology, both in undergraduate (Medicine, Biomedicine, Nutrition, Physiotherapy, Occupational Therapy, and Psychology) and postgraduate courses. She is an Associate Professor of Human Physiology at Universidade Santo Amaro (S. Paulo, Brazil). Her original research field was neural plasticity, but recently she has dedicated herself to studying the relationship between spirituality and human health.

Contents

Preface

An important principle of the Hippocratic precept is "Vis Medicatrix Naturae" (the curative power of nature), meaning the organism can often heal itself. Under this view, most of the physician's role is to support this innate tendency. Mind and body relations indubitably play important roles in human health, disease and healing. Safe, low-cost mind-body interventions have shown potential to support clinical treatment, and clinicians could encourage them more often. In 2017, the editors wrote a paper [1] with thoughts on mind-body dynamics. We reproduce below some highlights of the text:

- The next medical frontier will certainly involve questions: What are all the relationships between mind and body, and how can they be explored in clinical practice?

- An earlier interpretation placed mind and body as two distinct entities, with a few minor relationships, emphasizing biology.

- Today, the concept has evolved to consider mind and body as two components of the same entity, with many significant relationships.

- Mind and body may have deeper connections, such as those supported by ancient practices, religious traditions, and contemplative approaches.

- To paraphrase Shakespeare (in Hamlet): we could say "there are more things in mind and body than are dreamt of in our philosophy".

The purpose of this work is to contribute to progress towards a more integrative future. The current book aims to present academically reliable and clinically useful information. All the chapters closely correlate with the book's theme, making a valuable contribution to our project. Most texts address subjects rarely discussed in the academic environment and seldom forgotten in healthcare education. Some chapters present theoretical frameworks, supported by pertinent scientific literature, while others present original empirical results and professional experience. The academic world will benefit from such contributions by authors from diverse continents and different cultural perspectives.

The first book section, entitled "Mind-Body Modalities", aims to introduce techniques that may be unfamiliar to many readers. The description of contents below is in the order of the chapters in the summary:

- Kakumanu presents a theoretical framework that reinforces a holistic mind paradigm and foresees clinical applications. The author discusses how Abhidhamma, a Buddhist doctrine, offers a new perspective for cognitive processing and sensory perception.

- Saha, Pathak and Gogoi address the treatment of substance use disorders. The authors examine the intersections between conventional therapeutics and holistic approaches. The work is constructed on a scholarly framework that is corroborated by pertinent scientific literature.

- Ahuja, Pathania and Bhardwaj made a literature review on the physiological and clinical benefits of Yoga Nidra. The authors prospect the ancestral history of the technique and accumulated empirical knowledge. A valuable collaboration with the Indian perspective on a health-promoting practice.

- Saad and de Medeiros wrote a chapter based on the authors' experience of 25 years of study in spirituality in healthcare, sustained by recent literature about this issue. The text suggests objective guidelines for practical use for healthcare professionals and institutions.

- Pelling reviews the challenges of people with communication disorders practicing meditation. The author explores the sensory characteristics in different techniques and suggests alternatives that provide inclusion.

The second book section, entitled "Clinical Outcomes", aims to present results with potential clinical applications. The description of contents below is in the order of the chapters in the summary:

- Patil presents the results of a spiritual practice for mental health. The author examines the impact of Sahaja Yoga, suggesting that the self-realization it fosters could be a mechanism for increasing resilience among young adults.

- Gitler, Kula, Katz and Gidron approach techniques for stress management in children and adolescents under anxiogenic situations. It has the merit of suggesting and explaining accessible techniques for clinical practice. The knowledge could be helpful for caregivers in war zones or developing countries.

- Hagen and Bhavanani address the therapeutic potential of a specific yoga stream. The authors discuss their experience with a university course based on the principles they studied. The work is a theoretical framework grounded in personal experience and supported by previous publications.

- Anderson ventures into the relationship between biology and sociology in trauma healing for war crimes victims. The author advocates incorporating this knowledge to create effective interventions and preventions. The author's professional experience corroborates the data.

- Pyatin, Borodulina, Kozlova and Maslova wrote on an original, prospective, quantitative study, exploring factors associated with procedural pain in children. A better knowledge of this issue should favor therapeutic acceptance and may have immediate clinical application.

- Büyüköksüz advocates for the role of Acceptance and Commitment Therapy and self-compassion as interventions for psychosomatic disorders. The author synthesizes current literature, offering a structure for incorporating these approaches for practical purposes.

- Tchienga and Heavens address a way of offering mind-body interventions for patients with neurodegenerative disorders. The authors discuss the role of neuropsychological assessments in individualizing the choice of the most viable techniques for each case.

In short, congratulations on your interest in this work, which the editors hope readers will find helpful and enjoyable!

Marcelo Saad
Director,
Spiritist Medical Association,
Sao Paulo, Brazil

Roberta de Medeiros
Universidade de Santo Amaro,
Sao Paulo, Brazil

References

[1] Saad M, de Medeiros R. The continuum of mind-body interplay—from placebo effect to unexplained cures. Medical Science and Healthcare Practice. 2017;**1**(1):1-9. DOI: 10.22158/mshp.v1n1p1

Section 1

Mind-Body Modalities

Chapter 1

Perspective Chapter: Consciousness as Cause or Effect? Buddhist Abhidhamma Insights into Mind–Brain Dynamics and Wellbeing

Ratna Jyothi Kakumanu

Abstract

The *Abhidhamma*, a classical Buddhist doctrine, offers a profound understanding of *cognitive processing* and *sensory perception*, concepts formulated over 2700 years ago and recently reflected in modern *neuroscience*. It presents a sophisticated cognitive model in which consciousness (*citta*), mental factors (*cetasika*), and materiality (*rūpa*) co-arise and function in a causally interdependent manner. Central to this is the principle of *Paṭicca Samuppāda* (Dependent Origination), which articulates the reciprocal conditioning of mind and body across experiential and physiological dimensions. This chapter explores the convergence between *Abhidhamma's cognitive sequences* (*vīthi-citta*) and modern *neuroscientific models* of *sensory processing* and *motor responses*. By aligning *neural mechanisms* with traditional cognitive stages, it proposes an integrative framework bridging *contemplative insight* and *empirical science*. This synthesis reinforces a *holistic mind-body paradigm* and offers promising clinical applications, particularly for *psychosomatic disorders* and *altered states of consciousness*. Additionally, the Abhidhamma's emphasis on *mental training*—such as *Vipassana meditation*—aligns with findings in *neuroplasticity*, showing how *intentional mental states* reshape *neural architecture*. This integrated perspective contributes to evolving discussions on *consciousness*, *mental health*, and *well-being*, advocating for *ethically grounded therapeutic approaches* and inviting a rethinking of cognitive health through a *contemplative-scientific lens.*

Keywords: information processing, consciousness, cognition, neuroplasticity, mind-brain correlations, mind, Abhidhamma, cognitive neuroscience, Vipassana, mindfulness, psychosomatic, dependent origination, Tipitika, Buddhist doctrine, mind-matter relations

1. Introduction

This chapter explores the convergence between *Abhidhamma*—a classical *Buddhist doctrine*—and contemporary *neuroscience* in understanding *sensory perception, cognitive processing*, and *mind-body dynamics*. The *Abhidhamma* presents a refined model wherein *consciousness (citta), mental factors* (*cetasika*), and *materiality (rūpa)* co-arise through *Dependent Origination* (*Paṭicca Samuppāda*), emphasizing the *causal precedence of mind over matter*. By mapping its *cognitive sequences (vīthi-citta)* onto *neural pathways* involved in *sensory* and *motor processing*, this study proposes an *integrative framework* bridging *contemplative insight* and *empirical science*. It invites a rethinking of the *mind-brain relationship*, challenging *materialist assumptions* by questioning whether *consciousness* is the *cause or effect of brain activity*. The synthesis highlights *Abhidhamma's* relevance to *neuroplasticity*, particularly through *mental training practices* like *Vipassana*—and its implications for *psychosomatic medicine*. The study positions *consciousness* not merely as an epiphenomenon, but as a dynamic agent in shaping *neural* and *experiential realities*, inviting empirical inquiry into this *mind-over-matter hypothesis*.

1.1 The chapter outline

This chapter explores the parallels between neural mechanisms of sensory perception and motor responses, as described in contemporary neuroscience, and the cognitive sequences (*vīthi-citta*) elaborated in the Abhidhamma, the classical Buddhist analytical treatise on mind. Positioned within the growing scientific discourse on mind-matter interdependence, the chapter underscores Abhidhamma's conceptual depth and its relevance to modern neurobiological models. It further examines the potential of these ancient insights to inform integrative approaches to psychosomatic medicine, emphasizing the synergy between contemplative traditions and empirical science in promoting holistic health and well-being.

The chapter unfolds through the following sections:

- Doctrine of Abhidhamma
- Mind and Cognition in Abhidhamma
- Mind As the Sixth Sense Faculty
- Brain and Cognitive Processing in Neuroscience
- Consciousness and Cognitive Processing in Abhidhamma
- Neuroscience Meets Abhidhamma: Mapping Cognitive Processing
- Mind and Matter: A Converging View
- Summary and Implications

2. Doctrine of Abhidhamma: Introduction and significance

Pāḷi Canon, also known as the *Pāḷi Tipiṭaka* (meaning "three baskets"), is the canonical collection of scriptures in the Theravāda Buddhist tradition, preserved in the Pāḷi[1] language. This comprehensive repository contains the teachings and discourses attributed to the historical Buddha, which were initially transmitted orally and later written down in Pāḷi. The Canon is divided into three primary "baskets" or sections: the *Vinaya Piṭaka* (Doctrine of Monastic Rules), the *Sutta Piṭaka* (Doctrine of Conventional Teachings or Discourses), and the *Abhidhamma Piṭaka* (Doctrine of Higher Teachings), collectively known as the *Tipiṭaka*.

The *Abhidhamma Piṭaka* (translated as "Basket of Higher Doctrine") is the third division of the *Tipiṭaka*. For deep thinkers and scholars, it holds particular importance, as it contains the profound and complex philosophy behind the Buddha's teachings. This contrasts with the more accessible and practical discourses found in the Sutta Piṭaka. According to Bhikkhu Bodhi [1], a modern Theravāda scholar, the Abhidhamma is not only a philosophy but also a psychology and an ethics, all woven into a comprehensive framework aimed at liberation from suffering, whether gross or subtle. As the third basket, it provides a theoretical and analytical understanding of the Buddhist path, while the Vinaya and Sutta Piṭakas offer practical guidelines and teachings for monastics and lay practitioners. The Abhidhamma delves into the foundational principles governing mental and physical processes, offering a systematic analysis of Buddhist philosophy.

3. The role of the Abhidhamma Piṭaka in complementing the Sutta and Vinaya

A Deeper Theoretical and Practical Understanding of Buddhist Teachings.

- *Theoretical framework*:
    - The *Sutta Piṭaka* contains the Buddha's discourses (*sutta* meaning discourse), while the *Vinaya Piṭaka* focuses on monastic rules and practices (*Vinaya* meaning discipline). The *Abhidhamma Piṭaka*, in contrast, offers a deeper, more theoretical understanding of these teachings, elucidating the fundamental principles and processes that govern mental and physical reality.
- *Detailed analysis:*
    - The *Abhidhamma* provides a meticulous analysis of the Buddha's teachings, exploring the finer points of mental and physical phenomena. It offers a more systematic, detailed, and scholarly approach compared to the Suttas, addressing the intricate workings of the mind and matter.
- *Bridging theory and practice:*
    - The *Abhidhamma Piṭaka* acts as a bridge between the practical teachings found in the *Suttas* and *Vinaya* and the theoretical understanding of how these teachings function in practice. It provides the framework for understanding how mental processes and physical phenomena interact in the context of the Buddhist path [1].

[1] This chapter includes original Pāḷi terms with their closest English translations. Diacritics are used for Pāḷi words, guiding accurate pronunciation.

3.1 Significance of Abhidhamma Piṭaka in Theravāda Buddhism

- *Foundation for meditation and wisdom*:
    - The *Abhidhamma Piṭaka* is regarded as a crucial text for those seeking a deeper understanding and cultivation of wisdom through meditation. It offers a systematic analysis of the mind's workings, which is essential for advancing along the path of liberation.
- *Specialty for monks*:
    - Many Theravāda monks dedicate significant time to the study of the *Abhidhamma Piṭaka*, as it is considered an essential resource for developing a profound understanding of the *Dhamma* (the Law of Nature). Abhidhamma's analytical depth supports monastic discipline and meditation practice.

3.2 Key differences between the Abhidhamma Piṭaka and other Piṭakas

- *Not direct teachings*:
    - Unlike the *Sutta Piṭaka*, which contains direct discourses of the Buddha, the *Abhidhamma Piṭaka* is more focused on commentaries, analysis, and discussions that provide a detailed breakdown of the Buddha's teachings.
    - In the *Sutta Piṭaka*, terms like "individual," "being," "I," "you," and "man" are used terms that are familiar to laypersons. These terms serve as conventional labels to discuss the world. In contrast, the *Abhidhamma* uses more precise, scientific terminology to describe the definitive realities (paramāttha dhamma), preventing misinterpretations and ensuring clarity [2]
- *Four absolute "realities"*: The *Abhidhamma Piṭaka* focuses on the ultimate nature of reality, breaking down the components of existence into four essential factors:
    - *Citta*: Consciousness—defined as "knows" or "experiences" an object. Different types of *citta* represent distinct momentary states of consciousness.
    - *Cetasika*: Mental concomitants—these are the various mental factors that arise alongside *citta*, such as compassion, jealousy, anger, kindness, and generosity.
    - *Rūpa*: Physical phenomena or material form—this refers to the material elements or the physical body.
    - *Nibbāna*: The unconditioned mental state of liberation—the final goal of Buddhist practice, representing freedom from suffering and attachment [3].

3.3 Scholastic approach

The Abhidhamma stands out for its rational and scholastic methodology. Unlike the more narrative and contextual style of the Suttas, it adopts a systematic and analytical approach, examining mental and physical phenomena in meticulous detail. This tradition of inquiry is known as Vibajja Vāda—the Doctrine of Analysis [2].

It presents a thorough examination of the individual as a composite of mind[2] (Nāma) and body (Rūpa). Nāma encompasses all mental phenomena, including consciousness (Citta[3]) and associated mental factors (Cetasikas[4]), while Rūpa refers to the physical body, including the brain and other material elements, from the gross to the subtle. This analytical framework allows for a deep understanding of the mind-body process. When realized through introspective meditation, it leads to a liberated state—*Nibbāna*, the ultimate reality beyond suffering.

3.4 Focus on philosophical and psychological concepts

- The *Abhidhamma Piṭaka* delves deeper into philosophical and psychological concepts, offering an in-depth exploration of the nature of mind, consciousness, and material phenomena. Its meticulous examination of mental states and processes makes it an invaluable text for understanding the complexities of human experience, far beyond the more straightforward teachings in the Suttas.

4. Mind and cognition in Abhidhamma

Renowned for its analytical depth and clarity, the *Abhidhamma* offers a detailed and systematic model of the mind—one that intriguingly parallels insights from modern cognitive neuroscience. Integrating elements of philosophy, psychology, neurobiology, psychiatry, and ethics, it provides a comprehensive framework aimed at understanding and ultimately alleviating psychological suffering such as dissatisfaction, anxiety, and mental distress.

At its heart, the *Abhidhamma* delves deeply into conscious experience, examining awareness and its sensory and mental objects through precise introspection—resembling phenomenological methods. It emphasizes *vipassanā* (direct experiential insight) into how cognition, emotion, and perception operate, revealing the inner processes that shape our subjective reality [4].

A central feature of this model is the classification of discrete mental events known as *cittas*—individual moments of consciousness. Each *citta* represents the mind's basic unit of knowing or cognizing an object. However, *citta* never arises alone; it always co-arises with mental factors (*cetasikas*) and is shaped by both internal and external conditions.

Though each *citta* lasts for just a fleeting instant—performing a function such as seeing, hearing, or thinking, it is immediately followed by another, forming a rapid, continuous stream. This seamless succession creates the illusion of a stable, unified mind.

---

[2] Abhidhamma regards the mind as an inseparable blend of consciousness (citta) and mental factors (cetasika-s), which co-arise and function in unison.

[3] In the *Abhidhamma*, *citta* means *consciousness*—the moment the mind becomes aware of something. It's the knowing aspect of the mind—whether that's a sight, a sound, a thought, or a feeling.

[4] Cetasika-s are mental factors that accompany citta (consciousness) and shape cognition based on its type. Abhidhamma identifies 52 such factors, including seven universal (sādhāraṇa) ones present in all forms of consciousness (sabba-citta). Each cetasika has a distinct role in the cognitive process. Examples include perception, feeling, decision, energy, attention, wisdom, greed, compassion, and delusion.

Each *citta* is:

- *Ethically variable*: It may be wholesome (*kusala*), unwholesome (*akusala*), or result-bearing (*vipāka*) [5, 6].
- *Object-oriented:* Every *citta* takes an object—whether sight, sound, bodily sensation, or thought.
- *Function-specific:* Different *cittas* perform different roles in the cognitive process, such as adverting, receiving, investigating, judging, or responding.

The five sensory modalities—vision, hearing, smell, taste, and touch—serve as primary input channels, each associated with a corresponding *sense-door consciousness* (*dvāracitta*) that initiates information processing. This model offers a dynamic account of perception as a sequence of causally linked mental events, aligning introspective Buddhist psychology with modern principles of embodied cognition and brain-mind interdependence.

The *Abhidhamma* traditionally identifies *89 distinct cittas*, expanding to *121* when refined meditative absorptions and supramundane states are included.

5. The mind as the sixth sense faculty: A neurophenomenological insight from the Abhidhamma

A particularly distinctive contribution of the *Abhidhamma* lies in its identification of the mind (*manas*) as the sixth sense faculty (*mana-indriya*), which not only regulates but also integrates the functions of the five external sensory modalities: hearing, olfaction, gustation, and tactile sensation. This concept, while deeply rooted in early Buddhist psychology, anticipates certain aspects of contemporary theories in cognitive neuroscience, especially those related to central executive functions and multisensory integration. Yet, the centrality of the mind as a unifying perceptual faculty remains underrecognized in mainstream medical science.

The *Abhidhamma* goes beyond a mere enumeration of the senses; it offers a rigorous analysis of how consciousness (*citta*) interacts with material phenomena (*rūpa*) to produce a seamless, dynamic stream of subjective experience. This continuous interaction between mind and matter forms the very basis of perceptual reality. As Bhikkhu Bodhi *(2006c)* emphasizes, this process is essential for comprehending how the mind participates in the construction of the experiential world—a concept now echoed in enactive and embodied cognition theories in the philosophy of mind and neuroscience.

Unlike traditional Western science, which often prioritizes third-person objectivity and empirical detachment, the *Abhidhamma* advocates for direct, first-person inquiry. It invites practitioners to turn inward, using disciplined introspection and meditative observation to investigate the mind and body as the primary instruments of truth-seeking. The purpose is not theoretical abstraction but practical liberation (*vimutti*), freedom from suffering (*dukkha*) through experiential wisdom (*paññā*) [7]. Thus, its epistemology is fundamentally ethical and transformative.

The *Abhidhamma*'s portrayal of reality is not a speculative metaphysics but a phenomenological map—one shaped and validated by the purified cognition of an awakened mind. Its intricate breakdown of mental factors, cognitive processes, and sensory consciousness parallels many contemporary insights in neuropsychology, neurophenomenology, and affective neuroscience [8]. Remarkably, these insights were systematically outlined over 2800 years ago, underscoring the text's enduring relevance.

By positioning the mind as a central and integrative sense faculty, Abhidhamma offers a holistic framework for understanding perception, consciousness, and the construction of reality. Its convergence with modern scientific paradigms—particularly in the domains of sensory processing, self-modeling, and the embodiment of experience—reveals a deep compatibility between ancient contemplative science and cutting-edge neuroscience. This convergence opens new avenues for interdisciplinary dialog and offers a compelling vision for uniting inner experience with external observation in the study of consciousness.

6. Brain and cognitive processing in neuroscience

Neuroscience is the scientific study of the nervous system, focusing on how sensory systems—such as sight, hearing, touch, taste, and smell—process information from the environment. It delves into sensory information processing, examining the neural pathways and brain regions responsible for interpreting sensory input. Pioneers like Charles Sherrington and Santiago Ramón y Cajal have significantly advanced our understanding of how sensory signals are transmitted and integrated with the brain.

Information from both the internal and external environment activates the central nervous system through various sensory receptors located in the sense organs. These receptors function as transducers, converting different forms of environmental energy into action potentials in neurons. These energy forms include mechanical (e.g., touch or pressure), thermal (e.g., temperature), electromagnetic (e.g., light), and chemical energy (e.g., odor or taste). Each receptor is most sensitive to a specific form of energy, known as its "adequate stimulus." For example, the adequate stimulus for the photoreceptors in the eye is light [9].

In the context of vision, when an object enters the visual field, the light-sensitive photoreceptors (rods and cones) in the eye absorb light and trigger a sequence of events, initiating neural activity. This visual stimulus is converted into nerve signals that travel from the retina through the afferent pathways—the optic nerve, optic chiasm, and optic radiation—toward the primary visual cortex in the brain. Here, sensory information is processed, analyzed, and integrated with both cortical and subcortical brain areas. The motor areas then issue appropriate commands *via* efferent pathways, leading to motor responses through effector organs.

However, it is important to note that sensory impulses do not always lead to immediate motor responses; instead, they can be stored as part of the brain's learning and memory processes [9].

7. Consciousness and cognitive processing in Abhidhamma

In Abhidhamma, cognition is a dynamic process driven by a series of mental phenomena known as *citta*-s (moments of consciousness) and *cetasika*-s (mental factors). These elements work together to perceive and interpret objects. When no active cognitive process is occurring, the mind remains in a passive state, sustained by a continuous stream of *citta*-s called *bhavaṅga*-s.[5] This state functions as the resting or default mode of consciousness, maintaining mental continuity in the absence of external stimuli.

7.1 Citta-Vīthi: The cognitive process in Abhidhamma

In the *Abhidhamma*, *citta-vīthi* refers to the detailed sequence by which consciousness arises and flows when we experience an object—whether it is seen, heard, thought about, or felt. Every moment of experience involves a rapid succession of different *cittas* (moments of consciousness), each performing a specific function. Though each *citta* arises and ceases in a flash, together, they form a highly coordinated and purposeful cognitive sequence [10].

7.2 Two primary types of cognitive processes

- Sense-door process (pañca-dvāra-vīthi):

  Involves perception through the five senses—sight, sound, smell, taste, and touch.

- Mind-door process (mano-dvāra-vīthi):

  Involves mental objects such as thoughts, memories, emotions, and concept.

7.3 Cognitive sequence in the context of vision

When a stimulus—such as a visual form—appears, the ongoing stream of *bhavaṅga* (background or passive consciousness) is momentarily interrupted. This disruption marks the beginning of an *active cognitive process* called *vīthi-citta*, initiating a transition from passive awareness to active engagement.

For visual cognition to occur, four essential conditions must be met:

- *Eye sensitivity (Cakkhupasāda):* The visual faculty must be intact and receptive.
- *Visible object (Rūpārammaṇa):* An external form must be present to be seen.
- *Light (Āloka):* Adequate illumination is necessary for visual perception.
- *Attention (Manasikāra):* The mind must be directed toward the object.

If any of these factors are missing or compromised, visual cognition cannot take place. This illustrates the precision with which *Abhidhamma* analyzes perceptual mechanisms.

[5] *Bhavaṅga*, or life-continuum consciousness, is the passive flow of mind (bhavaṅga-sota) present when no active cognition occurs. During a cognitive process, this flow is momentarily disturbed (calana) and then cut off (upaccheda) by an arising stimulus. This interruption allows active consciousness to engage with the object. Once the process concludes, the mind returns to the bhavaṅga state until the next stimulus arises.

7.4 Stages of the visual cognitive process

- Five-door adverting consciousness (pañca-dvārāvajjana-citta)[6]:

  This marks the initial phase of the mental process, where the mind identifies the nature of a stimulus and determines which sense faculty it pertains to. The mind first directs its attention toward the sensory input, recognizing whether the stimulus is visual, auditory, or of another type, and then focuses on the corresponding sense door.

- Eye consciousness (cakkhu-viññāṇa):

  This citta arises in coordination with the visual faculty to register the incoming image in its raw form—without interpretation or meaning.

- Receiving consciousness (sampaṭicchana):

  Accepts and holds the sensory data for preliminary processing.

- Investigating consciousness (santīraṇa):

  Analyzes and inspects the object more deeply.

- Determining consciousness (votthapana):

  Makes a final evaluation, categorizing the object and preparing for an emotional or volitional response.

- The Javana phase: Ethical and Volitional Response

  Once the object has been identified, the Javana[7] cittas arise in rapid succession. These are the most ethically significant cittas, as they initiate volitional actions. Depending on the mental state, these actions can be:

  o *Wholesome (kusala)* – rooted in generosity, compassion, or wisdom

[6] *Pañca-dvārāvajjana-citta (Five-Door Adverting Consciousness) and mano-dvāra-vajjana-citta (Mind-Door Consciousness)* represent distinct yet interrelated mental functions within the cognitive process. Pañca-dvārāvajjana-citta (Five-Door Adverting Consciousness) and mano-dvāra-vajjana-citta (Mind-Door Adverting Consciousness) are distinct yet interrelated stages in cognition. The Five-Door Consciousness arises when an external stimulus contacts a sense door, identifies the type of stimulus, and directs attention to the relevant sense faculty, thereby initiating the corresponding sensory consciousness. Acting as a gatekeeper, it orients awareness toward external input. Mind-Door Consciousness follows, processing and experiencing the registered sensory input. It arises in response to purely mental phenomena and plays a crucial role in revisiting past experiences, attending to internally generated content, and engaging with ideas, thoughts, and mental images.

[7] *The javana phase* refers to the impulsive or decisive stage in a cognitive process, where the mind responds to an object with full force and ethical intention. In a typical process, this phase consists of seven consecutive javana cittas (mind-moments), each capable of generating kārmic results.

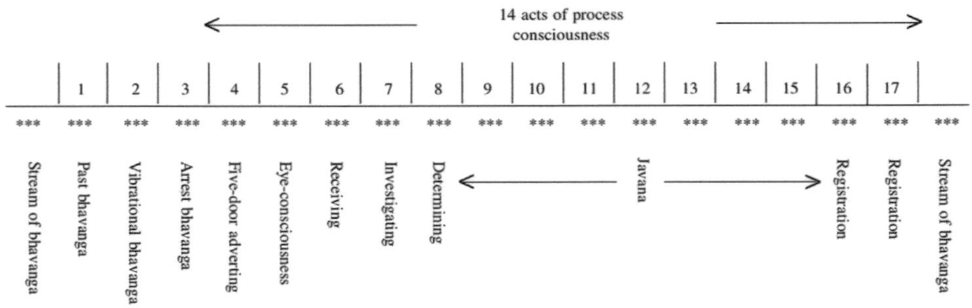

Figure 1.
A complete eye-door process [1]: In response to a visual stimulus, the continuous flow of the default consciousness (bhavanga) is momentarily interrupted, initiating a series of 17 citta (mind) moments. These cittas sequentially perform functions ranging from initial awareness and recognition to reaction or storage in memory. The number of cittas involved may vary depending on the significance and clarity of the visual object. Note: The triple asterisks (***) beneath the numbers represent the three sub-moments of each mind-moment: arising, presence, and dissolution.

- o *Unwholesome (akusala)* – driven by greed, aversion, or delusion

  The Javana phase gives rise to thoughts, speech, or bodily actions, each carrying kārmic consequences that shape future experiences.

- *Registering Consciousness*: *Final Phase* If the stimulus is significant, a *registering consciousness (tadārammaṇa-citta)* may arise briefly to retain the object in awareness. However, if the stimulus is deemed trivial, this stage might not occur. Once the entire process concludes, the mind naturally returns to its passive resting state—the *bhavaṅga* stream—until another stimulus interrupts it [11]

The *Abhidhamma*'s explanation of *citta-vīthi* offers a nuanced and systematic account of how perception unfolds—from sensory contact to ethical response. It captures both the structural and functional aspects of cognition, providing a sophisticated inner model of the mind. By tracing the emergence of awareness moment-by-moment, it reveals the layered complexity of perception, attention, evaluation, and volition (**Figure 1**).

This structured framework in the Abhidhamma provides a precise account of how visual perception evolves—from basic sensory contact to complex cognitive engagement and ethical response [2].

8. Neuroscience meets Abhidhamma: Mapping cognitive processing across traditions

Abhidhamma's portrayal of cognitive processes shows a striking alignment with contemporary neuroscience's understanding of sensory perception and cognition. Both frameworks begin with sensory input that triggers recognition and response, but while the Abhidhamma emphasizes mental activity through direct experience, neuroscience addresses these processes at the neural level.

In neuroscience, sensory processing initiates with afferent neural activity, starting with physiological changes in sensory organs like the retina. These changes generate nerve impulses that are transmitted to respective cortical regions for processing.

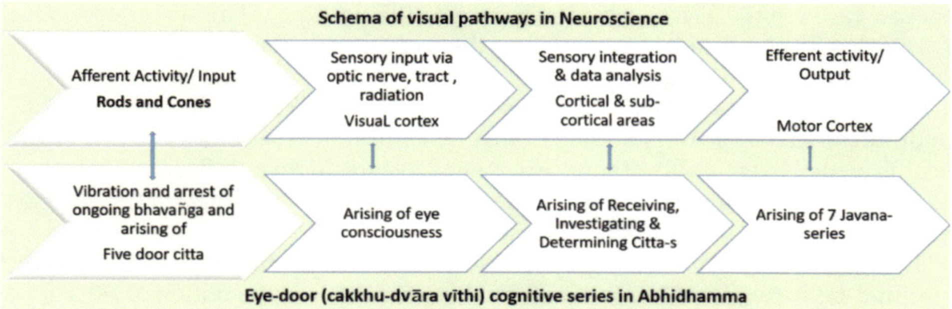

Figure 2.
Mapping of visual pathways with eye-door cognitive series [12]. The top row of the figure shows the visual sensory process as per neurosciences. The bottom row shows the corresponding cognitive series occurring for a visual object as per Abhidhamma tradition (Schematic representation).

This mirrors Abhidhamma's concept of the *citta* series, where sensory input culminates in the emergence of *eye-consciousness*, perceiving visual form.

As the brain integrates sensory information across cortical and subcortical regions, it mirrors the sequential processes outlined in the Abhidhamma: receiving, investigating, and determining *citta-s*. These stages reflect how the brain processes, evaluates, and interprets sensory input.

The efferent system, which transmits signals from the brain's motor areas to initiate physical actions, corresponds to the *Javana* series in the Abhidhamma. This series is central to the enactment of *kamma* (karma-action) through thoughts, bodily movements, or speech. Just as motor circuits in the brain control physical action, the *Javana* series drives the initiation of actions, both mental and physical, with corresponding outcomes.

Furthermore, the neural circuits involved in learning and memory work in harmony with the *registering function* of the *citta-s*, which consolidates and retains experiences. This process solidifies memories and shapes future responses based on prior experiences.

This mapping extends beyond vision to encompass all sensory modalities—smell, taste, hearing, and touch. Abhidhamma's comprehensive model of cognition thus resonates deeply with modern neuroscience, demonstrating its relevance across sensory processing. Its insights into consciousness, mind, and matter not only align with but often precede contemporary scientific findings (**Figure 2**) [12].

8.1 Mind and matter: A converging view from Abhidhamma and neuroscience

8.1.1 Interdependence of mind and body in Abhidhamma thought

Recent advances in neuroscience and embodied cognition have rekindled interest in the intricate interdependence between mental processes and bodily states. In Buddhist philosophy, this profound relationship is articulated through the doctrine of *Paṭicca Samuppāda* (Dependent Origination). While acknowledging the ontological distinction between mind and body, this foundational teaching asserts their dynamic and reciprocal co-arising [13, 14].

According to the Abhidhamma, a human being is composed of consciousness (*citta*), associated mental factors (*cetasika*), and material phenomena (*rūpa*), together forming the psycho-physical aggregate (*nāma-rūpa*). This integrated model affirms that lived experience is shaped by the mutual conditioning of mental and physical processes.

Paṭicca Samuppāda elaborates on this interdependence by showing how material conditions—such as sensory stimuli or neurochemical fluctuations—can give rise to specific mental events, while those very mental events, in turn, influence physiological responses, behaviors, and neural states. Thus, mentality and materiality exist in a loop of co-evolution, where neither exists in isolation.

The Abhidhamma offers a highly refined introspective framework that explores this mind-body relationship down to the subatomic level *via* the notion of *rūpa kalāpa*-s—fundamental units of materiality [15]. While a detailed exposition of these microstructures lies beyond this summary, their inclusion demonstrates how Buddhist thought seeks to understand consciousness as both embodied and dynamic.

8.1.2 A testable hypothesis: Do mental processes precede neural activity?

The prevailing view in neuroscience suggests that mental phenomena emerge from neural activity. In contrast, early Buddhist teachings—particularly the assertion that "mind precedes matter"—propose a compelling alternative: mental processes may precede, and even generate, neural activity [16–18]. Though the temporal gap may be infinitesimally small, this reversal of causality introduces a paradigm-shifting hypothesis.

In this model, mental events, whether they are consciously recognized or not—can give rise to patterns of neural activation. These patterns are not random but align with the nature and quality of the preceding mental process. Over time, repetition of specific mental states leads to deeply entrenched neural pathways, resulting in automatic, habitual, or instinctual responses—mental, verbal, or physical. What often appears as "hardwired" behavior may, in fact, be the cumulative product of sustained mental conditioning.

An apt analogy is that of a candle flame and its shadow. Although the flame and shadow appear to co-exist, the shadow is wholly dependent on the flame. Similarly, neural activity may represent the responsive "shadow" of a prior mental event rather than its origin.

This hypothesis harmonizes with current findings in neuroplasticity, which demonstrate that deliberate mental training can reshape the brain's structure and function. Practices such as *Vipassana* (Insight) meditation and Mindfulness practices—rooted in introspective and observation-sustained attention—gradually transform reactive patterns and rewire brain circuits [19, 20]. As mental phenomena evolve, so does neural architecture, indicating a bidirectional, and possibly asymmetric, influence between mind and brain.

8.1.3 Toward an integrative framework

Bridging the explanatory models of Abhidhamma and neuroscience brings us closer to resolving a foundational mystery of science: how conscious experience arises and interacts with material processes. By aligning Buddhist cognitive maps with empirical models of perception and integration, we gain deeper insights into how the mind processes sensory input, constructs reality, and regulates bodily responses.

This integrative framework has broad implications. In fields such as neuropsychiatry, contemplative psychology, and cognitive neuroscience, the mind-body relationship is increasingly seen as central to understanding health and behavior. Comparative studies between Abhidhamma and modern neuroscience offer nuanced interpretations of consciousness across its spectrum—from wakefulness and sleep to altered and near-death states.

Furthermore, this synergy opens promising therapeutic pathways. Understanding how mental processes influence neural activity can inform novel approaches for managing disturbed states such as insomnia, delirium, stupor, and coma. It also sheds light on affective dysregulation and maladaptive behaviors, offering new strategies rooted in both ancient wisdom and contemporary science.

9. Summary and future directions

Synthesizing insights from Abhidhamma and modern neuroscience reveals a compelling framework in which mind and brain are not merely co-existent phenomena but dynamically interlinked through potentially causal relationships. The proposition that *mental processes precede and shape neural activity* challenges dominant materialist paradigms and invites a paradigm shift in the study of consciousness.

This integrative model encourages interdisciplinary exploration—bringing together contemplative traditions, cognitive science, neurobiology, and philosophy of mind. If empirically supported, it could fundamentally reshape how we understand consciousness, volition, mental health, and the intricate dance between subjective experience and brain function.

Moreover, this hypothesis offers not only theoretical depth but also practical implications. It enriches the dialog between science and spirituality, paving the way for innovative clinical approaches grounded in both introspective wisdom and neuroscientific evidence. As we deepen our understanding of how consciousness functions, we move closer to cultivating holistic models of healing, resilience, and human flourishing.

9.1 Applications for clinical therapeutics, scientific innovation, education, and contemplative training programs

This model also holds significant potential for transforming education and therapeutic practices. By incorporating mindfulness and mental training techniques—such as Vipassana meditation—into educational curricula and therapeutic interventions, we can cultivate more adaptive and resilient neural pathways in individuals. These practices may enhance emotional regulation, cognitive flexibility, and mental well-being, offering valuable tools in mental health management, particularly for addressing psychosomatic conditions where mental processes influence physical health. Additionally, a deeper integration of mind-body principles in contemplative training can enhance self-awareness, emotional intelligence, and a profound understanding of the interconnectedness between mental and physical health. This approach also offers an alternative model, suggesting that a healthy body rests in a healthy mind, challenging the popular notion that it is the other way around.

Acknowledgements

I extend my heartfelt gratitude to Mr. Satyanarayana Raju Jampana, Chairman of Na-Uyana Monastery, Andhra Pradesh, India, for his generous support of this book chapter. Nestled in the serene landscape of Chekkapalli Village, Na-Uyana Monastery is not only a retreat but also a living embodiment of the forest monastic tradition rooted in the revered Sri Lankan lineage. Serving as both a training center for monastics and a refuge for lay practitioners, it harmonizes ancient wisdom with disciplined practice, offering a rare sanctuary for inner transformation. Under Mr. Jampana's visionary leadership, the monastery has become a beacon of India's spiritual resurgence, drawing an international community and rekindling the country's monastic legacy. Anchored in meditative discipline and ethical clarity, Na-Uyana bridges timeless Dhamma teachings with modern inquiry, standing as a vital nexus for preserving and transmitting the Buddha's path in its land of origin.

Author details

Ratna Jyothi Kakumanu
Medical Advisor, Innovation Incubator Inc., NY, USA

*Address all correspondence to: jyothi.maanu@gmail.com

References

[1] Bodhi B. Comprehensive Manual of Abhidhamma. Vol. 109. Kandy, Sri Lanka: Buddhist Publication Society; 2006. p. 13

[2] Dhammananda K. What Buddhists Believe. Fifth ed. Taipei, Taiwan: The Corporate Body of the Buddha Educational Foundation; 1993

[3] Nyanatiloka M. Guide through the Abhidhamma Pitaka. Kandy, Sri Lanka: BPS; 1971

[4] Goenka SN. Buddha's path is to experience reality. Sayagyi U Ba Khin Journal. 1991;**109**:13

[5] Mendis N. Access to Insight, BCBS Ed. 2013. Available from: https://www.accesstoinsight.org/lib/authors/mendis/index.html

[6] Sucitto A. Kamma & the end of Kamma. Taipei, Taiwan: Buddha Educational Foundation; 2008

[7] van Gorkom N. Abhidhamma in Daily Life. 4th Revision ed. London: Zolag; 2022

[8] Gordon S. In: Gordon S, editor. Neurophenomenology and its Applications to Psychology. New York, NY: Springer; 2013

[9] Barrett KE, Boitano S, Barman SM, Brooks HL. Ganong's Review of Medical Physiology. New York: McGraw-Hill Education; 2012

[10] Thera NM. A Manual of Abhidhamma, Kuala Lumpur. Malaysia: The Buddhist Missionary Society; 1987

[11] Nyanaponika and Bhikku Bodhi. Abhidhamma Studies: Buddhist Explorations of Consciousness and Time, Kandy. Sri Lanka: BPS; 1998

[12] Kakumanu RJ. Vipassana Meditation & Well-Being: A Neuro-Psycho-Physiological Study. Bangalore, India: National Institute of Mental Health and Neuro Sciences (NIMHANS); 2016

[13] Goenka SN. Discourse Summaries, Igatpuri. India: Vipassana Research Institute; 1987

[14] Piyadassi T. Dependent Origination, Kandy. Sri Lanka: Buddhist Publication Society; 1981

[15] Ven. Pa-Auk Tawya Sayadaw, Knowing and Seeing. 4th ed. North Charleston, South Carolina: CreateSpace Independent Publishing Platform; 2010

[16] Buddharakkhita B. Dhammapadam. 2nd ed. Telangana, India: Mokshananda Buddhavihara; 2018

[17] Pali Learning Centre. Pāli Course Program. 2011. Available from: http://learning.pariyatti.org

[18] Fronsdal G. The Dhammapada: A Translation of the Buddhist Classic with Annotations, Boulder. Colorado: Shambhala Publications; 2023

[19] Lutz A, Dunne JD, Richard RJ. Meditation and the neuroscience of consciousness: An introduction. In: The Cambridge Handbook of Consciousness. New York: Cambridge University Press; 2007. p. 499

[20] Tang Y-Y, Hölzel BK, Posner MI. The neuroscience of mindfulness meditation. Nature Reviews Neuroscience. 2015;**16**(4):213-225

Chapter 2

Perspective Chapter: Healing Pathways in Northeast India – Integrating Traditional Wisdom with Modern Approaches to Substance Use Disorders

Proshanto Kr. Saha, Priyanka Pathak and Simi Gogoi

Abstract

The term "substance use" refers to the consumption of psychoactive substances-both legal and illegal-outside of medical prescriptions. In Northeast India (NEI), regional differences in drug use are underexplored. This chapter examines how modern therapies, movement arts, and traditional healing practices can be integrated to address substance use disorders (SUDs) in the region. It emphasizes SUDs as a significant public health challenge and investigates how Indigenous psycho-spiritual practices and medicinal plants like *Centella asiatica* and *Rauvolfia serpentina* contribute to mental health care in the region. By integrating these traditional and contemporary approaches, the chapter aims to provide a unique understanding of SUD management within the sociocultural fabric of NEI. The chapter expands on modern interventions including rehabilitation facilities with a holistic approach including dance therapy, education, and extracurricular activities, and community-based interventions *viz.*, Manipur and Nagaland's Opioid Substitution Therapy (OST) emphasizing their effectiveness in addressing emotional regulation and recovery challenges. The chapter also explores a culturally relevant recovery model from Assam, which outlines the cyclical nature of addiction recovery through phases like recreational use, chaotic addiction, and support recovery. Community initiatives, such as women's empowerment programs, are highlighted as key to tackling addiction's social dimensions. It advocates for a holistic approach combining traditional wisdom, movement arts, and modern psychiatry in treating SUDs.

Keywords: substance use disorders, traditional healing, Northeast India, integrative therapies, psycho-spiritual interventions, medicinal plants

1. Introduction

Substance use disorder (SUD) is a mental health disorder that alters human behavior and brain functions, making it difficult to restrain the use of psychotropic substances, including drugs, alcohol, and various pharmaceutical tablets that change moods and make an individual difficult to manage their daily lives. Addiction is the ultimate and most extreme form of SUD and the intensity is highly variable, as reported by the National Institute of Mental Health [1]. According to the reports from The National Institute of Mental Health, SUD commonly co-occurs with other mental health conditions like stress, anxiety, depression, ADHD, bipolar disorder, personality disorders, and schizophrenia. Three board categories explain the link. Firstly, there can be found common risk factors for mental health disorders and SUD, such as genetics, environment. Secondly, various substances are used as coping strategies for mood stabilizing, which can provide instant short-term palliation over some time which leads to addiction. Thirdly prolonged substance use does alter the morphology and physiology of the brain and entire physic, which is more susceptible to psychological alignments. So, through these links, their correlation can be understood [1].

The Diagnostic and Statistical Manual of Mental Disorders (DSM-IV-TR) edition was replaced by the DSM-5 published in 2013. The revision demonstrated progress in both knowledge and treatments for mental health disorders. The DSM-IV substance dependence and abuse were combined into a single diagnosis in the DSM-5 [2]. Substance-use disorder severity was categorized as mild, moderate, and severe. The Global Burden of Disease 2010 (GBD 2010) has outlooked and potentially underestimated the true burden of mental, neurological, and substance use disorders (MNSDs) and may have failed to look at the significant reduction in life expectancy for those who are affected by these disorders due to its focus on traditional cause-specific deaths. This discrepancy demonstrates the urgent requirement for structural and evidence-based interventions to bridge the lifespan gap between individuals with MNSDs and the general population [3].

The development of economic corridors in the NEI region is an important part of India's Look-East policy to promote foreign trade and economic development. The political unrest of the bordering countries such as Myanmar, Thailand, China's western markets, and Afghanistan created NEI as a hotspot for trafficking drugs and other narcotics in these regions across Arunachal Pradesh, Manipur, Mizoram, and Nagaland. In Northeastern India, regarding illegal consumption of drugs, the unauthorized use of narcotics, opiates, and proxyvon has enhanced despite legal prohibitions. In Meghalaya and Upper Assam, a 1997–1998 survey of 1831 people aged 10 and up revealed substance use rates of 4.9% for opium, 12.5% for alcohol, and 29.4% for tobacco. Assam, which is near the border with Arunachal Pradesh, had higher rates of morphine and marijuana use, while Meghalaya had the highest rate of tobacco use (41.7%). While tobacco use was influenced by religion and ethnic background, substance use patterns were influenced by sexual orientation, maturity level, labor, and academic achievement. The initial minimum ages for alcohol, opium, and tobacco were 18.5, 21.8, and 25.8, respectively. These results highlight the necessity of prevention and intervention initiatives tailored to a given region [4].

2. Traditions and drug use in Northeast India

Throughout India's history, drug use has been deeply ingrained in both religious and cultural customs, especially in the North Indian tribal communities. During social events and religious rituals, people frequently drank alcohol, ganja, bhang, and raw opium. Rituals such as "Madak" and "Chandu" ingrained these drugs deeply into society and normalized their use. During festivals, cannabis preparations—particularly bhang and majun—were even offered in temples, demonstrating the spiritual importance attached to these drugs [5].

Nevertheless, the advent of "modern" drugs such as heroin, brown sugar, and amphetamines has drastically changed the drug use landscape in NEI. Results of a complex interaction between psychological factors (such as stress reduction and pleasure-seeking behaviors), socioeconomic pressures (such as peer pressure and social status), and physiological needs (such as fatigue relief and sexual enhancement), and this shift has caused a rise in the prevalence of addiction among young people. The Golden Triangle, weak security, political conflicts, and drug trafficking have all led to this issue. NEI has much higher rates of drug use than the rest of the country. While 50.37% of people in other Indian states report using narcotics of some kind, 70.83% of people in the NEI do so. At 46.74%, the percentage of NEIs who consume alcohol is much higher than the national average of 29.51% [6, 7].

3. Rehabilitation for substance use disorder in Northeast India

A systematic and reasonable pathway to recover from SUD is the rehabilitation services that help patients with SUD to recover, achieve the path, and maintain sobriety. These centers follow all the guidelines for therapy that are specific to each patient while taking their regional social and cultural setting into respect. The process initially started in a way where the family or the caretaker contacts the facility and shows consent, to begin with the process for the patients or patients willingly show concern to begin the process. Then, the stage of admission starts with medical and psychological evaluation. This is carried out to measure the addiction level, the substances being used, and the associated mental health issues. This evaluation assists in creating a treatment plan to yield the maximum likelihood of recovery. The plan is regularly modified and planned by changing individual needs. The next step is the detoxification, or "detox." In detox, the dangerous chemicals of the substances are removed from the body with the help of the supervision of an attending medical professional. The main goal of this phase is to help manage the intoxication and the withdrawal symptoms so the patient is prepared for therapy. It is an important step as it helps to detect the extent of addiction and co-occurring disorders. Then begins with the therapy session and the medication which is holistic in nature where continuous support can be provided across a range of treatments.

This phase places a strong emphasis on maintaining sobriety, developing new skills, and assisting patients in a gradual transition out of inpatient care. The last phase, aftercare and alumni involvement, guarantees long-term recovery by offering continuing assistance *via* peer support groups, 12-step meetings, and therapy sessions. To help people sustain their sobriety over time, many rehabilitation facilities provide alumni programs that encourage a sense of motivation. Recovery facilities offer several organized and in-depth procedures essential, as more people become addicted to drugs like NEI. Through these institutions, these people will receive vital help, which, in turn, will help them to recover because the addiction-induced psychological and physical changes will also be treated there and through this, the social adaptation deficit will be fulfilled [8]. Rehabilitation is a process that takes place throughout one's life and ways include hard work, a network of supportive friends and family, and aftercare, which is the most dependable source of the recovery process. One becomes addicted to substances because they change how the brain functions. Reasonable decision-making is altered by decreased prefrontal cortex activity, which makes it difficult to stop even if there are bad consequences. These are the milestones you have to reach (technological advances) to address these neurobiological changes and continue to provide support for the person.

4. Innovative approaches to addressing substance use disorders in Northeast India

Researcher have identified SUDs as significant public health concerns, linking them to Indigenous psycho-spiritual practices involving plant medicine, psycho-spiritual praxis, and the community's role in the successful implementation of these healing modalities [9]. By introducing a comprehensive and practical process, this work demonstrates how modern science can be blend with traditional methods to treat SUDs.

The growing popularity of *Centella asiatica* as a psychopharmacological herb largely stems from its properties that help relieve anxiety and other symptoms associated with SUDs. The co-occurrence of anxiety and SUDs reflects a dynamic interplay and mutual reinforcement, explaining the long-standing connection between them.

Anxiety-like symptoms often emerge during periods of chronic intoxication or withdrawal, where the substance itself becomes the central issue. Moreover, individuals with anxiety are more vulnerable to developing SUDs due to specific predispositions that influence the onset, pattern, and characteristics of substance use [10]. Research states that the herb *C. asiatica* helps relieve symptoms of anxiety, relaxes immediately after use, and if used regularly, induces its long-term effects. This makes it a useful adjunct therapy in SUD treatment that addresses withdrawal-related anxiety and reduces chances of relapse. Yet, previous studies have been limited in scope, with small sample sizes and short duration of active treatment, requiring further investigation to elucidate its effects in SUD treatment regimens. *C. asiatica*'s protective properties against sleep deprivation are associated with SUDs [11].

Sleep deprivation (SD) is the result of inadequate or poor-quality sleep, and SD adversely affects the brain and body functioning. In clinical practice, treatment providers frequently underestimate persistent sleep disturbances, which play an important role in the recovery of individuals with SUD. Studies show that sleep disturbances are a significant barrier to achieving sobriety among some individuals who experience psychological distress or have no structured daily routines. Poor sleep can trigger drug use events, increasing relapse vulnerability; thus, routine screening and evidence-based sleep interventions should be an integral part of standard SUD treatment [12].

Centella asiatica (CA) is a medicinal plant used to enhance cognition and healing. It has demonstrated the ability to counteract some of the deleterious effects associated with sleep deprivation. This study examined the protection offered by CA against SD-induced anxiety, brain cell damage (oxidative stress), and inflammation. There was also an examination of the effects of NO through the administration of CA in combination with agents that elevated or lowered NO levels in the brain. Results indicated CA improved locomotion, diminished anxiety-like behaviors, and protected neuronal cells from oxidative stress and inflammation. Its protective effects were

DOI: http://dx.doi.org/10.5772/intechopen.1009874

potentiated in the presence of NO blockade and diminished when co-administered along with drugs that amplify NO, supporting the concept that the beneficial effects of CA are, at least in part, mediated by NO signaling. These observations point to the potential of CA as an adjunct therapy in treating SUDs, especially in addressing concomitant sleep disorders that heighten relapse risk [13].

5. Dance therapy in substance use disorder recovery

Based on traditional Indian Classical and Folk dances, dance therapy is a very important means of physical and emotional healing. Classical Indian dance forms such as Kathak and Manipuri have therapeutic roles—while the rapid footwork of Kathak releases strong emotional tension and anger, the gentle, fluid movements of Manipuri invoke calmness and inner peace. They are by Ayurvedic principles, which see dance as a means to achieve holistic wellness and equilibrium.

Modern dance therapy has evolved to address a wide range of health problems, including stress, high blood pressure, diabetes, arthritis, asthma, and gynecological issues. Dance/movement therapists (DMT) are an essential part of inpatient care, guiding patients in creative group therapy and serving as communication bridges to the treatment team. They connect patients with evidence-based SUD strategies by encouraging them to think about how drug and alcohol use have affected their lives. In accordance with respect for the patient's level of recovery, DMT offers movement experience and reflective conversation intended to lead to insight and change. The process emphasizes non-judgmental acceptance to ensure the patient feels seen and cared for. Therapists also provide important observations to the treatment team to enhance improved treatment planning [14]. Dance therapy is also an important part of reintegration for people, as it provides them with an opportunity to interact with a supportive community, which is so important during the recovery process. The use of traditional dances from Northeast India in therapy programs brings an element of cultural importance, providing participants with something they can relate to and find meaningful as they go through their recovery. This integrated process not only encourages physical and emotional healing but also a deeper understanding of one's cultural heritage, thus aiding the general efficacy of substance use disorder treatment [15]. Also, various other dance forms from NEI like Sattriya Dance and Bihu from Assam, Laho from Meghalaya, and Khantumm bamboo from Mizoram have various health and psychological benefits like improved spatial awareness, increased physical confidence, improved psychological well-being, better self-confidence, self-esteem, and also better social skills and together have a therapeutic effectiveness [16].

6. Education and activities as shields against substance abuse

A study from Northeast India concludes that substance use prevalence in the northeastern states is significantly high. Key contributing factors include early initiation of substance use among younger age groups, gender differences, economic status, social background, and lower levels of education [17]. Thus, education and extracurricular activities, like sports and music, have a transformative impact on safeguarding youth against substance abuse in North Eastern States in India for Substance use disorder [18].

7. Traditional healing practices for mental health in Nagaland: Bridging tradition and modern care

Research conducted in 2017 on Nagaland's Traditional ways of treating mental health carried out in-depth interviews with 510 rural and 300 urban households. The study states that three primary traditional treatment methods were identified, namely herbal remedies, mechanical methods such as massage, and psycho-spiritual rituals—used individually or in combination. The research established that nearly 30% of the respondents went to traditional healers, which reflected a high rural-urban disparity—34.8% in rural areas versus only 16.5% in urban areas. Out of the people who employed traditional remedies, 58.9% claimed beneficial results, with rural respondents reporting higher satisfaction (60%) than their urban peers (24%). Traditional healers continue to be essential in rural communities due to their cultural relevance, respect for their knowledge, and valued expertise, although their numbers are declining gradually. Traditional healing is used more frequently for daily illness, but it remains the first line of assistance for mood disorders. Psycho-spiritual therapies were the most frequent intervention used for treating mental disorders. Rural areas showed greater reliance on and satisfaction with these indigenous practices compared to urban dwellers. The study shows the possible benefits of mixing modern mental care in Nagaland with the traditional healing methods. Access to holistic mental health therapy would be improved by combining old healing methods with contemporary mental health services as well as culturally appropriate counseling treatments. This would combine the benefits of both modern and traditional approaches for complete therapy [19].

8. Multidirectional pathways to substance use disorder recovery in Northeast India

People find it difficult to overcome substance use disorders (SUDs) because of the interaction of mental, social, and physical factors. Traditional recovery approaches frequently promote complete abstinence or harm reduction simply.

Recent research highlights the need for more holistic, culturally relevant approaches that represent people's challenging real-life experiences. The basis for understanding addiction and recovery has been established by popular theories such as the Disease Model and the Biopsychosocial Model. The Transtheoretical Model of Change, another used approach, describes recovery as a step-by-step process that moves from not thinking about change to maintaining new behaviors. While enlightening, such models are less culturally nuanced and fail to address recovery's nonlinear, bidirectional nature, especially in multicultural populations. The study in Assam presents a novel multi-route, multidirectional pathway to recovery model that breaks away from conventional linear models. It has three phases, Recreational Use, Addiction (Relaxed, Chaotic, Strategic), and Supported Recovery, each phase consists of cycling between, or transitioning through, a series of stages.

This model sees recovery as an active, person-focused journey that influences cultural, social, psychological, and spiritual aspects. It recognizes that recovery does not follow a straight line—individuals can progress, regress, or move sideways as they recover. Experts agree there are many ways to recover such as quitting using in a controlled way trying to cut down on harm and following spiritual routines. The model further emphasizes cultural context as significant, including neighborhood beliefs, neighborhood support systems, and Indigenous practices with strong influences on recovery experiences. Emotional regulation, cognitive functioning, personality traits, and sociodemographic factors all interact in complex ways and influence the recovery process. Interestingly, the model even normalizes relapse during recovery, seeing it as a chance for development and learning rather than a failure. This method promotes resilience and the development of adaptive ways of coping.

The multi-route, multidirectional model has significant implications for Northeast Indian SUD research and intervention.

In summary, this model is an important step ahead in the understanding of SUD recovery in culturally diverse settings. Breaking linear trends and showcasing the diversity of lived experiences creates new opportunities for person-centered, more successful treatments that reflect Northeast India's unique cultural and socioeconomic setting.

9. Empowering women through self-help groups: Overcoming social barriers and combating substance abuse in India

Women Empowerment and self-help groups (SHGs) in India have been successful but still, there is a great scope of development and the quality of training programs for skill development. So, there is an urgent need to uplift these programs per standards. One of the biggest challenges is the geographical isolation of most training programs, which often fails to enable facilitators to provide consistent, high-quality training. This calls for defining clear criteria for trainer recruitment and developing a well-thought-out, comprehensive curriculum to guarantee consistency and efficiency. Aside from logistical barriers, social barriers continue to hamper the broader empowerment process. Addictions such as alcohol and drug addiction, along with deeply rooted cultural and societal beliefs, are major challenges. Despite all this, women's organizations have taken the initiative in addressing social issues. The Naga Mothers' Association, for instance, has played a crucial role in minimizing addiction in Indian society, although their efforts could be strengthened with more legislative support. Just so, the women's branch of the Koch Rajbongshi Student Union has been instrumental in mobilizing the community and building awareness around addiction as a potential threat. This at last highlights the importance of mindfulness as an impetus to revolutionary social change. With the practice of mindfulness combined with compassion and introspection, there lies a valuable aid to confronting even the most nuanced of social issues. Women's association leaders play a central role in developing this attitude, employing it to direct action against social ills and drug abuse [20].

10. Northeast India's community-based interventions for substance use disorders

Manipur and Nagaland's Opioid Substitution Therapy (OST) program played a crucial role in addressing opioid dependence among injecting drug users (IDUs) in zones like underdevelopment, conflict, and heroine-abundant regions.

Utilizing sub-lingual buprenorphine a partial opioid agonist the program sought to reduce cravings and withdrawal symptoms without inducing the euphoric "high" resulting from heroin. In addition to decreasing rates of relapse and overdose, this strategy assists harm-reduction efforts within these frequently neglected communities.

The NGO-run program focused on sustained treatment retention, given the evidence that longer retention in treatment has been shown to reduce the risk for HIV, including needle sharing and unprotected sex. Another major element of the program was an emphasis on family involvement, which served as a critical source of support, improving compliance with treatment and reducing relapse rates.

However, beyond the medical treatment, routine counseling and examination classes were conducted to address psychological and social issues linked with the addiction in order to provide holistic treatment to the patients. The results showed significant improvements in quality of life for the participants and a decrease in risky behavior [21].

A community-based tobacco cessation program done in Guwahati (2009–2010) used a uniquely disciplined and individualized approach to assist 800 tobacco consumers quit, which was successful. Door-to-door surveys were conducted by trained Medical social workers and educational material was provided along with counseling sessions to enhance behavior change for health awareness.

There was a consistent follow-up, every month for 8 months, to maintain support, and zero loss to follow-up and a 47% quit rate were observed. The program has proven successful and demonstrates that community involvement and long-term counseling can be effective, suggesting that it could have wider applicability in terms of addressing substance use disorder (SUD) in resource-poor settings [22].

11. Conclusion

In North East India, substance use disorder is a severe public health concern that results from a combination of sociocultural and mental health variables. Integrated methods must be applied to address both substance dependence and psychological well-being since the relationship between SUD and mental health conditions correlates. Despite improvements in diagnostic methods, the global prevalence of SUD is still not reliably estimated. Despite advancements in diagnostic techniques, the global scale of SUD remains inaccurately assessed. The challenges and the unique socioeconomic conditions of Northeast India, and its closeness touching the Golden Triangle, have given rise to high trafficking and hotspots for narcotics and drug abuse. These changes in society which make easy access to the various contemporary drugs and also different mental problems led to addiction issues among youths in Northeast India. Rehabilitation programs have been initiated with a touch of holistic model which is therapeutic and effective along with indigenous practices, modern psychological therapies, and medicinal detoxification. In addition to this, NEI regions also depend on various herbal medicines that offer various existing benefits. Manipuri and Kathak, two forms of Indian classical dance, can be used as emotional well-being therapy. NEI has various forms of arts and culture which are divine, various soothing music from all the different cultures such as Sattriya Dance and Bihu from Assam, Laho from Meghalaya, and Khantumm bamboo from Mizoram has various therapeutic effectiveness on mental health.

The combination of modern psychological treatments with indigenous healing methods promotes culturally sensitive mental health interventions in areas such as Nagaland. To recognize the unpredictable nature of recovery, new recovery models such as the Multi-Path Multidirectional model incorporate spiritual treatments, harm reduction, and abstinence. Women Empowerment groups from Nagaland and community-led programs like Manipur and Nagaland's Opioid Substitution Therapy (OST), and community-based tobacco cessation from Guwahati are helpful and effective. To address SUD as a mental health issue for development and to promote resilience in the area, an integrated, culturally appropriate strategy for prevention, identification, and intervention is required. Therefore, to address SUD and related mental health in North East India the approach should include a holistic community-based, traditional aspects, contemporary psychological treatments, and medicinal therapies.

Author details

Proshanto Kr. Saha*, Priyanka Pathak and Simi Gogoi
Department of Psychology, Rajiv Gandhi University-A Central University, Arunachal Pradesh, India

*Address all correspondence to: saha.csl@gmail.com

References

[1] US Department of Health and Human Services. Substance use and cooccurring mental disorders. National Institute of Mental Health. Retrieved. June 22 2021;**2022**

[2] Guha M. Diagnostic and statistical manual of mental disorders: DSM-5 (5th edition). Reference Reviews. 2014;**28**(3):36-37. DOI: 10.1108/RR-10-2013-0256 ISSN 0950-4125

[3] Charlson FJ, Baxter AJ, Dua T, Degenhardt L, Whiteford HA, Vos T. Excessmortalityfrommental,neurological and substance use disorders in the global burden of disease study 2010. Epidemiology and Psychiatric Sciences. 2015;**24**(2):121-140

[4] Chaturvedi HK, Phukan RK, Mahanta J. The association of selected sociodemographic factors and differences in patterns of substance use: A pilot study in selected areas of Northeast India. Substance Use & Misuse. 2003;**38**(9):1305-1322

[5] Arya K, Kumar RR. Traditions, globalization and drug abuse in North-East India: Highlighting the renewed concerns of an organized drug crime. In Globalisation and the concerns of social landscape in India (Renu Publishers). 2018. pp. 109-120

[6] Goswami N. Drugs and the Golden Triangle: Renewed Concerns for Northeast India. New Delhi, India: Institute for Defence Studies and Analyses; 2014

[7] Saikia N, Debbarma B. The socioeconomic correlates of substance use among male adults in Northeast India. Clinical Epidemiology and Global Health. 2020;**8**(1):149-157

[8] Ningombam SK, Hazarika R. Ancient remedies: Exploring the traditional medicine systems of Northeast Indian tribes. The International Journal of Bharatiya Knowledge System. 2024;**1**:67-78

[9] Back SE, Brady KT. Anxiety disorders with comorbid substance use disorders: Diagnostic and treatment considerations. Psychiatric Annals. 2008;**38**(11):724-729. DOI: 10.3928/00485713-20081101-01

[10] Sarris J, McIntyre E, Camfield DA. Plant-based medicines for anxiety disorders, part 2: A review of clinical studies with supporting preclinical evidence. CNS Drugs. 2013;**27**(4):301-319. DOI: 10.1007/s40263-013-0059-9

[11] Erga AH, Nesvåg S, Dahlberg IE, McKay JR. Persistent sleep problems among people in recovery from substance use disorders: A mixed methods study. Addiction Research & Theory. 2022;**30**(6):422-430. DOI: 10.1080/16066359.2022.2074406

[12] Chanana P, Kumar A. Possible involvement of nitric oxide modulatory mechanisms in the neuroprotective effect of Centella Asiatica against sleep deprivation induced anxiety like behaviour, oxidative damage and neuroinflammation. Phytotherapy Research: PTR. 2016;**30**(4):671-680. DOI: 10.1002/ptr.5582

[13] Kirane K. Dance/movement therapy: A unique response to the opioid crisis. American Journal of Dance Therapy. 2018;**40**:12-17. DOI: 10.1007/s10465-018-9268-6

[14] Chatterjee A. The therapeutic value of Indian classical, folk, and innovative dance forms. Rupkatha Journal on

Interdisciplinary Studies in Humanities. 2013;**5**(1):75-83

[15] Deekshitulu PVB. Physical & Mental Health for Indian Classical Dance. American Journal of History and Culture. 2024;**2**:1-8

[16] Yadav J, Singh JK, Gautam S. Correlates of substance use in northeast states, India. International Journal of Community Medicine and Public Health. 2016;**3**(6):1531

[17] Ningsangrenla L, Rao PSS. Traditional healing practices and perspectives of mental health in Nagaland. Journal of North East India Studies. 2019;**9**(2):33-56

[18] Nidecker M, DiClemente CC, Bennett ME, Bellack AS. Application of the transtheoretical model of change: Psychometric properties of leading measures in patients with co-occurring drug abuse and severe mental illness. Addictive Behaviors. 2008;**33**(8):1021-1030

[19] Madill A, Duara R, Goswami S, Graber R, Hugh-Jones S. Pathways to recovery model of youth substance misuse in Assam, India. Health Expectations: An International Journal of Public Participation in Health Care and Health Policy. 2023;**26**(1):318-328. DOI: 10.1111/hex.13658

[20] Mcap TPL. Drug and alcohol addiction treatment – everything you need to know. Addiction Center. Brentwood, TN, USA: 18 February 2025, Available from: https://www.addictioncenter.com/treatment/

[21] Armstrong G, Kermode M, Sharma C, Langkham B, Crofts N. Opioid substitution therapy in Manipur and Nagaland, North-East India: Operational research in action. Harm Reduction Journal. 2010;**7**:1-7

[22] Bhagabaty SM, Kataki AC, Kalita M, Salkar S. Community based intervention for tobacco cessation: A pilot study experience, north East India. Asian Pacific Journal of Cancer Prevention. 2015;**16**(2):811-814

Chapter 3

Yoga Nidra: A Potential Preventive and Therapeutic Intervention

Navdeep Ahuja, Monika Pathania and Praag Bhardwaj

Abstract

Yoga Nidra (YN) is a conscious relaxation practice that, while drawing on the philosophical foundations of yoga laid out in Patanjali's Yoga Sutras, was first explained in the twentieth century by the Bihar School of Yoga and later refined by spiritual teachers and organizations such as the Art of Living. It elicits deep physiological rest while maintaining awareness. Evidence from cardiovascular, metabolic, sleep-related, and psychological research shows that routine YN practice can lower resting blood pressure, shift autonomic balance toward parasympathetic activity, and support glycemic control when paired with usual care. Controlled trials in insomnia report shorter sleep-onset latency and longer total sleep time, while both healthy and clinical cohorts demonstrate reductions in perceived stress, anxiety, and depressive symptoms. These benefits appear to arise from reduced hypothalamic-pituitary-adrenal reactivity, enhanced vagal tone, and reduced limbic-cortical activation. With minimal equipment needs and suitability for group or digital delivery, YN is especially practical for low- and middle-income countries, where its low cost and easy scalability could help curb the growing burden of non-communicable diseases (NCDs). Overall, YN stands out as a relatively safe, accessible intervention with potential preventive, and therapeutic value across multiple body systems. Continued research should provide optimal dosing and delivery and confirm the reliability of these effects.

Keywords: Yoga Nidra, therapeutic relaxation, heart rate variability (HRV), autonomic nervous system, mind-body intervention, stress, hypertension

1. Introduction

Yoga Nidra, often translated as "yogic sleep," is a practice that has attracted increasing attention from the scientific community for its potential effects on psychological well-being and physiological functions. While traditionally described as a state of conscious relaxation which is performed in an awake state, modern research seeks to understand its mechanisms through empirical investigation. It seems to have evolved from the confluence of early Upaniṣad texts, Tantric methods (especially Nyasa), and the sensory-withdrawal step (Pratyahara) articulated in Patanjali's Yoga Sutras [1, 2]. Practiced almost exclusively in Savasana (Supine) while the teacher guides the mind through a sequence of body-focused cues, Yoga Nidra aims to elicit physiological rest without reducing awareness of the inner or outer environment.

IntechOpen

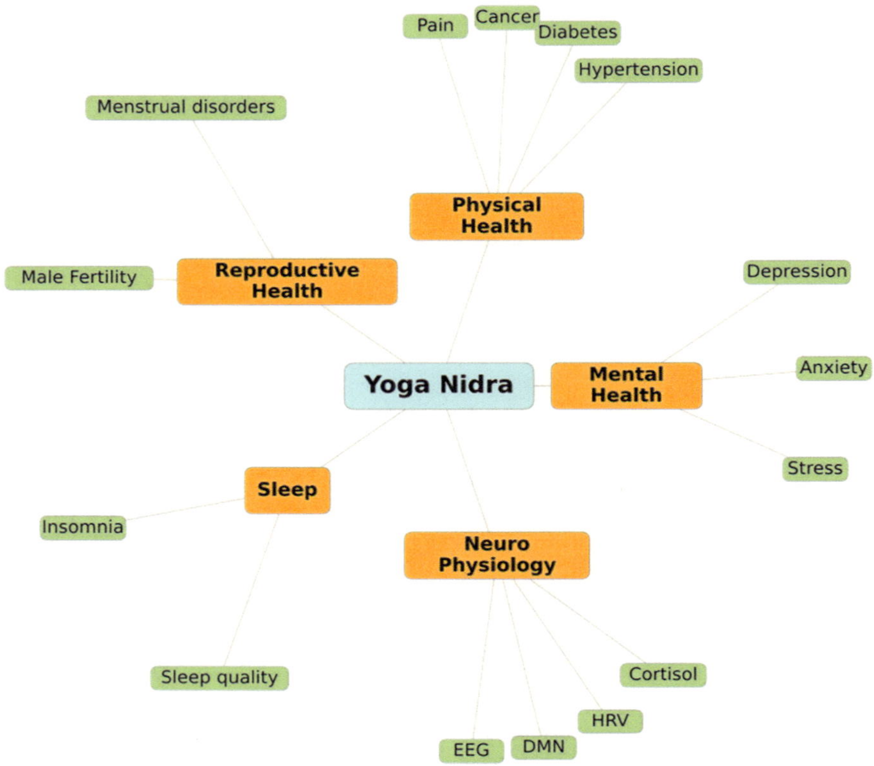

Figure 1.
Overview of effects and evidence of Yoga Nidra on physiology and in diseases.

Outwardly, the practitioner appears asleep, but the internal consciousness is maintained [2]. The overview of the physiological effects of Yoga Nidra on the systemic level and the potential mechanisms are depicted in a schematic diagram (**Figure 1**).

2. Historical and traditional perspectives

2.1 From Pratyahara to modern Yoga Nidra

Patanjali has explained Astanga Yoga having eight components/steps in his seminal work Yoga Sutras. It is a comprehensive framework described to achieve a healthy state at both physical and mental levels. Each step serves as a tool for making the body and mind healthy. The first two, Yama (ethical restraints) and Niyama (personal observances) lay the moral foundation. Asana refers to the practice of a stable and comfortable seated posture, while Pranayama involves the conscious regulation of breath (Prana). Pratyahara, the fifth limb, marks a pivotal shift inward as the senses withdraw from external objects, allowing the practitioner to enter the subtler states of awareness. The last three, Dharana (focused concentration), Dhyana (uninterrupted meditation), and Samadhi (absorption in pure awareness) constitute the internal limbs that refine consciousness toward liberation (kaivalya). It is within this schema that Pratyahara forms the theoretical and experiential foundations for what later probably evolved into the modern practice of Yoga Nidra [3].

DOI: http://dx.doi.org/10.5772/intechopen.1011437

Yoga Nidra operationalizes these sutras step by step. Subject is guided to withdraw attention from the environment, then from proprioception, and finally from the stream of thought, yet awareness of being aware in the present moment is preserved. This internalized conscious awareness distinguishes Yoga Nidra from ordinary sleep, in which conscious perception of external surroundings is totally lost functionally [1]. In a commentary on the Patanjali Yoga Sutras by global spiritual leader and teacher of yoga, Sri Sri Ravi Shankar, he has given a contemporary explanation and emphasizes that the Patanjali Yoga Sutras are one of the few classical treatises that elaborate on the phenomenon of sleep, offering insights [4].

A second ancient practice is Nyasa ("placing"), a Tantric practice in which mantras, seed syllables, or deities are mentally installed in specific body loci, kara-nyasa on the fingers, anga-nyasa on the limbs, hṛdayadi-nyasa on vital organs. The practice serves to integrate external and internal perception, and anchors awareness internally [5]. The rotation of consciousness through different parts of the body in modern Yoga Nidra is similar to Nyasa but performed supine in Savasana instead of seated ritual.

2.2 Systematization by Swami Satyananada

Despite the previous knowledge, Yoga Nidra remained an esoteric practice until Swami Satyananda Saraswati of the Bihar School of Yoga described its components into an multi-stage protocol. He described a sequence of steps, which includes rotation of consciousness through different body parts. Thus, the whole process is to guide the practitioners from muscular relaxation to subtle mental imagination, while ensuring they remain awake and aware. He also described the resulting state in which waking, dream, and deep sleep pass like clouds, yet awareness of Self remains [2]. The term Yoga Nidra, commonly translated as "yogic sleep," has been interpreted in deeper spiritual contexts as well.

3. Physiological and clinical relevance

A defining trait of Yoga Nidra is that its primary intention is relaxation. Neurophysiological data suggest that this state has distinctive signatures. PET imaging shows increased dopamine release in the ventral striatum and redistributed cerebral blood flow during Yoga Nidra compared to normal resting state [6, 7]. Clinically, the practice has been associated with improved hemoglobin levels [8], better glycemic control in diabetes [9], favorable hormonal profile in menstrual disorders [10, 11], and lowered blood pressure in hypertension [12]. Randomized trials show alleviation of mild depression and anxiety [10] and mitigation of chronic insomnia with reductions in salivary cortisol [13]. Taken together, these evidences depict Yoga Nidra as a technique that could have a potential role in preventive and therapeutic aspects.

While rigorous mechanism-oriented studies are still emerging, convergent evidence, from endocrinology to functional neuroimaging, suggests that the practice engages neural circuits of interoception, emotional regulation, and parasympathetic dominance. An overview of probable mechanisms is shown in **Figure** 2.

3.1 Electrophysiology and fMRI

One of the primary areas of scientific inquiry has been to characterize the state of consciousness experienced during Yoga Nidra using electrophysiological methods

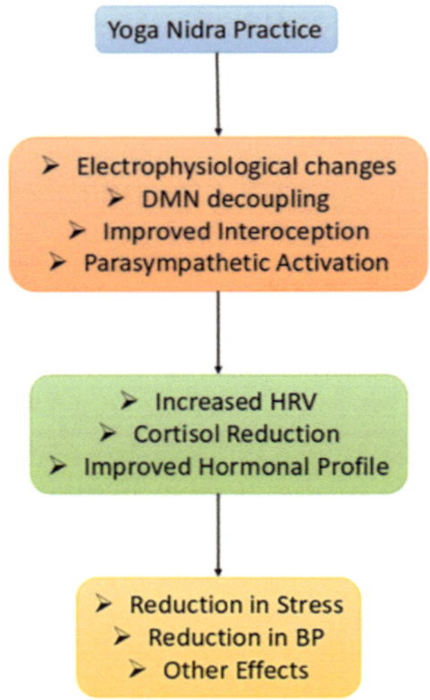

Figure 2.
Probable mechanisms of the effects of Yoga Nidra.

like electroencephalography (EEG) and polysomnography. Studies involving novice practitioners have indicated that during Yoga Nidra sessions, individuals are largely in an electrophysiologically awake state [14, 15]. Furthermore, preliminary EEG data in volunteers did not detect characteristic sleep hallmarks such as K-complexes and sleep spindles during the practice. However, study reported significant changes in certain frequency bands such as over central scalp area, an increase in delta power, and a decrease in the delta band over prefrontal area during Yoga Nidra. The authors have described the presence of local slow waves as local sleep [14]. However, the traditional understanding and the subjective experience aimed for in Yoga Nidra involves inducing a deeply relaxed state similar to sleep as observed from an external observer, while maintaining awareness [16, 17]. It is also hypothesized to be phenomenologically distinct from lucid dreaming, offering access to subtler states of consciousness as the awareness is maintained throughout, but according to the current evidence, this state is not similar to physiological sleep and needs to be investigated in depth, as such states were demonstrated only in specific studies, in which awareness is maintained while having electrophysiological signatures of non-REM sleep [17, 18]. Thus, a scientific validation of this specific phenomenology, particularly conscious awareness during a state of relaxed mind and body, is noted as an area requiring further sleep studies and experimental methodologies. Beyond electrophysiology, fMRI studies have begun to explore the neural correlates of Yoga Nidra, focusing on functional connectivity. A study examined the neurophysiological state attained during Yoga Nidra in experienced meditators compared to novice controls [16]. There was a significant reduction in DMN functional connectivity, distinct DMN decoupling among meditators compared to controls [16]. The reduced DMN connectivity during Yoga Nidra and the meditators' self-reported cumulative hours of meditation and yoga practice were found to be correlated. These findings suggest a unique neural modulation of the DMN occurs in experienced practitioners during Yoga Nidra, which aligns with their subjective experience of being restful yet aware.

3.2 HRV and cortisol

The scientific investigation also extends to the physiological effects on the autonomic nervous system (ANS) and stress hormones. Heart rate variability (HRV), a measure reflecting ANS balance, has been studied in the context of Yoga Nidra [19]. Yoga Nidra has been shown to increase HRV, indicating an increase in parasympathetic activity. It was found that Yoga Nidra intervention alone and the intervention along with Hatha yoga caused significant changes in heart rate and various HRV indices. Cortisol is considered a stress hormone and its levels have been studied as a marker of effect of the intervention on Stress. A study found that Yoga Nidra practice caused a reduction in serum cortisol [20]. A longer (30-minute) form of Yoga Nidra practice was found to result in a flatter cortisol wake-up reaction compared to controls and a shorter (11-minute) form. Regular practice, regardless of duration, was associated with the beneficial changes in cortisol patterns.

One of the probable mechanisms of increasing parasympathetic dominance is that adopting a supine posture leads to baroreceptor loading due to increased central blood volume, which reflexively suppresses sympathetic outflow. This postural shift is associated with immediate reductions in heart rate and muscle sympathetic nerve activity [21]. Also, slow and deep breathing enhances respiratory sinus arrhythmia and activates vagal output, resulting in increased parasympathetic tone. This autonomic shift is associated with reduced anxiety and improved emotional regulation. Although Yoga Nidra only involves an awareness of breathing, it could result in slowing of breathing due to relaxation, which could cause this effect. However, experimental data would be needed to explore this mechanism as well [22].

3.3 Neurophysiology

During Yoga Nidra, the instructor guides attention sequentially through every-body region, a "rotation of consciousness" that resembles the body scan used in mindfulness-based stress reduction. Neuro-imaging shows that during Mindfulness and body scan practices, attentional shift produces modulatory alpha activity in the corresponding strips of the primary somatosensory cortex [23, 24]. This has been thought to be beneficial as training to modulate alpha in chronic pain and depression, the attention could be taken away from pain and rumination toward the focus on the body part or sensation. Repeating practice strengthens functional connectivity between the salience network with frontal gyri and the Default Mode Network [25–27], which may be the mechanisms underlying the practice of Yoga Nidra. Greater interoceptive practice in body scan practice may increase the ability to detect subtle physiological processes such as heartbeat, breath, and visceral sensations [25]. This ability could equip subjects with the information needed to interpret and consciously regulate those feelings. However, some of these mechanisms have been studied in Mindfulness-based practices and need to be replicated specifically in Yoga Nidra, while more studies will be required to understand the exact mechanisms underlying the interoceptive awareness.

During Yoga Nidra, positron-emission studies show a surge of dopamine in the ventral striatum, a neurochemical signature of reward and a redistribution of blood flow in executive areas [6, 7]. The prefrontal regions could result in inhibition of the central autonomic network, and that could reduce the sympathetic outflow, a mechanism postulated in neuro-visceral integration models [28]. It posits that HRV is not only a marker of cardiac function but also reflects the health of top-down cortical regulation, particularly by the prefrontal cortex over the brainstem and autonomic nervous system [29]. Smith et al. [29] expanded on this model, describing an eight-level neuroanatomical hierarchy through which emotional and attentional regulation influence cardiovascular dynamics. During Yoga Nidra, the intentional withdrawal of attention from external stimuli and re-direction toward internal bodily sensations (interoception) can be hypothesized to activate this neural cascade, enhancing vagal output and suppressing sympathetic arousal, which, in turn, causes beneficial effects in cardiovascular disorders such as hypertension, endocrine and metabolic abnormalities such as diabetes mellitus, metabolic syndrome and psychiatric disorders such as anxiety and depression. Consistent with this theory, single-session trials report immediate falls in heart rate, systolic blood pressure, and LF/HF ratio after the practice [19].

4. Yoga Nidra and mental health

It is suggested that the relaxation generated through Yoga Nidra can serve as an effective intervention for managing various aspects of mental health. Studies have provided evidence of the effects of Yoga Nidra on multiple aspects of mental health, including stress, anxiety symptoms, depressive symptoms, worry, and overall well-being. A review of studies found it to be effective in addressing several aspects related to mental health, such as stress, mood, well-being, and psychological dysfunction [30].

4.1 Effects on perceived stress

Stress is a commonly studied outcome in Yoga Nidra research. An experimental study involving university students found that there was a reduction in life stress intensity levels after practicing Yoga Nidra for 8 weeks [31]. Similarly, the iRest program, having a Yoga Nidra intervention for college students, showed statistically significant improvements in perceived stress [32]. Yoga Nidra has also been found to mitigate psychosocial stress in adolescents. A study on students who practiced Yoga Nidra for 21 consecutive days showed a significant decrease in total stress compared to a control group [33]. They reported that they had reductions of stress across many domains of life including work, home, and future worries. Research on college professors also suggests that Yoga Nidra can be an effective therapeutic approach in reducing stress levels [34].

4.2 Effects on anxiety disorders and depression

Anxiety disorders and depressive disorders are highly prevalent conditions that have been investigated in relation to Yoga Nidra practice. Studies have shown that Yoga Nidra can lead to reductions in indices of mild depression and anxiety [1]. In a randomized controlled trial, Yoga Nidra interventions of different time durations were examined [20]. Significant improvements were observed for the short form of intervention consisting of an 11-minute Yoga Nidra group compared to a waitlist control group in relation to anxiety. The short form Yoga Nidra specifically showed a reduction in depression. Similar types of reductions in anxiety levels were also found in college professors [34]. These results show that Yoga Nidra could be utilized as a potential intervention for the therapeutic reduction in anxiety. Yoga Nidra intervention for a period of 8 weeks, mentioned earlier, for college students also found statistically significant improvements in depression [32].

4.3 Effects on worry and well-being

Beyond stress, anxiety, and depression, Yoga Nidra has shown effects on worry and overall well-being. The study examining different lengths of online Yoga Nidra described earlier found significant improvements on measures of worry and satisfaction with life [20]. The iRest yoga-nidra intervention with college students also found statistically significant improvements in worry [32].

4.4 Yoga Nidra and psychological trauma

Psychological trauma can manifest in the form of Post-Traumatic Stress Disorder (PTSD) or other symptoms such as sleep disturbances. While Yoga Nidra is a potential intervention that could reduce these symptoms, authors speculate that Yoga Nidra could enhance some of these symptoms if not conducted in a proper manner [35]. The authors have provided a framework of 10 principles to be followed while conducting the intervention of Yoga Nidra for such patients. These principles include paying attention to safety, appropriateness, and providing choice to the practitioner by maintaining openness. Thoughtful decisions based on context should prioritize the safety and benefit of practitioners. Another study utilizing iRest intervention as described earlier, which includes Yoga Nidra, has also studied its effect on patients of PTSD, especially those who had developed these symptoms after combat in the military [36]. There was a reduction in symptoms such as rage, anxiety, and emotional reactivity. Other positive feelings, such as relaxation and peace, were reported to be increased.

4.5 Mindfulness

Yoga Nidra practice may also contribute to improvements in mindfulness-based skills [32]. An increase in acting with awareness was noted with the longer duration of online Yoga Nidra [20]. Furthermore, a modulation of individual alpha peak frequency values was observed in athletes after Yoga Nidra [37].

5. Yoga Nidra and physical health

The practice of Yoga Nidra has shown a potential for its therapeutic benefits, not only for psychological distress but also for various aspects of physical health, often acting as a complementary therapy alongside conventional medical care. Research suggests that Yoga Nidra may influence physiological processes and contribute to improved physical well-being in individuals facing chronic conditions or treatment-related challenges.

5.1 Cardiovascular effects

One area where Yoga Nidra shows promise is in the management of hypertension, which is a significant contributor to cardiovascular morbidity and mortality [12]. A recent systematic review and meta-analysis synthesized findings from multiple clinical trials, concluding that there was a significant reduction in both systolic blood pressure (SBP) and diastolic blood pressure (DBP) in patients with hypertension who had undergone Yoga Nidra Intervention. The meta-analysis included five RCTs and three non-RCTs. The potential mechanisms by which these types of results could be brought about have been discussed in earlier sections. In one such study to find out the potential mechanisms, a single-arm intervention trial was conducted on hypertensive adults, which demonstrated that a single 16-minute session of Yoga Nidra resulted in a reduction in BP [38]. Importantly, the study also found significant increases in heart rate variability (HRV) parameters following the session. Regression analysis indicated that the observed reduction in blood pressure could be explained by these increases in HRV, suggesting a link mediated by the Neurovisceral Integration Model. HRV is an indicator of autonomic nervous system function, and increased variability is generally associated with better cardiovascular health.

Further randomized controlled trials investigating the combined effects of OM chanting and Yoga Nidra in hypertensive patients have also reported the significant physical health improvements. A 2-month intervention showed a significant reduction in both systolic and diastolic BP [39]. It was also reported that LDL cholesterol levels had reduced and HDL cholesterol levels had increased. Another similar study using Yoga Nidra and Om chanting as interventions found that these interventions caused a reduction in mental symptoms such as stress, anxiety, improved sleep quality, and autonomic parameters among the patients of hypertension [40]. These findings collectively highlight Yoga Nidra's potential role in addressing the multifactorial nature of hypertension by influencing stress levels, autonomic balance, and even lipid metabolism. While promising, research suggests that further studies with larger sample sizes, longer follow-up periods, and more homogenous populations are needed to fully understand and standardize the optimal application of Yoga Nidra for hypertension.

5.2 Diabetes mellitus

The practice may also offer benefits for metabolic conditions, specifically diabetes mellitus. A study evaluated the effect of Yoga Nidra on levels of blood glucose in middle-aged patients of type-2 diabetes mellitus, with concomitant oral hypoglycemic therapy [9]. After 90 days of intervention, there was a significant reduction in blood glucose levels. Additionally, most of the symptoms associated with diabetes significantly subsided in the Yoga Nidra group. The study concluded that integrating Yoga Nidra with concomitant drug therapy leads to better control of blood glucose and associated symptoms compared to drug therapy alone.

5.3 Pain

Yoga Nidra has also been explored as a mind-body intervention for individuals experiencing persistent pain [41]. A pilot qualitative study examined the experiences of patients with persistent pain who participated in a six-week iRest Yoga Nidra program within a multidisciplinary pain management service. The iRest program included various aspects of the practice of the Yoga Nidra, such as breath awareness and rotation of Consciousness. Participants described the practice in detail and found that it could actually relieve some of the symptoms they were previously experiencing. They felt that their pain severity had reduced. One of the important perceptions that they explained was that the practice made them feel disidentified from the pain. This disidentification has been described in contemplative practice, which helps the practitioner in a way that the intensity of emotional experiences gets reduced. These feelings led to an increase in motivation among the participants, and they felt that it reduced their dependence on drugs such as opioids. This suggests that Yoga Nidra may offer a valuable nonpharmacological approach to managing chronic pain by enhancing coping mechanisms and promoting relaxation.

5.4 Cancer

In the context of cancer care, patients often face significant physical challenges and side effects from treatments such as chemotherapy and radiotherapy, which can exacerbate distress and impact physical well-being [42]. One study noted that Yoga Nidra can potentially reduce the psychological aftereffects of chemotherapy and radiotherapy in patients with cervical cancer [43]. While research often focuses on the psychological benefits of Yoga Nidra in this population (such as reducing anxiety and depression [43]), the research should also focus on the physical effects of this intervention. Given its noninvasive and gentle nature, Yoga Nidra can be considered particularly efficacious for cancer patients undergoing intensive treatments.

6. Yoga Nidra and reproductive health

The section explores the application of Yoga Nidra across several aspects relevant to reproductive health, from addressing psychological distress and hormonal imbalances associated with menstrual disorders in women of reproductive age to potentially supporting male fertility and improving overall well-being in the post-menopausal phase.

6.1 Menstrual disorders

Menstrual disorders are often accompanied by emotional alterations, stress, and symptoms of anxiety and depression [44]. Several studies have investigated the effects of Yoga Nidra as an intervention for menstrual irregularities [11, 45–47]. Yoga Nidra has been assessed for its impact on psychological problems associated with menstrual disorders. A systematic review of randomized controlled trials found evidence that Yoga Nidra may have favorable effects in terms of reducing problems such as anxiety and depression in women with menstrual disorders [46]. Multiple randomized controlled trials support this, showing a significant decrease in anxiety and depression scores in intervention groups practicing Yoga Nidra compared to control groups receiving only medication or no yogic intervention [10, 44, 45]. Beyond psychological symptoms, Yoga Nidra has been studied for its effects on physiological and biological factors related to menstrual irregularities. One RCT studied the effect of Yoga Nidra on hormone levels in patients with menstrual irregularities [11]. After practicing Yoga Nidra for 6 months, the study found that levels of various hormones such as TSH, FSH, LH, and prolactin were decreased significantly which was interpreted by the authors that Yoga Nidra practice was helpful in patients with hormone imbalances associated with menstrual disorders. Another study reported significant differences in hormonal levels in the intervention group after 6 months of Yoga Nidra and medication compared to their pretest levels [10]. Furthermore, Yoga Nidra appears to impact somatoform symptoms and autonomic functions in women with menstrual disturbances. A study found that after 6 months of Yoga Nidra, there was a significant improvement in pain and other symptoms related to other organ systems as well [45]. Another study focused on autonomic functions, observing significant positive effects when Yoga Nidra was used as an adjunct in patients with menstrual disturbances [47]. Significant improvements were noted in variables related to autonomic functions after 6 months of Yoga Nidra practice.

6.2 Male fertility

While research primarily focused on women's health, the effect of Yoga Nidra on male fertility has also been studied. One case study explored the potential role of Yoga and Yoga Nidra for a patient having abnormal semen analysis [48]. The patient practiced a customized yoga regimen, which had included Yoga Nidra for 12 weeks. The male participant had improvement in semen analysis, showing the improvements in sperm count and motility, and reduced morphological abnormalities. However, it is important to note that this was a single case report, and more evidence would be required to understand the effects and their mechanisms.

6.3 Postmenopausal phase

Although not directly related to reproductive capacity, the postmenopausal phase is a significant stage in women's health following the reproductive years. Yoga Nidra has been highlighted as a promising nonpharmacological technique for the management of insomnia and overall health in postmenopausal women [49]. Regular practice can potentially help reduce anxiety and pain in this phase of life, and has therapeutic potential to improve sleep quality and quantity.

6.4 Psychological well-being

Psychological well-being is intrinsically linked to reproductive health and overall quality of life. Yoga Nidra has been reviewed to improve psychological well-being [50]. A pilot study using iRest, a form of guided mindfulness meditation similar to Yoga Nidra, with women who experienced sexual trauma (including military sexual trauma) showed promising results [51]. Participants reported significant decreases in symptoms of Post-Traumatic Stress Disorder.

In summary, the section collectively presents Yoga Nidra as a potentially valuable complementary approach to reproductive health, particularly for managing psychological distress, hormonal imbalances, somatoform symptoms, and autonomic dysfunctions associated with menstrual disorders. While preliminary, there is also emerging evidence from a case study suggesting its potential benefit for stress-related male infertility factors. Furthermore, its documented positive impact on overall wellbeing, sleep, and psychological health in phases like postmenopause and the context of trauma underscores its broader relevance to health across the reproductive lifespan and beyond. However, more extensive research, particularly large-scale controlled trials, is needed to validate these findings and establish definitive clinical guidelines [46, 48, 51].

7. Sleep and cognition

Emerging research, including randomized controlled trials and pilot studies, is exploring how this ancient practice might serve as a complementary or alternative approach to address common issues like insomnia and improve mental processing.

7.1 Effects on sleep

Studies have investigated its effects in various populations, including individuals with chronic insomnia and healthy novices. The traditional treatments for chronic insomnia may have limitations, so relaxation practices such as Yoga Nidra may be useful in such cases. Research has been conducted using subjective measures such as sleep diaries and objective measures, like polysomnography (PSG). A randomized controlled trial compared Yoga Nidra [13] with CBT as therapies for patients with chronic insomnia, found that both interventions led to significant improvements in parameters of sleep and in subjective sleep quality. Objectively, both interventions improved some of the parameters, and an improvement in N2 and N3 sleep stages. A study involving novices also utilized objective parameters, including overnight PSG and sleep diaries, to assess the effects of Yoga Nidra. After 4 weeks of practice, participants showed significant improvement in sleep efficiency [52]. They also experienced a reduction in wake after sleep onset. Objectively measured delta wave activity during deep sleep also saw a significant increase, further supporting the finding of improved deep sleep. Feasibility studies have also explored the potential of Yoga Nidra specifically for adults reporting insomnia. A preliminary clinical trial found Yoga Nidra to be a well-tolerated and feasible intervention for this population [53]. While this specific study did not find significant between-group changes in objective measures like sleep onset latency or alpha EEG power, it did observe a statistically significant decrease in respiratory rate during and after the practice compared to a control group. Although the link between respiratory rate and sleep needs further confirmation in larger studies, a reduced respiratory rate is often associated with relaxation states that can be conducive to sleep. Qualitative findings from another study exploring the experience of a single Yoga Nidra practice for patients of insomnia suggested it was useful for facilitating sleep [54]. Participants in focus groups reported feelings of relaxation and perceived improvements in sleep. Subjective reports on sleep improvement have also been noted in other populations practicing Yoga Nidra. In a pilot study, Yoga Nidra sessions were associated with the positive findings for sleep measures [55]. Health care workers participating in an 8-week Yoga Nidra program, a specific form of the practice, did not show a statistically significant difference in average Epworth Sleepiness Scale scores at baseline and follow-up, but there was a negative correlation between the number of weeks of intervention and the degree of improvement in sleepiness. This shows that more consistent practice might yield better results [56]. Furthermore, stress and cortisol levels, a study on insomnia patients showed a reduction in salivary cortisol levels [13]. In a randomized controlled trial, regular practice of an 11-minute version of Yoga Nidra was associated with reductions in total cortisol and steeper diurnal slopes compared to a waitlist control group [20]. The 30-minute version exceeded the effects of the shorter form and controls, including showing a flatter cortisol wake-up reaction [20]. Reducing stress and regulating cortisol patterns through Yoga Nidra may contribute to its positive effects on sleep.

7.2 Effects on cognition

Beyond sleep, Yoga Nidra practice has also been investigated for its effects on cognitive processing and performance. The study involving novices practicing Yoga Nidra utilized a comprehensive cognition testing battery (CTB) to objectively assess various cognitive functions. There was an improvement in reaction times after the practice of Yoga Nidra [52]. Thus, it provides evidence that Yoga Nidra practice can improve cognitive processing. Another cognitive aspect examined in relation to Yoga Nidra is mindfulness, which shows improvement after the practice is performed, especially in awareness scores [20]. Similarly, health care workers participating in an iRest Yoga Nidra program showed significantly higher post-intervention scores on the Five-Facet Mindfulness Questionnaire (FFMQ) [56]. While not a direct measure of cognitive performance in the same way as reaction times or task accuracy, increased mindfulness, particularly acting with awareness, is a cognitive skill that can influence attention, focus, and overall mental clarity. The findings suggest that Yoga Nidra practice can positively impact both fundamental cognitive processes like reaction time and accuracy in complex tasks, as well as the aspects of mindfulness related to awareness and non-judgment.

8. Yoga Nidra in specific populations

Yoga Nidra has emerged as a promising nonpharmacological approach with potential benefits across various specific populations facing unique physical, mental, and emotional challenges. The studies explore its application and observed effects in groups ranging from children with behavioral concerns to frontline healthcare workers, burn patients, adolescents, and individuals undergoing medical procedures. One significant area of investigation is the potential of Yoga Nidra for behavioral disorders in pediatric age group. These disorders include anxiety, hyperactivity, and emotional dysregulation [57]. While traditional interventions such as behavioral modification or medication are often used, their success can vary, and they may have potential side effects. The profound impact of the COVID-19 pandemic on mental health led to an increased interest in various mind-body therapies [58]. COVID-19 had a significant impact on mental health during the pandemic due to social isolation enforced due to quarantine and protocols related to the prevention of the spread of the disease. A randomized controlled trial was conducted on frontline COVID-19 workers to compare the effects of Yoga Nidra intervention and music as relaxation therapy on various mental health parameters such as depression, anxiety, stress, and insomnia. The workers were provided with YouTube links to perform the practices at their homes for 2 weeks, as the authors found that it was not feasible to provide an intervention in a physical setup under direct supervision. Both groups had around 40 workers each. It was found that the Yoga Nidra group had a significant reduction in the described markers of mental health as compared to the music group. Thus, it demonstrates that the underlying neurological effects by the practices of Yoga Nidra are not simply relaxation, but may have more elaborate mechanisms that are yet to be explored. Another specific population studied was burn patients, where the effect of Yoga Nidra on self-esteem and body image was investigated [59]. YN can have a role in psychological recovery in serious traumatic illnesses such as burns. A study conducted on burn patients (>30% burns) found that YN practice could improve the self-esteem and body image of the patients after 4 weeks of regular practice. Although long-term or follow-up data were not taken, an improvement in these parameters could have positive outcomes in recovery from a serious physical illness.

The well-being of adolescents is identified as a priority area for healthcare interventions [60]. Not only in the adult population, positive effects of YN have also been documented in the adolescent population of the age group 13–15 years. It was found that after a month-long YN sessions in which participants conducted YN for 3 days per week, their measures of well-being improved significantly. The tested measures included happiness, perceived stress, general well-being and also some experiential measures that were included by the authors themselves such as clarity of thought, enthusiasm, self-confidence, alertness. So, it seems that the practice of yoga nidra has evidence of positive effects across all age groups from adolescence to adulthood.

Finally, guided Yoga Nidra recordings were explored for pain management in patients undergoing colonoscopy [61]. The study compared the effects of a Yoga Nidra and relaxation music for pain management during this procedure. There were three groups of patients including Yoga Nidra group and a relaxation music group. The findings revealed that both the music and the Yoga Nidra recording significantly reduced the patients' perceptions of pain and the endoscopist's perceived colonoscope insertion difficulty and overall patient satisfaction. Also, patients' willingness to repeat the procedure was improved. Thus, it was concluded that both the Yoga Nidra recording and relaxation music helped reduce the pain during colonoscopy. This demonstrates the potential of Yoga Nidra as an adjunct therapy for managing discomfort and improving the patient experience during medical procedures.

9. Conclusion

Yoga Nidra emerges not merely as a relaxation technique but as a structured practice rooted in the ancient yogic traditions, rearticulated in the modern era to address challenges of healthcare. Contemporary research increasingly validates what ancient seers intuitively knew that the conscious withdrawal of sensory attention while maintaining awareness, generates potential physiological and psychological benefits. This is evident in the measurable effects of Yoga Nidra on autonomic tone, endocrine profiles, and central nervous system activity. The practice, when pursued regularly, not only modulates blood pressure and glycemic control in metabolic disorders such as hypertension and diabetes but also helps to restore hormonal homeostasis in menstrual irregularities.

In the domain of mental health, Yoga Nidra offers a nonpharmacological intervention for reducing stress, anxiety, and depression, the conditions that increasingly pervade modern life and have significant prevalence. It can empower practitioners by facilitating non-effortful awareness, thereby potentially bypassing the usual resistance encountered in cognitive or behavioral therapies.

Moreover, Yoga Nidra's benefits extend to sleep architecture, showing improvements in insomnia and sleep quality, while simultaneously enhancing cognitive function and emotional resilience. Its adaptability makes it a viable modality for specific and vulnerable populations ranging from adolescents and students to individuals with chronic illnesses, underscoring its inclusivity and therapeutic flexibility.

Ultimately, Yoga Nidra exemplifies the unification of ancient contemplative wisdom with modern evidence-based health practices. It represents a paradigm shift from managing disease to cultivating embodied awareness as a means of restoring systemic physiological balance.

10. Limitations and future directions

While Yoga Nidra shows significant promise as a preventive and therapeutic intervention, several limitations in the current body of research need attention. Many studies suffer from small sample sizes, short durations, and methodological inconsistencies, which limit the generalizability of their findings. The heterogeneity in intervention protocols, including variations in session length, frequency, and instructional content, makes it difficult to standardize Yoga Nidra for clinical application. Additionally, the subjective nature of outcome measures, particularly in domains like stress, well-being, and sleep, can introduce bias and reduce the reliability of findings.

A large proportion of the existing evidence comes from single-center studies or those conducted in homogenous populations, often within specific cultural or sociodemographic contexts. This raises questions about the cross-cultural applicability of the results. Furthermore, while physiological metrics such as heart rate variability (HRV), salivary cortisol, and EEG parameters provide encouraging objective support, the mechanistic pathways underlying Yoga Nidra's effects on neuroendocrine and autonomic regulation remain inadequately understood.

Future research should prioritize multicentric, randomized controlled trials (RCTs) with larger and more diverse cohorts to strengthen the evidence base. Longitudinal studies examining the sustained effects of Yoga Nidra over months or years are also needed, particularly to explore its role in chronic disease prevention and relapse reduction. In addition, well-designed studies that integrate neuroimaging (e.g., fMRI and PET) and neurophysiological techniques (e.g., high-density EEG and polysomnography) can help clarify the states of consciousness induced by Yoga Nidra and differentiate or explain the underlying mechanisms w.r.t. rest, sleep, or meditation [6, 14, 16, 17].

Another future direction involves developing standardized Yoga Nidra protocols suitable for clinical settings. Establishing contraindications and safety guidelines, especially in vulnerable individuals with psychiatric comorbidities, is also essential. Integration of wearable biosensors and mobile health platforms may further support real-time monitoring and personalized delivery of Yoga Nidra interventions [20].

Overall, while Yoga Nidra holds a lot of potential, rigorous scientific inquiry is required to transform this ancient practice into a universally accepted evidence-based modality in modern healthcare.

Author details

Navdeep Ahuja[1], Monika Pathania[2*] and Praag Bhardwaj[3,4]

1 Department of Physiology, AIIMS, Bilaspur, HP, India

2 Department of Internal Medicine, Ayush, AIIMS, Rishikesh, India

3 Faculty of Health and Wellness, Sri Sri University, Cuttack, Odisha, India

4 Department of Medicine, All India Institute of Medical Sciences (AIIMS), Rishikesh, Uttarakhand, India

*Address all correspondence to: anshupathania27@gmail.com

References

[1] Pandi-Perumal SR, Spence DW, Srivastava N, Kanchibhotla D, Kumar K, Sharma GS, et al. The origin and clinical relevance of yoga nidra. Sleep and Vigilance. 2022;**6**(1):61-84

[2] Saraswati SS. Yoga Nidra. 6th ed. Munger, Bihar, India: Yoga Publications Trust; 1998

[3] Satchidananda S. The Yoga Sutras of Patanjali. Buckingham, Virginia, USA: Integral Yoga Publications; 1978. Commentary by Swami Satchidananda

[4] Shankar SSR. Patanjali Yoga Sutras. 1st ed. Bangalore: Sri Sri Publications Trust; 2022. 280 p. ISBN: 9789391598068

[5] Bodri W. Nyasa Yoga: Kundalini, Prana, Chakra and Nadi Cultivation Techniques. USA: Top Shape Publishing LLC; 2017

[6] Kjaer TW, Bertelsen C, Piccini P, Brooks D, Alving J, Lou HC. Increased dopamine tone during meditation-induced change of consciousness. Brain Research. Cognitive Brain Research. 2002;**13**(2):255-259

[7] Lou HC, Kjaer TW, Friberg L, Wildschiodtz G, Holm S, Nowak M. A 15O-H2O pet study of meditation and the resting state of normal consciousness. Human Brain Mapping. 1999;**7**(2):98-105

[8] Kumar K. Changes in hemoglobin among house wives through yoga: A pilot study. International Journal of Yoga and Allied Sciences. 2018;**7**(2):113-117. Available from: https://indianyoga.org/wp-content/uploads/2020/09/v7-issue2-article22.pdf

[9] Amita S, Prabhakar S, Manoj I, Harminder S, Pavan T. Effect of yoga-nidra on blood glucose level in diabetic patients. Indian Journal of Physiology and Pharmacology. 2009;**53**(1):97-101

[10] Rani K, Tiwari SC, Kumar S, Singh U, Prakash J, Srivastava N. Psycho-biological changes with add on yoga nidra in patients with menstrual disorders: A randomized clinical trial. Journal of Caring Sciences. 2016;**5**(1):1-9

[11] Rani M, Singh U, Agrawal GG, Natu SM, Kala S, Ghildiyal A, et al. Impact of yoga nidra on menstrual abnormalities in females of reproductive age. Journal of Alternative and Complementary Medicine. 2013;**19**(12):925-929

[12] Ahuja N, Bhardwaj P, Pathania M, Sethi D, Kumar A, Parchani A, et al. Yoga Nidra for hypertension: A systematic review and meta-analysis. Journal of Ayurveda and Integrative Medicine. 2024;**15**(2):100882

[13] Datta K, Tripathi M, Verma M, Masiwal D, Mallick HN. Yoga Nidra practice shows improvement in sleep in patients with chronic insomnia: A randomized controlled trial. National Medical Journal of India. 2021;**34**(3):143-150

[14] Datta K, Mallick HN, Tripathi M, Ahuja N, Deepak KK. Electrophysiological evidence of local sleep during yoga nidra practice. Frontiers in Neurology. 2022;**13**:910794

[15] Zaccaro A, Riehl A, Piarulli A, Alfì G, Neri B, Menicucci D, et al. The consciousness state of traditional nidrâ yoga/modern yoga nidra: Phenomenological characterization and preliminary insights from an eeg study.

International Journal of Yoga Therapy. 2021;**31**(1)

[16] Fialoke S, Tripathi V, Thakral S, Dhawan A, Majahan V, Garg R. Functional connectivity changes in meditators and novices during yoga nidra practice. Scientific Reports. 2024;**14**(1):12957

[17] Kavi PC. Conscious entry into sleep: Yoga nidra and accessing subtler states of consciousness. Progress in Brain Research. 2023;**280**:43-60

[18] Parker S. Training attention for conscious non-rem sleep: The yogic practice of yoga-nidrā and its implications for neuroscience research. Progress in Brain Research. 2019;**244**:255-272

[19] Markil N, Whitehurst M, Jacobs PL, Zoeller RF. Yoga nidra relaxation increases heart rate variability and is unaffected by a prior bout of hatha yoga. Journal of Alternative and Complementary Medicine. 2012;**18**(10):953-958

[20] Moszeik EN, Rohleder N, Renner KH. The effects of an online yoga nidra meditation on subjective well-being and diurnal salivary cortisol: A randomised controlled trial. Stress and Health. 2025;**41**(3):e70049

[21] Notarius CF, Badrov MB, Tobushi T, Keir DA, Keys E, Floras JS. Cardiovascular reflex contributions to sympathetic inhibition during low-intensity dynamic leg exercise in healthy middle-age. Physiological Reports. 2023;**11**(17):e15821

[22] Magnon V, Dutheil F, Vallet GT. Benefits from one session of deep and slow breathing on vagal tone and anxiety in young and older adults. Scientific Reports. 2021;**11**(1):19267

[23] Kerr CE, Jones SR, Wan Q, Pritchett DL, Wasserman RH, Wexler A, et al. Effects of mindfulness meditation training on anticipatory alpha modulation in primary somatosensory cortex. Brain Research Bulletin. 2011;**85**(3-4):96-103

[24] Kerr CE, Sacchet MD, Lazar SW, Moore CI, Jones SR. Mindfulness starts with the body: Somatosensory attention and top–down modulation of cortical alpha rhythms in mindfulness meditation. Frontiers in Human Neuroscience. 2013;**7**:12

[25] Fischer D, Messner M, Pollatos O. Improvement of interoceptive processes after an 8–week body scan intervention. Frontiers in Human Neuroscience. 2017;**11**:452

[26] Doll A, Hölzel BK, Boucard CC, Wohlschläger AM, Sorg C. Mindfulness is associated with intrinsic functional connectivity between default mode and salience networks. Frontiers in Human Neuroscience. 2015;**9**:461

[27] Guu S-F, Chao Y-P, Huang F-Y, Cheng Y-T, Ng H-YH, Hsu C-F, et al. Interoceptive awareness: Mbsr training alters information processing of the salience network. Frontiers in Behavioral Neuroscience. 2023;**17**:1008086

[28] Thayer JF, Lane RD. A model of neurovisceral integration in emotion regulation and dysregulation. Journal of Affective Disorders. 2000;**61**(3):201-216

[29] Smith R, Thayer JF, Khalsa SS, Lane RD. The hierarchical basis of neurovisceral integration. Neuroscience & Biobehavioral Reviews. 2017;**75**:274-296

[30] Musto S, Hazard VA. Exploring the uses of yoga nidra: An integrative

review. Journal of Nursing Scholarship. 2023;**55**(6):1164-1178

[31] Dol KS. Effects of a yoga nidra on the life stress and self-esteem in university students. Complementary Therapies in Clinical Practice. 2019;**35**:232-236

[32] Eastman-Mueller H, Wilson T, Jung AK, Kimura A, Tarrant J. Irest yoga-nidra on the college campus: Changes in stress, depression, worry, and mindfulness. International Journal of Yoga Therapy. 2013;**23**:15-24

[33] D'souza OL, Jose AE, Suresh S, Baliga MS. Effectiveness of yoga nidra in reducing stress in school going adolescents: An experimental study. Complementary Therapies in Clinical Practice. 2021;**45**:101462

[34] Ferreira-Vorkapic C, Borba-Pinheiro CJ, Marchioro M, Santana D. The impact of yoga nidra and seated meditation on the mental health of college professors. International Journal of Yoga. 2018;**11**(3):215-223

[35] Luu K. Key components of trauma-informed yoga nidra. International Journal of Yoga Therapy. 2024;**34**:2024

[36] Stankovic L. Transforming trauma: A qualitative feasibility study of integrative restoration (irest) yoga nidra on combat-related post-traumatic stress disorder. International Journal of Yoga Therapy. 2011;**21**:23-37

[37] di Fronso S, Robazza C, Pompa D, Bertollo M. Dreaming while awake: The beneficial effects of yoga nidra on mental and physical recovery in two elite karate athletes. Heliyon. 2024;**10**(1):e24180

[38] Ahuja N, Pathania M, Mohan L, Mittal S, Bhardwaj P, Dhar M. The effect of yoga nidra intervention on blood pressure and heart rate variability among hypertensive adults: A single-arm intervention trial. Cureus. 2025;**17**(1):e77717

[39] Anjana K, Archana R, Mukkadan JK. Effect of om chanting and yoga nidra on blood pressure and lipid profile in hypertension - a randomized controlled trial. Journal of Ayurveda and Integrative Medicine. 2022;**13**(4):100657

[40] Rajagopalan A, Krishna A, Mukkadan JK. Effect of om chanting and yoga nidra on depression anxiety stress, sleep quality and autonomic functions of hypertensive subjects - A randomized controlled trial. Journal of Basic and Clinical Physiology and Pharmacology. 2023;**34**(1):69-75

[41] Barber M, Evans S, Marks R, Sheedy J, Miller R, Lopez S, et al. "I am not pain, I have pain": A pilot study examining irest yoga nidra as a mind-body intervention for persistent pain. Complementary Therapies in Clinical Practice. 2025;**59**:101955

[42] Giridharan S. Yoga nidra: A promising complementary therapy for enhancing cancer care. Cureus. 2024;**16**(9):e70536

[43] Nuzhath FJ, Patil NJ, Sheela SR, Manjunath GN. A randomized controlled trial on pranayama and yoga nidra for anxiety and depression in patients with cervical cancer undergoing standard of care. Cureus. 2024;**16**(3):e55871

[44] Rani K, Tiwari S, Singh U, Singh I, Srivastava N. Yoga nidra as a complementary treatment of anxiety and depressive symptoms in patients with menstrual disorder. International Journal of Yoga. 2012;**5**(1):52-56

[45] Rani K, Tiwari SC, Singh U, Agrawal GG, Srivastava N. Six-month trial of yoga nidra in menstrual disorder

patients: Effects on somatoform symptoms. Industrial Psychiatry Journal. 2011;**20**(2):97-102

[46] Kim SD. Psychological effects of yoga nidra in women with menstrual disorders: A systematic review of randomized controlled trials. Complementary Therapies in Clinical Practice. 2017;**28**:4-8

[47] Monika SU, Ghildiyal A, Kala S, Srivastava N. Effect of yoga nidra on physiological variables in patients of menstrual disturbances of reproductive age group. Indian Journal of Physiology and Pharmacology. 2012;**56**(2):161-167

[48] Jadhav R, More A, Dutta S, Gajabe G, Shrivastava J, Mehakar S. Improving semen quality in a male partner with abnormal seminal parameters through yoga and yoga nidra: A case report. Cureus. 2024;**16**(2):e54095

[49] Gulia KK, Sreedharan SE. Yoga nidra, a nonpharmacological technique in management of insomnia and overall health in postmenopausal women. Sleep Medicine Clinics. 2023;**18**(4):463-471

[50] Nayak K, Verma K. Yoga-nidra as a mental health booster: A narrative review. Journal of Ayurveda and Integrative Medicine. 2023;**14**(6):100842

[51] Pence PG, Katz LS, Huffman C, Cojucar G. Delivering integrative restoration-yoga nidra meditation (irest®) to women with sexual trauma at a veteran's medical center: A pilot study. International Journal of Yoga Therapy. 2014;**24**:53-62

[52] Datta K, Bhutambare A, Mamatha VL, Narawa Y, Srinath R, Kanitkar M. Improved sleep, cognitive processing and enhanced learning and memory task accuracy with yoga nidra practice in novices. PLoS One. 2023;**18**(12):e0294678

[53] Sharpe E, Butler MP, Clark-Stone J, Soltanzadeh R, Jindal R, Hanes D, et al. A closer look at yoga nidra-early randomized sleep lab investigations. Journal of Psychosomatic Research. 2023;**166**:111169

[54] Sharpe E, Tibbitts D, Wolfe B, Senders A, Bradley R. Qualitative impressions of a yoga nidra practice for insomnia: An exploratory mixed-methods design. Journal of Alternative and Complementary Medicine. 2021;**27**(10):884-892

[55] Anderson R, Mammen K, Paul P, Pletch A, Pulia K. Using yoga nidra to improve stress in psychiatric nurses in a pilot study. Journal of Alternative and Complementary Medicine. 2017;**23**(6):494-495

[56] Livingston E, Collette-Merrill K. Effectiveness of integrative restoration (irest) yoga nidra on mindfulness, sleep, and pain in health care workers. Holistic Nursing Practice. 2018;**32**(3):160-166

[57] Pandya PR. The potentials of yoga nidra for addressing pediatric behavioral concerns: A comprehensive review. International Journal of Yoga. 2024;**17**(2):76-82

[58] Gunjiganvi M, Rai S, Awale R, Mishra P, Gupta D, Gurjar M. Efficacy of yoga nidra on depression, anxiety, and insomnia in frontline covid-19 healthcare workers: A pilot randomized controlled trial. International Journal of Yoga Therapy. 2023;**33**:2023

[59] Ozdemir A, Saritas S. Effect of yoga nidra on the self-esteem and body image of burn patients. Complementary Therapies in Clinical Practice. 2019;**35**:86-91

[60] Vaishnav BS, Vaishnav SB, Vaishnav VS, Varma JR. Effect of

yoga-nidra on adolescents well-being: A mixed method study. International Journal of Yoga. 2018;**11**(3):245-248

[61] Li L, Shu W, Li Z, Liu Q, Wang H, Feng B, et al. Using yoga nidra recordings for pain management in patients undergoing colonoscopy. Pain Management Nursing. 2019;**20**(1):39-46

Chapter 4

Spiritual Support as a Component of the Whole Approach in Healthcare

Marcelo Saad and Roberta de Medeiros

Abstract

The patient's spiritual dimension has gained increasing relevance in healthcare. Countless studies over the past decades have shown causal associations between spiritual well-being and healthy physiological parameters. In turn, such association positively impacts physical and mental health, quality of life, and even longevity. The researchers note two significant challenges for the clinical application of this solid knowledge. First, it would be impractical to "prescribe" the promotion of spiritual well-being for health purposes. Second, spirituality is often linked to religiosity (although they are two different concepts), contaminating the technical discussion. This chapter was based on the authors' experience of 25 years of study in this field and supported by pertinent clinical literature. It suggests objective guidelines for practical usage for healthcare professionals and institutions.

Keywords: spirituality, spiritual coping, religiosity coping, existentialism, pastoral care, hospital chaplaincy, psychological well-being, mental health

1. Introduction

1.1 The dynamic evolution of health sciences

The World Health Organization has adopted this definition of health since its founding: "a state of complete physical, mental and social well-being and not merely the absence of disease or infirmity." However, in 1999, the 52nd WHO Assembly approved a revision to include spiritual well-being in its concept of health [1]. Although this adjustment was not implemented, the fact that it was proposed highlights the issue's significance. Thus, spiritual well-being is a strong candidate to be included as a general health dimension, enhancing the biopsychosocial model.

Healthcare is dynamic, with new knowledge and views reshaping clinical practices and valuing previously neglected needs. In the last 50 years, medicine has seen significant efforts to become more humanised. The humanisation of medicine broadened health understanding to a broader model, valuing the patient's subjective experience while empowering them in therapeutic decisions. This shift has transformed notions of health, disease, treatment, and cure, with spirituality becoming increasingly important for patient's health and quality of life.

1.2 Spirituality has a lot to do with healthcare

Everything "spiritual" was considered inseparable from religion for a long time. In ancient times, healthcare and spirituality were interconnected, with spiritual leaders often overseeing healing practices. After the modern technical-rationalistic development, the secular nature acquired by healthcare professions distanced spirituality from clinical attention. However, the appreciation of patient-centred care in recent decades has made a rapprochement mandatory.

Contemporary pluralistic societies and cultures allow each one to interpret personally what would mean "spiritual." Individuals often cultivate their spirituality through structured religions or belief systems, while others express their spiritual dimension with non-religious practices. The profile of religious affiliations is changing dynamically, with a trend towards secularisation for some people and multiculturalism for others. Western society increasingly expresses spirituality without basing it on specific religious pillars or delineated worldviews.

Recently, "secular spirituality" [2] emerged from non-religious, humanistic perspectives, liberal principles, and analytical considerations of what constitutes a meaningful life. The concept of secular spirituality is relatively new, and the designation "spiritual but not religious" has become an increasingly popular faith affiliation [3], though this group remains heterogeneous. Thus, spiritual support in healthcare has gradually shifted from a religiously based activity to a broader activity of caring for all existential needs.

Accordingly, spiritual care is not optional. It becomes an obligation and an ethical prerequisite for good healthcare practice. Integral healthcare inherently includes the spiritual dimension, where narratives of meaning are constructed, and internal coping resources emerge for health and disease situations [4].

1.3 State of the scientific literature

Before addressing the specific subject of this chapter, the reader must be familiar with some knowledge derived from scientific studies in recent decades, listed below [5–10]:

- Spiritual well-being is linked to better physical and mental health, quality of life, and longevity.
- Most research shows that this association is causal, positive, significant, and clinically relevant.
- Spiritual well-being helps balance physiologic functions mainly by reducing stress.
- Biological and psychological changes have been observed in prayer, rituals, and blessings.
- A patient with spiritual well-being is better equipped to manage the illness process.
- However, misinterpretations of faith can exacerbate stress and lead to adverse outcomes.

- Spiritual support should be a fundamental responsibility of the health institution.
- Understanding and applying these facts is important for increasing clinical practice standards.

2. Some important concepts

2.1 Spirituality

Among several definitions of spirituality for health purposes, the more inclusive types are used primarily in clinical practice, and others more restricted are used mainly in research. Due to the lack of a universal consensus, Sena et al. [11] systematically searched for definitions published in scientific journals, and they proposed a new framework in which spirituality is (a) a human individual, dynamic characteristic; (b) expressed through beliefs, practices, and experiences in the search for connection with something that promotes meaning and personal growth; and (c) leads to the development of values and positive feelings.

2.2 Religiosity

It refers to the extent to which an individual adheres to, follows, and practises a specific religious denomination. Such observance occurs in its inner facets (belief, private prayer, subjective experience) and outer ones (participation in public cults, congregational life). Many people find spirituality through their religiosity; however, some find it through non-religious elements, such as nature, art, or a set of values and principles. The concept of an individual belief system can transcend the limits of a specific religious doctrine. Personal perspectives can be blurred and not always logical or consistent. People may fluidly integrate a variety of ideas that they identify with into a mix of sources [12].

2.3 Spiritual-religious coping

It is the effort to find or maintain meaning, purpose, and connectedness in distressing situations [13]. The term refers to applying a personal belief system for dealing with stressful and traumatic circumstances. These strategies can be employed to manage a crisis or alleviate the associated emotional distress. Faith-related practices and concepts promote comfort, well-being, security, and idealism. A solid belief structure can be a valuable resource for well-being [14]. It is crucial to know that spiritual-religious coping can have a positive or negative impact on spiritual well-being. Some disruptive religious interpretations, such as questioning the theological justification for the present unfavourable condition, may give rise to spiritual struggle (described below).

2.4 Spiritual well-being

It refers to the capacity to integrate meaning and purpose in life through connections with oneself, others, or a higher power [15]. It is the dimension accessed through the subjective perception of well-being regarding beliefs, experienced through a sense of purpose in life. Another literature source defines it as a state comprising positive feelings, behaviours, and cognitions that provide the individual with a sense of identity, completeness, satisfaction, contentment, constructive attitudes, inner peace, harmony, and purpose in life [16].

2.5 Spiritual needs

They refer to human aspirations and anticipations to find meaning, purpose, and value in their life [17]. Such needs may be explicitly religious, but even individuals who do not adhere to any religious identity keep constructs that provide meaning and purpose to their lives. Spiritual needs differ from emotional and social ones, as the former pertains to the transcendental aspects of existence. These needs are addressed by focusing on the connection between existential concerns and life events. If spiritual needs are not contemplated, it may lead to spiritual distress.

2.6 Spiritual struggle

They are instances of tension, conflict, or strain that focus on what individuals consider sacred [18]. This state may adversely affect patients' health by worsening stress [19]. Specific religious interpretations may be harmful when elements of the doctrine are taken out of context. Sectarian or fundamentalist religious leaders can sometimes place patients in situations where medical and religious ethics conflict. A dysfunctional belief system might lead patients to rely on faith instead of seeking appropriate clinical care. Specific beliefs about the sanctity of life may result in dysthanasia, where futile treatments are continued in terminal conditions.

2.7 Spiritual support

This activity addresses the spiritual and religious perspectives of patients, focusing on how these beliefs relate to their illness, hospitalisation, and either their recovery or potential death [20]. Recognising patients' spiritual values and experiences is essential in delivering high-quality clinical practice. It can be promoted by immediate generalists (such as healthcare staff) or trained specialists (such as faith representatives). The "clients" (beneficiaries) of spiritual support in healthcare facilities include the patients, their families, the accompanying caregivers, and the healthcare professionals.

3. The role of the healthcare system and its professionals

3.1 Benefits for the healthcare institution

The future of healthcare quality is intrinsically linked to integrating humanistic values as an essential component of patient-centred attention, not just the incorporation of exorbitant new technologies. In this tendency, spiritual support is key in promoting compassionate care and improving the patient experience.

When patients feel that their spiritual needs are acknowledged and addressed, their treatment experience improves, and they are more likely to achieve positive outcomes [21]. A comprehensive humanisation programme incorporating spiritual support as part of the procedures promotes a more positive patient experience. Besides, it brings tangible benefits for the organisation by strengthening its mission of providing broad and compassionate health attention.

DOI: http://dx.doi.org/10.5772/intechopen.1010156

Certification companies for healthcare quality accreditation reinforce the importance of spiritual care by establishing some specific standards. Successfully implementing these standards requires a constant commitment to improvement and innovation. Many quality accreditation systems currently require healthcare services that respect patients' spiritual and religious values and attitudes. For hospital quality accreditation, the Joint Commission International demands standards such as [22]:

- PFR.1.2 The hospital provides care that supports patient dignity, respects the patient's intimate values and beliefs, and responds to requests for spiritual and religious observance.

- AOP.1.1 Each patient's initial assessment includes a physical examination and health history as well as an evaluation of psychological, spiritual/cultural (as appropriate), social, and economic factors.

Meeting the above standards requires awareness, resource investment, and a commitment to continuous improvement to attend to spiritual needs effectively and sensitively. However, there are still no precise specifications for structuring processes in institutions or qualifying their employees. Each facility must perform its own self-diagnostic and design its improvement.

3.2 Implementing a spiritual support infrastructure

To integrate spiritual support into healthcare, each institution must continuously devote itself to improvements that demand finance and energy. Managers must see such initiatives as an investment so that the project does not lose momentum over time. A first step may be done with staff orientation—professionals must know that spirituality is related to health and that the institution begins to value this. Staff must feel confident that the institution will provide them with the conditions for this initiative. Ideally, a specific committee should draw up a plan tailored to the reality of the service. Its work would include choosing validated screening questionnaires and instilling an atmosphere of cultural sensitivity and respect for diversity. Integrating spirituality into healthcare should be respectful, voluntary, and adapted.

Competition with other assistance priorities creates time and space restrictions for adequate spiritual screening. Secular norms in healthcare contribute to staff reluctance to engage with patients' spiritual histories. At times, staff may even face prejudice from colleagues or managers. Thus, services must foster staff confidence so that they can provide care that meets patients' spiritual needs. Training programmes and educational initiatives are institutional approaches to equip staff with the skills needed to address spiritual issues sensitively and effectively.

It is not necessary to have extensive resources to provide spiritual assistance in a healthcare facility. Having a multi-faith space, even if small and unpretentious, can be of great value for family members and employees to have a place of contemplation and peace. To ensure appropriate referral when necessary, the administration should have a contact list of religious leaders who could provide assistance. Regular evaluation feedback from staff and patients is essential to determine whether the programme meets its aims. The awareness and motivation must resist the stream of monotony and indifference when someone does something without remembering why.

Spiritual support must be provided not only to patients but also to any person involved with them, as the positive relationship between spiritual well-being and good health parameters applies. Healthcare professionals face significant challenges in their work, and spiritual support can be a valuable tool to help them cope. Implementing programmes targeted at this population is essential to ensure they have access to the support they need to maintain their well-being and technical performance, providing the conditions that enable them to fully exercise their potential and provide the best care and experience for patients and families.

3.3 Spiritual screening by healthcare professionals

All health professionals are also responsible for spiritual care. As a "generalist" in spiritual support, the health professional can perform a spiritual screening and anticipate the impacts of the patient's beliefs on treatment. From the perspective of this integral care, the professionals must do it in the same way that other spheres of the individual are systematically evaluated. This practice also becomes fundamental for establishing an empathetic bond, which produces better patient care results. Besides, early recognition of spiritual distress can promote a better quality of multidisciplinary care.

Religious affiliation is the first piece of information in spiritual history; however, doctrinal interpretations and observance levels tend to differ among believers. The way patients reflect their religious values in the health and illness process can be beneficial or harmful to them, depending on how they are used. Thus, spiritual care should be customised, avoiding labelling or stereotyping the recipient.

The professional must identify and contemplate the patient's spiritual needs in the treatment plan whenever possible. Before addressing spiritual aspects, the patient should be given context regarding the desire to undertake a comprehensive approach. The professional should explain that spiritual aspects are important to many people, and if the patient wishes, these issues will be addressed. The spiritual assessment can strengthen the professional-patient relationship, having an intrinsic therapeutic character.

Some questionnaires are available to guide the spiritual anamnesis; the most used are FICA, SPIRITual, HOPE, and FAITH [23]. Standardised screening scales are a practical and valuable tool that minimises barriers such as lack of knowledge or uncertainty about receptiveness.

Human connection is central through attitudes such as openness, respect, authenticity, non-judgement, hope, honesty, empathy, kindness, and spiritual awareness. The professional must act impartially, without imposing their own values, at the risk of resulting in proselytism and breaking the professional bond.

The professional's spirituality must also be developed since entering the R/S of individuals in distress is a challenge subject to adversities that can lead to conflicts with one's uncertainties of meaning and purpose. Consequently, the professional may suffer stress, compassion fatigue, and burnout. Thus, self-care is also essential for the sustainability of this holistic care. Here are two brief pieces of advice taken from a previous publication by the present authors [24]:

- Religiously orientated professionals can maintain their faith to gain strength to face professional challenges. However, most of the time, clinical practice requires lay premises and standard methods. They can always follow their personal commitments by referring the patient to another colleague in delicate cases, such as abortion or euthanasia.

- The secularly orientated professionals must remember that their role is to give the patient the best information and allow patients to decide, even when some religious interpretations are detrimental to health. Recognising the patient's religious values is key to cultural sensitivity, and respecting such background is important to a patient-centred approach.

3.4 Hospitals and admissions facilities

For inpatients, chaplains are not the only professionals, although they are the most qualified and experienced to provide spiritual assistance to the entire hospital community. They are part of the interdisciplinary care team in many developed countries. The institutional chaplain can create a care plan, record it in the clinical chart, and discuss it with the multidisciplinary team. In religiously pluralised societies, chaplains often care for patients with a different faith orientation than their own.

Many hospitalised patients have restrictions on some religious/spiritual practices, such as restricted diet, mobility constraints by invasive devices (accesses, tubes, probes, or catheters), and isolation due to contagious disease, among others. These should not prevent the performance of practices, prayers, and/or rites, and they can often be adapted using creativity and available equivalents. For religiously observant inpatients, the community's religious minister can come to the hospital to offer pastoral care specific to his or her tradition.

4. Spiritual support for any belief system

4.1 The patient with a "secular spirituality"

With the diversity of the spiritual landscape, meeting spiritual needs has become a complex process that involves patients of any faith or even no faith. The spiritual caregiver must support people with different traditions and worldviews. Parallel to the plurality of worldviews and spiritual traditions, people with secular views also search for meaning in their lives. Secular spirituality, like religious spirituality, may strongly relate to mental health [25]. Some examples of secular resources for spiritual health are [26]:

- Feeling connected to something bigger, awakening the unconditional love.

- Being open to inspiration from insights and inner voice.

- Investing in moral growth through personal reflection and life choices.

- Getting strength from philosophical and humanistic worldviews.

- Spending more time with nature, art, and contemplative practices.

- Identifying what is intimately significant and making room for it.

- Cultivating optimism, hope, gratitude, and a good mood.

- Seeking out the awesomeness in everyday tiny miracles.

- Practising philanthropical actions with solidarity and compassion.
- Finding expanded consciousness in a secular form of meditation.

On one hand, freedom of creed is guaranteed as a patient's right and a duty of institutions; on the other hand, legal provisions maintain the separation between churches and civil society. In Western countries, some laws seek to ensure the secularity of the State to combat religious discrimination. However, the State's laicity cannot be an obstacle to providing spiritual support.

4.2 The interfaith model

Spiritual support can be delivered through an interfaith model when the provider is trained to address universal needs that go beyond specific religious doctrines. An interfaith chaplain can offer support irrespective of religious affiliation, thereby connecting the patient to their fundamental spiritual framework. In some countries, professional organisations certify health chaplains with well-systematised training. Interfaith support requires both a recognition of the person as a human being and an understanding of that person's spiritual path. The goal of interfaith support includes an appreciation of all faiths, including non-religious ones such as secular humanism. Spiritual support providers can initiate interactions with patients and use some strategies when working with someone with a religious background different from their own.

Atheists, agnostics, and the like may have fundamental values and enquiries about worth and purpose and be undergoing an existential crisis. Individuals can enhance their spiritual well-being through non-religious elements, philosophical reasoning, or contemplative practices. Among the philosophical approaches to achieving this goal, Stoicism presents a framework centred on virtue and pursuing the highest good. Living wisely and virtuously can enhance strength and character, leading to ultimate harmony [27].

5. Can spirituality-religiosity do harm?

5.1 Disruption of the patient's belief system

The subject has already been previously introduced in the section "Some important concepts," especially in the topics of COPING, WELL-BEING and STRUGGLE. The dictates of any belief system are open to individual interpretations regarding their meaning for the facts of life. When theological expectations do not correspond to clinical outcomes, the patient may be overcome by distress and disorientation. The reaction may include feelings of incoherence ("why did God do this to me?"), injustice ("I did everything that was expected of me") that may culminate in anger. The persistence of these states tends to aggravate stress, consequently damaging mental-emotional balance. Patients open to specialised doctrinal counselling may have a chance to reframe the facts and rebuild the comforting role of their beliefs.

5.2 Conflicts between belief systems and clinical planning

In some situations, creed values can conflict with clinical decisions, challenging the intersection between patient autonomy and professional ethics. Each country that recognises patient autonomy would allow individual objection to treatment for creed reasons. However, the potential consequences of such autonomy pose a delicate legal challenge, especially in critical situations and serious illnesses. Conflicts in medical decision-making can be characterised by verbalisation of uncertainty, indecision between different options, delay in decision-making, and questioning of inner values. Some religious interpretations can affect end-of-life decisions in which life is the ultimate value and its quality is secondary. In extreme cases, the problem is worsened when decisions need to be made by family members or patient representatives.

Open dialogue can help to dispel misunderstandings that could affect treatment. Sometimes, clinical information is conveyed in a way that inadvertently offends or confuses the patient. The interfaith chaplain can assess how the patient's or a family member's religious or spiritual values may interfere with their decisions about medical care and can also mediate dialogue between patients, families, and clinical teams. Despite the potential drawbacks, understanding the meaning of spirituality is vital for healthcare professionals. Recognising cultural aspects and respecting beliefs are crucial. Overall, embracing the importance of spirituality promotes compassionate healthcare.

5.3 Patient waiting for a miracle

Many patients believe that miracles can occur, and then an unexpected cure may happen to them. This belief may generate conflict when the expectations of the patient or family interfere with clinical decision-making. In extreme situations, resolute and unshakeable believers would energetically oppose any rational argument. In these cases, the presence of a religious authority recognised by them may be necessary. Thus, the expectation of a miraculous cure poses a challenge for treatment planning if this expectancy is a form of denial masked as hope. Intermediation is necessary if this belief is a source of distress or a reason for risk, such as treatment abandonment. Some proposals on identifying and managing this situation have already been published [28]. Healthcare workers must keep in mind that their biases related to patients' spiritual-religious perspectives can be disrespectful, posing a risk of harming their relationship.

6. Future perspectives for spiritual support

6.1 Teaching the subject in healthcare colleges

Most health schools do not prepare their graduates in this area of knowledge. Health education rarely includes specifically the spiritual dimension in its curriculum. Thus, professionals do not feel trained to address these sensitive issues and subjective discomforts. Another challenge health professionals face when learning spiritual issues is the traditional difficulty in defining spirituality and related terms, which can hinder communication. Furthermore, once spirituality is defined, graduates would still face the complexity of cultural competence. Professionals must also navigate their biases, as discomfort in discussing spirituality may stem from a lack of personal spiritual grounding.

A common concern for professionals is the fear of overstepping their professional boundaries when discussing a patient's spiritual values. The resulting reluctance may arise from this concern about causing offence or cultural differences. Approaching a patient's spiritual values without imposing personal beliefs requires specific training. The professional may end up taking refuge under the argument that spiritual assessment "is not my professional role."

There is still much to be done to introduce teaching about spirituality and health in colleges. College courses must evolve from merely teaching professional skills to personal development in a humanistic model. Finally, beyond undergraduate courses, the subject must continue to be explored in post-graduation courses and professional societies.

6.2 Interaction between clinicians and clergies

Healthcare professionals are still reluctant to discuss aspects of patients' spiritual and religious culture with clergy. Due to prejudice or lack of knowledge, some health professionals believe that acting apart from the clergy is a way of avoiding bad practices. However, clinicians and clergy would have more power as a team than as individuals to identify and remedy existential pain. However, it is important to understand the difference between multi-confessional secularism and religiously neutral secularism. Multi-confessional secularism allows for allocating a prayer space adapted to various religious symbols. In the idea of religiously neutral secularism, religious issues are something that should be avoided in the public space, given their potential to generate conflicts. This "separation with cooperation" of multi-confessional secularism can and should be present in health services.

In order to advance this issue, further research should explore care delivery models in synergistic collaboration. Developing this dynamic of spiritual support could provide ethically appropriate and disciplinarily integrated care. In this way, relationships between clinicians and clergy, previously viewed with distrust and separation, could serve an expanded need for spiritual healing. Of course, such a model of spiritually integrated care would be restricted to selected patients after obtaining the necessary consent.

6.3 Demonstrating cost-effectiveness of spiritual support

There is a need to explore further the benefits for a health system in providing spiritual care. More research is required to show that the benefits of spiritual support for patients are therapeutically helpful rather than merely comforting. Going further, it is necessary to demonstrate that spiritual support not only leads to improved patient and family satisfaction outcomes but also brings economic benefits, with the potential to minimise costs. However, demonstrating the cost-effectiveness of spiritual support is a complex task, as some benefits would be intangible because they follow an indirect route.

One study [29] showed that more patient-centred hospitals had significantly better outcomes than those without such initiatives. However, patient-centredness was also associated with higher costs. Thus, administrators must determine whether the resulting benefits are worth the investment, considering both the short and long term.

A literature review [30] indicated a need for more rigorous studies on the effectiveness of spiritual support. Former studies have not clearly described chaplain interventions or thoroughly documented this practice. According to the authors, there is a lack of description of what contributions are unique to chaplains, identification of best practices to optimise outcomes, and testing of the effectiveness of this care. Current research does not conclusively identify the most effective practices for different types of clients across various settings.

6.4 Non-in-person forms of spiritual assistance

Primary care providers and major healthcare institutions are increasingly adopting telehealth-based care models. Recently, the COVID-19 pandemic forced people to isolate themselves and caused great insecurity. Access to religious and spiritual resources was limited, while serious mental health problems were also reported. People who could maintain support from religious and spiritual resources tended to have better psychological outcomes [31]. The experience highlighted the need to adopt a more comprehensive view of health that includes forms of spiritual support.

Efforts to provide this service remotely have demonstrated significant promise, although telechaplaincy remains nascent. A recent study [32] analysed data from an international congress concerning aspects of telechaplaincy. The authors noted that although telechaplaincy has become more prominent since the COVID-19 pandemic, maintaining professional standards in digital care settings remains challenging. Furthermore, one of the main disadvantages of remote spiritual support is that it does not allow for the principle of "ministry of presence," a characteristic of chaplaincy.

6.5 New appreciation of spiritual experiences

Certain patients might exhibit unusual mental phenomena that include spiritual elements in their presentation. Health professionals should understand how patients integrate these experiences into their spiritual framework. The objective is not to validate or disapprove the reality of these experiences but to remain receptive to the sacred experiences of patients. Practitioners should not change their practice based on these experiences but rather maintain an open mind and show interest and respect for these beliefs and values.

It is crucial to offer a secure environment where patients can articulate and examine their perspectives. This approach can enhance the patient-professional relationship by acknowledging what is important to the individual. Some experiences deserve attention as they are related to physical or mental health parameters: communication after death, memories of supposed past lives, near-death experiences, and end-of-life experiences [33].

7. Conclusion

Although challenges persist, an individualised approach to a patient's spirituality can enrich healthcare and promote the overall well-being of those receiving care. Through open dialogue, rigorous research, and a compassionate approach, healthcare systems can better understand and address the spiritual needs of their patients. Despite the enduring difficulties of issues raised by past religious misunderstandings, the professional's role is to provide patients with the best practice and empower them to make decisions based on their values.

Conflict of interest

The authors declare no conflict of interest.

Author details

Marcelo Saad[1*] and Roberta de Medeiros[2]

1 Brazilian Spiritist Medical Association, São Paulo, Brazil

2 University Santo Amaro, São Paulo, Brazil

*Address all correspondence to: msaad@uol.com.br

References

[1] World Health Organization. Fifty-Second World Health Assembly. Amendments to the Constitution of WHO [Web Page]. 1999. Available from: http://apps.who.int/gb/archive/pdf_files/WHA52/ew24.pdf

[2] Walach H. Secular spirituality–what it is. Why we need it. How to proceed. Journal for the Study of Spirituality. 2017;**7**(1):7-20. DOI: 10.1080/20440243.2017.1290028

[3] Wixwat M, Saucier G. Being spiritual but not religious. Current Opinion in Psychology. 2020;**40**:121-125. DOI: 10.1016/j.copsyc.2020.09.003

[4] Hvidt NC, Nielsen KT, Kørup AK, Prinds C, Hansen DG, Viftrup DT, et al. What is spiritual care? Professional perspectives on the concept of spiritual care identified through group concept mapping. BMJ Open. 2020;**10**(12):e042142. DOI: 10.1136/bmjopen-2020-042142

[5] Saad M, de Medeiros R. Implications for public health of the religiosity-longevity relation. Revista da Associação Médica Brasileira. 2017;**63**(10):837-841. DOI: 10.1590/1806-9282.63.10.837

[6] Schachter AB, Argentieri MA, Seddighzadeh B, Isehunwa OO, Kent BV, Trevvett P, et al. R|S Atlas: Identifying existing cohort study data resources to accelerate epidemiological research on the influence of religion and spirituality on human health. BMJ Open. 2021;**11**(10):e043830. DOI: 10.1136/bmjopen-2020-043830

[7] Garssen B, Visser A, Pool G. Does spirituality or religion positively affect mental health? Meta-analysis of longitudinal studies. The International Journal for the Psychology of Religion. 2021;**31**(1):4-20. DOI: 10.1080/10508619.2020.1729570

[8] Christopoulos K. Religion and survival among European older adults. European Journal of Ageing. 2023;**20**(1):42. DOI: 10.1007/s10433-023-00789-4

[9] The Lancet Regional Health-Europe. Time to integrate spiritual needs in health care. The Lancet Regional Health. Europe. 2023;**28**:100648. DOI: 10.1016/j.lanepe.2023.100648

[10] Dominguez LJ, Veronese N, Barbagallo M. The link between spirituality and longevity. Aging Clinical and Experimental Research. 2024;**36**(1):32. DOI: 10.1007/s40520-023-02684-5

[11] Sena MAB, Damiano RF, Lucchetti G, Peres MFP. Defining spirituality in healthcare: A systematic review and conceptual framework. Frontiers in Psychology. 2021;**12**:756080. DOI: 10.3389/fpsyg.2021.756080

[12] Miller C, Beaman LG. Non-religious afterlife: Emerging understandings of death and dying. Religions. 2024;**15**(1):104. DOI: 10.3390/rel15010104

[13] Clark CC, Hunter J. Spirituality, spiritual well-being, and spiritual coping in advanced heart failure: Review of the literature. Journal of Holistic Nursing. 2019;**37**:56-73. DOI: 10.1177/0898010118761401

[14] Pargament KI, Koenig HG, Tarakeshwar N, Hahn J. Religious coping methods as predictors of psychological, physical and spiritual outcomes among

medically ill elderly patients: A two-year longitudinal study. Journal of Health Psychology. 2004;**9**(6):713-730. DOI: 10.1177/1359105304045366

[15] Unterrainer HF, Ladenhauf KH, Moazedi ML, Wallner-Liebmann SJ, Fink A. Dimensions of religious/spiritual well-being and their relation to personality and psychological well-being. Personality and Individual Differences. 2010;**49**(3):192-197. DOI: 10.1016/j.paid.2010.03.032

[16] Gomez R, Fisher JW. Domains of spiritual well-being and development and validation of the spiritual well-being questionnaire. Personality and Individual Differences. 2003;**35**:1975-1991. DOI: 10.1016/S0191-8869(03)00045-X

[17] Murray SA, Kendall M, Boyd K, Worth A, Benton TF. Exploring the spiritual needs of people dying of lung cancer or heart failure: A prospective qualitative interview study of patients and their carers. Palliative Medicine. 2004;**18**(1):39-45. DOI: 10.1191/0269216304pm837oa

[18] Pargament KI, Exline JJ. The Psychology of Spiritual Struggle. USA: John Templeton Foundation; 2021. 42 p. Available from: https://www.templeton.org/discoveries/the-psychology-of-spiritual-struggle

[19] Saad M, Medeiros R. Religion and health: Most of times, an excellent combination. Einstein (São Paulo). 2021;**19**:eCE6382. DOI: 10.31744/einstein_journal/2021CE6382

[20] VandeCreek L. Defining and advocating for spiritual care in the hospital. The Journal of Pastoral Care & Counseling. 2010;**64**:1-10. DOI: 10.1177/154230501006400205

[21] Saad M, de Medeiros R. Programs of religious/spiritual support in hospitals—Five "Whies" and five "Hows". Philosophy, Ethics, and Humanities in Medicine. 2016;**11**(1):5. DOI: 10.1186/s13010-016-0039-z

[22] Joint Commission International Accreditation Standards for Hospitals, 6th Edition. 2017. Available from: https://store.jointcommissioninternational.org/assets/3/7/JCI_Hosp_Standards_6th_STANDARDS_ONLY_14Jan2018.pdf

[23] Lucchetti G, Bassi RM, Lucchetti AL. Taking spiritual history in clinical practice: A systematic review of instruments. Explore (New York, N.Y.). 2013;**9**(3):159-170. DOI: 10.1016/j.explore.2013.02.004

[24] Saad M, de Medeiros R. Spirituality and healthcare—Common grounds for the secular and religious worlds and its clinical implications. Religions. 2021;**12**(1):22. DOI: 10.3390/rel12010022

[25] Moore JT. Multicultural and idiosyncratic considerations for measuring the relationship between religious and secular forms of spirituality with positive global mental health. Psychology of Religion and Spirituality. 2017;**9**(1):21-33. DOI: 10.1037/rel0000083

[26] Saad M, de Medeiros R. Advocating for the concept of spiritual health. The American Journal of Emergency Medicine. 2021;**45**:563-564. DOI: 10.1016/j.ajem.2020.11.080

[27] Daigle DA, Goff DV, Koenig HG. Holistic health as a twenty-first-century military strategy: Stoic philosophy and spiritual fitness for optimising warfighter readiness. In: Expeditions With MCUP. Vol. 2023. 2023. 46 p. DOI: 10.36304/expwmcup.2023.03. Available from: https://muse.jhu.edu/pub/419/article/887023/pdf

[28] Saad M, de Medeiros R. The patient with overestimated faith, expecting for a miraculous healing—Approaches from the physician. Sumerianz Journal of Medical and Healthcare. 2018;**1**(1):31-35. Available from: www.sumerianz.com/pdf-files/sjmh1(1)31-35.pdf

[29] Bechel DL, Myers WA, Smith DG. Does patient-centered care pay off? The Joint Commission Journal on Quality Improvement. 2000;**26**(7):400-409. DOI: 10.1016/S1070-3241(00)26033-1

[30] Jankowski KR, Handzo GF, Flannelly KJ. Testing the efficacy of chaplaincy care. Journal of Health Care Chaplaincy. 2011;**17**(3-4):100-125. DOI: 10.1080/08854726.2011.616166

[31] Ferrell BR, Handzo G, Picchi T, Puchalski C, Rosa WE. The urgency of spiritual care: COVID-19 and the critical need for whole-person palliation. Journal of Pain and Symptom Management. 2020;**60**(3):e7-e11. DOI: 10.1016/j.jpainsymman.2020.06.034

[32] Winiger F, Sprik P. Navigating challenges in telechaplaincy: A thematic analysis of an international conference. Journal of Health Care Chaplaincy. 2024;**30**(3):186-201. DOI: 10.1080/08854726.2023.2294680

[33] Saad M, de Medeiros R. Non-ordinary spiritual experiences- some phenomena without a satisfactory explanation. Avicenna Journal of Neuro Psycho Physiology. 2023;**10**(1):1-7. DOI: 10.32592/ajnpp.2023.10.1.100

Chapter 5

Accessible Meditation: Culturally Inclusive Practices for Deaf and Hard of Hearing Communities

Nadine J. Pelling

Abstract

Meditation offers a range of psychological, emotional, physical, and spiritual benefits. However, traditional practices often rely heavily on auditory cues—such as spoken guidance, bells, or music—which can create barriers to access for Deaf, deaf, and hard of hearing individuals. This chapter introduces the purposes and techniques of meditation, then explores key variations across cultural and spiritual traditions, highlighting how auditory reliance can limit participation. Foundational terminology and ethical considerations are discussed, with attention to audism, cultural safety, and the importance of respectful language. The chapter outlines specific psychological and cognitive benefits of meditation for Deaf participants, particularly when practices are adapted to accommodate visual and tactile communication. Inclusive and culturally aligned design strategies are presented, including visual anchors, signed or tactile guidance, and storytelling methods that resonate with Deaf culture. Facilitator communication techniques, co-design with Deaf community members, and long-term sustainability strategies are also explored. The role of interpreters is discussed in depth, along with recommendations for ensuring high-quality, culturally attuned communication access. By integrating ethical reflection, applied adaptations, and Deaf-led perspectives, this chapter offers a framework for culturally inclusive and sustainable meditation practice—one that affirms sensory diversity and enables long-term contemplative wellbeing.

Keywords: meditation, Deaf, inclusive, visual, disability, psychology, counselling, audism

1. Introduction

Meditation has been practised for centuries across cultures and traditions, offering individuals pathways to relaxation, mindfulness, and spiritual exploration. Despite its diverse forms, meditation typically involves certain core purposes and techniques that transcend individual traditions or belief systems. This section introduces the primary aims of meditation, describes common techniques and elements used across traditions, and highlights important variations shaped by cultural and religious contexts.

It also addresses the ways in which traditional meditation's reliance on auditory cues creates accessibility challenges for Deaf, deaf, and hard of hearing individuals, laying the foundation for exploring more inclusive meditative adaptations.

1.1 Purposes of meditation

Meditation is widely recognised for its positive impact on physical, emotional, and psychological wellbeing [1, 2]. Meditative techniques are frequently integrated into evidence-based therapeutic programmes. For example, mindfulness-based relapse prevention (MBRP) combines meditation and mindfulness practices with cognitive therapy to support substance use treatment [3–5]. Similarly, mindfulness-based cognitive therapy (MBCT) promotes overall wellbeing and improved mental health [6].

Given the broad range of meditative practices, clearly identifying an individual's purpose or intention is essential to ensure techniques align effectively with personal needs and goals [7, 8].

Broadly, meditation can be categorised according to three primary purposes:

1. Relaxation-based meditation, which aims to promote calm, reduce stress, and support emotional and physical restoration [9];

2. Mindfulness-centred meditation, which encourages heightened awareness of the present moment in a non-judgemental way [10];

3. Spiritual or contemplative meditation, which seeks deeper connection with something sacred—whether defined within a Buddhist, Christian, or other spiritual framework [11].

The differentiation between purpose and technique is crucial. For instance, a breathing technique might be used to promote relaxation in a secular context or to support contemplative prayer in a religious context. The underlying purpose informs how the practice is framed and experienced [8, 12].

Clarity of purpose can also help avoid misunderstandings when integrating meditation into different cultural or religious settings. Some advocates of Christian contemplative traditions, for example, caution against secular meditation programmes that focus solely on personal wellbeing, arguing that such approaches can conflict with the theological aims of Christian prayer practices [13–16].

When adapting meditation practices for Deaf and hard of hearing individuals, understanding the underlying purpose helps guide appropriate adaptations that preserve the intended benefits of the practice without unnecessary alteration of its core goals.

In recent years, mindfulness-based programmes, such as Mindfulness-Based Stress Reduction (MBSR) and Mindfulness-Based Cognitive Therapy (MBCT), have highlighted the importance of clearly identifying the purpose of meditation within therapeutic frameworks [3, 5]. In these programmes, meditation is primarily used to cultivate present-moment awareness and emotional regulation rather than to achieve a spiritual outcome [3, 5]. However, the personal meaning that individuals bring to their practice—whether secular, spiritual, or therapeutic—remains significant in shaping their experience and outcomes [6].

1.2 Techniques and common elements

Meditative techniques vary widely across traditions, cultures, and individual preferences. Techniques may focus on internal sensations, visualisation, verbal repetition, breath control, or movement, among other anchors [17–19].

The techniques used in meditation may include visualisation, repetition, breath awareness, or movement. Visualisation practices can take the form of guided meditation [17, 19], as well as variations of Visio Divina [20, 21] and Ignatian meditation [22–24].

Some approaches involve repetition of a mantra or sacred word—such as "So Hum," a transliteration of the Sanskrit phrase Soham, meaning "I am That" [25–27]—or the repeated use of the name of Jesus in Christian meditation [15]. In secular contexts, individuals may instead focus on a neutral, grounding word such as calm, repeated silently to support relaxation and attention.

Breath awareness may be used in practices such as yoga [28], centring prayer [29], or focused breathing [30]. Finally, meditation can include movement-based practices, including Tai Chi, yoga, or walking meditation [28, 31].

Despite their differences, most meditative techniques share several common elements:

- Focused attention on a chosen anchor (such as the breath or a repeated phrase),
- Calm and slow breathing,
- A quiet or comfortable setting,
- A posture that is both relaxed and alert,
- An open, non-judgemental attitude that allows for observation of thoughts, emotions, and bodily sensations [32].

Techniques may be selected based on individual needs or preferences. For example, movement-based forms of meditation, such as walking or rhythmic tapping, may be especially helpful for individuals with autism spectrum disorder or attention-deficit/hyperactivity disorder [31, 33], who may find seated stillness more difficult to sustain.

However, these common elements can also introduce unintended barriers for individuals who rely on visual or tactile communication methods, particularly given that many traditional meditation programmes rely heavily on spoken instructions, auditory cues, or guided verbal meditation [34, 35].

1.3 Variations across traditions

Meditation is a part of most world religions and can be categorised in many ways [18]. Commonly, meditation is divided into focused attention, open-monitoring-based practices [7], and loving-kindness or compassion-based meditation [1, 13, 36]. Some authors suggest novice meditators start with focused attention meditation to reduce mind-wandering [3, 4]. Others classify meditative practices by their originating spiritual tradition—such as Eastern, Western, or Christian forms [37, 38].

1.3.1 Eastern traditions

Eastern meditation, often associated with Buddhism, also includes Hindu and Taoist traditions [12]. Buddhist meditations align with teachings attributed to Buddha [7, 8, 19]. Key aims are to understand the true nature of existence (including the non-self) and cultivate wisdom and compassion [11]. Yoga may connect with meditation [39], and mindfulness also has roots in Buddhism [1].

1.3.2 Christian meditation

According to Pope Francis, Christian meditation is "to seek meaning" through engaging with divine revelation and "an encounter with the Other, with a capital 'O': the transcendent encounter with God" [38]. This framing affirms meditation as a spiritually relational act rather than a technique for inner calm alone. Meditation on God moves one from an intellectual knowledge of scripture to a practice that guides life [16]. Although practised in secular ways, meditation must ultimately be understood within a spiritual framework [40]. Christian meditation seeks a relationship rather than a mere state of being. Although calm and contentment can result, so too can redemptive experience and liberation [16, 41]. Christian meditation is therefore always seen as highly spiritual. It is not just about stopping but replenishing.

St Teresa of Avila wrote about developing a deeper union with God through meditation [16]. Other authors describe the purpose of contemplative spirituality as bringing into reality our union with God, as most do not generally feel such intimacy with the Divine [13]. Some Christians shy away from meditation despite Scripture encouraging believers to meditate on God's word. Perhaps this is due to Buddhist associations [14]. Some fear contemplation and mystical experiences [13, 16, 40]. However, others—including Deaf, deaf, or hard of hearing Christians—have explored ways in which spiritual connection and contemplation can deepen through embodied or non-verbal prayer practices [42]. Ways to adapt mindfulness for conservative Christians include reminding individuals of their connection to God [14].

1.3.3 Western secular approaches

Western meditation is generally secular, focusing on mental and physical, rather than spiritual, benefits. Thus, Western forms often emphasise mindset and prosperity, a sense of physical calm, and health-related outcomes [12].

These variations in meditation practices reflect diverse sensory modalities—verbal, visual, tactile, and kinaesthetic—that can be drawn upon when creating inclusive and Deaf-accessible meditation offerings. Recognising the range of traditional forms provides valuable models for adapting meditation to meet different sensory and cultural needs.

1.4 Auditory challenges and deaf-accessible adaptations

Despite the diverse techniques and traditions of meditation, many practices—especially in contemporary settings—continue to rely heavily on auditory elements. Spoken guidance, background music, chimes, gongs, and bells are common features of guided meditations, meditation apps, yoga classes, and contemplative retreats [17, 35]. These auditory cues are often integral to signalling transitions, providing pacing, and fostering a sense of atmosphere.

For individuals who are Deaf, deaf, or hard of hearing, such reliance on sound can create significant accessibility barriers. Auditory-based practices may exclude those who primarily engage with the world through visual, tactile, or other non-auditory modalities. In digital meditation spaces, many popular apps and recordings lack captions or sign language interpretation, further limiting accessibility and reinforcing spoken language as the default [43, 44].

Emerging adaptations aim to make meditation more inclusive. In Australia, initiatives such as Auslan Soul Yoga [39] and Carers Australia's Auslan mindfulness sessions [45] demonstrate how meditation can be adapted for Auslan users. These programmes integrate Auslan-interpreted guidance, visual cues, and clear pacing strategies to support inclusive participation.

Deaf-accessible meditation often involves replacing or supplementing auditory elements with visual and tactile alternatives. For example:

- *Visual cues:* Use of visual timers, gradual light changes, or on-screen text to indicate transitions

- *Auslan or signed guidance:* Meditation instructions delivered through sign language rather than speech [46]

- *Written scripts:* Providing captions, subtitles, or pre-session transcripts for guided practices

- *Tactile signals:* Gentle taps, vibration devices, or light tactile cues—referred to here as feather gestures—may be used as transitions or to cue breathing rhythms [44, 47].

Research shows that meditation offers psychological benefits for hearing individuals [48], and accessible adaptations—such as visual or tactile approaches—are increasingly being explored for use with Deaf participants [46]. While more targeted research is needed, these adaptations hold promise for offering comparable benefits by aligning with the visual and embodied nature of Deaf communication and culture.

By recognising the auditory challenges in traditional meditation and adopting inclusive sensory adaptations, practitioners and organisations can ensure that meditation becomes a welcoming and meaningful practice that honours diverse ways of experiencing the world.

2. Terminology

In discussing meditation practices for Deaf, deaf, and hard of hearing individuals, it is important to establish clear and respectful terminology. The capitalised term "Deaf" refers to individuals who identify as culturally Deaf, using sign language as their primary language and participating in Deaf culture and community [49, 50]. In contrast, "deaf" (lowercase) typically describes individuals with significant hearing loss who may not identify with the cultural aspects of the Deaf community. "Hard of hearing" generally refers to individuals who have partial hearing loss and who may communicate primarily through spoken language, sign language, or both [51].

Terms such as "hearing impaired" are generally rejected by the Deaf community because they frame deafness as a deficit. Preferred terminology reflects identity-first language and respects the cultural and linguistic richness of Deaf experience [49, 52].

Understanding the distinction between Deaf and deaf is essential when designing culturally inclusive meditation programmes, as communication preferences and cultural identity may differ significantly. Culturally Deaf individuals may have specific communication preferences—such as Auslan (Australian Sign Language) or American Sign Language (ASL)—and unique sensory experiences that differ from those who are deaf but more closely aligned with hearing cultural norms. Recognising these differences allows for more effective and respectful adaptations of meditation practices [52, 53].

It is also important to consider the concept of audism—the belief that hearing is inherently superior to deafness. The term combines "audio" with the suffix "-ism" and is sometimes mistakenly read or corrected as "autism," though it refers specifically to discrimination against Deaf individuals and signed language. Audism manifests in assumptions, systems, or behaviours that marginalise Deaf individuals by prioritising spoken language and auditory norms [54, 55]. This form of discrimination can influence how meditation programmes are structured, especially if they assume that all participants can hear verbal instructions or respond to auditory cues.

Terminology relating to meditation traditions also requires care. Terms such as "mindfulness," "meditation," and "contemplative practice" are sometimes used interchangeably in popular usage, but they carry distinct meanings in academic, therapeutic, and spiritual contexts. Mindfulness typically refers to present-moment, non-judgemental awareness cultivated through exercises such as breath observation, body scanning, or noticing thoughts without attachment [10, 56]. Meditation is a broader term encompassing a wide range of techniques, including mantra repetition, visualisation, breath awareness, and movement-based practices like yoga or Tai Chi [18, 19].

In sign languages such as Auslan, related variation also exists. Signs used to express "meditation" in Auslan (and other sign languages) may vary, including MIND-f-u-l, AWARE, and MIND-FOCUS, reflecting different conceptual and linguistic emphases across settings [44, 46].

Finally, the term inclusive meditation in this chapter refers to meditative practices that intentionally adapt methods, delivery formats, and environments to accommodate the diverse sensory needs of participants. Inclusive meditation considers variations in sensory processing, communication styles, and cultural identities—moving beyond traditional auditory reliance to foster broader participation and accessibility [44, 46, 57].

3. Ethical responsibilities and systemic barriers to access

Although meditation draws from diverse techniques and traditions, many contemporary practices continue to rely heavily on auditory elements. Spoken guidance, background music, chimes, gongs, and bells are common features of guided meditations, meditation apps, yoga classes, and contemplative retreats [17, 35]. These auditory cues often serve to signal transitions, establish pacing, and create a meditative atmosphere.

For individuals who are Deaf, deaf, or hard of hearing, such reliance on sound can create significant accessibility barriers. Meditation practices often assume that participants have typical sensory experiences—especially the ability to hear verbal instruction. For those who engage with the world through visual, tactile, or signed communication, these assumptions may lead to partial or total exclusion from meditative activities. In digital meditation spaces, many popular apps and recordings lack captions, transcripts, or sign language interpretation. This reinforces spoken language as the default and limiting full participation [43, 44]. National bodies such as Meditation Australia also encourage member practitioners to uphold accessibility and cultural safety as core ethical commitments in the delivery of meditation programmes [58].

Some researchers note that hard-of-hearing individuals experience more stress than their hearing peers [59]. Rates of anxiety and depression are also elevated among Deaf and deaf adults. These challenges are often associated with social, linguistic, and systemic barriers and are compounded by limited culturally appropriate mental health services [44, 60]. For Deaf individuals, persistent exclusion from wellness and therapeutic spaces contributes to ongoing health inequities [61]. Meditation practices that rely on auditory assumptions may inadvertently intensify these disparities.

Additionally, meditation programmes in healthcare and community settings often overlook the visual monitoring demands faced by Deaf individuals—for example, the need to maintain eye contact with interpreters or facilitators, or to scan for visual cues in group settings [57]. These unique cognitive and sensory demands are rarely addressed in conventional program design.

Offering meditation that is inclusive of Deaf, deaf, and hard of hearing communities is not merely a matter of good practice, but also of ethical responsibility. In psychological and allied health contexts, the principles of beneficence, justice, and autonomy offer a clear framework for inclusive design. Beneficence calls practitioners to actively support others' wellbeing through culturally safe and accessible services. Justice demands equitable access to care and the removal of barriers embedded in systemic norms—such as auditory reliance. Autonomy supports individuals' right to make informed choices about participation in health-promoting activities—choices that require access to culturally appropriate and accessible options [62, 63].

In allied health and psychological disciplines, ethical practice includes a duty to promote equitable access to effective interventions. Designing accessible meditation programmes is not simply a logistical consideration, but a professional responsibility grounded in the ethical principles of justice, beneficence, and respect for autonomy [57, 62–64]. Accessibility must be integrated from the outset, rather than retrofitted as an afterthought.

In Australia, accessibility in mental health and meditation contexts is supported through government-funded services such as the National Auslan Interpreter Booking Service (NABS) and the newer National Sign Language Program (NSLP). These programmes help Deaf individuals access interpreters during medical and allied health appointments [65]. Most Deaf individuals who use Auslan and are eligible for the National Disability Insurance Scheme (NDIS) now receive funding for interpreter access through that scheme. However, despite these provisions, many Deaf Australians report inconsistent interpreter availability and a lack of accessible wellness information—highlighting the importance of proactive inclusive design, especially in preventive and self-care programmes like meditation.

4. Meditation benefits

Meditation has long been associated with a broad range of physical, psychological, emotional, and relational benefits. Contemporary research supports these traditional claims, showing that meditation can improve mental health outcomes, enhance cognitive functioning, and support healthier interpersonal relationships [9, 66, 67]. For Deaf, deaf, and hard of hearing individuals, accessible meditation offers not only these general benefits but also unique psychological advantages, such as reducing stress associated with communication barriers and promoting greater self-regulation [44, 48].

The benefits of meditation can be grouped into three major categories: psychological and emotional outcomes, cognitive and workplace benefits, and relational and spiritual benefits. Each is discussed below.

4.1 Psychological and emotional benefits

Meditation is widely recognised as a tool for reducing anxiety, depression, and emotional dysregulation [1, 10, 67, 68]. Programmes such as Mindfulness-Based Stress Reduction (MBSR) and Mindfulness-Based Cognitive Therapy (MBCT) have demonstrated effectiveness in alleviating psychological distress across diverse populations. While most of this research has been conducted with hearing participants, early studies suggest that, when properly adapted, these approaches are likely to be effective for Deaf and hard of hearing individuals as well [3–6].

Deaf adolescents have been found to report higher rates of anxiety and distress than their hearing peers, often linked to systemic barriers and limited access to culturally appropriate support [59]. Deaf participants in accessible meditation programmes often report increased emotional resilience, reduced symptoms of anxiety and depression, and enhanced self-awareness [44, 48]. Practices that emphasise mindfulness, acceptance, and non-judgemental awareness are particularly supportive in fostering emotional wellbeing [10, 56, 67, 69, 70].

In addition, meditation may help reduce the chronic stress that Deaf individuals often face due to systemic barriers in communication, education, and healthcare [44, 59, 60].

4.2 Cognitive and professional benefits

While direct research on mindfulness among Deaf students and professionals is limited, some studies suggest potential benefits. For example, Brown and Cornes [59] explore mental health experiences among Deaf adolescents, highlighting the need for accessible psychological supports. More broadly, mindfulness training has been associated with increased academic focus and better self-regulation in general populations, including students and professionals [67]. These findings suggest that, when appropriately adapted, mindfulness practices may also support Deaf individuals in similar ways.

Meditation techniques such as breath-focused awareness and body scanning exercises can improve cognitive flexibility and working memory, both important skills in educational and workplace settings [30, 71]. For Deaf individuals navigating environments where cognitive load is increased by the need for constant visual monitoring—such as interpreting multiple visual stimuli during group conversations—mindfulness-based cognitive strategies can support better concentration and reduced mental fatigue [44, 57].

4.3 Relational, ethical, and spiritual benefits

Meditative practices can also nurture relational skills such as empathy, patience, and communication attunement [67]. Mindfulness-based practices encourage individuals to remain present and attentive in interactions, qualities that can be particularly beneficial in Deaf/hearing relationships where communication modalities differ [44].

Spiritual forms of meditation—whether practised within Buddhist, Christian, or secular humanist traditions—offer Deaf individuals pathways to inner peace and meaning that are not dependent on auditory experience [11, 40]. Visual contemplative practices such as Visio Divina (sacred seeing) [20] or tactile prayer approaches can create rich, embodied spiritual experiences without reliance on spoken or chanted word. Ignatian spirituality has been explored as a therapeutic resource, with its structured practices and rich imagery offering meditative grounding, particularly in clinical and therapeutic contexts where clients are receptive to integrating spiritual elements into therapy [72].

For example, in both therapeutic and religious contexts, the use of tactile tools such as prayer beads has been explored as a way to support embodied spiritual focus [73]. For some Deaf practitioners, accessible meditation is more than a wellness tool—it becomes a deeply affirming spiritual or existential practice that honours their embodied, visual, and sensory ways of being.

5. Inclusive and culturally aligned practice design

Creating a Deaf-inclusive meditation environment requires deliberate adaptations that honour visual, tactile, and embodied communication. These adaptations are not merely technical substitutions for sound, but are grounded in cultural, linguistic, and sensory preferences. Inclusive design considers not only how meditation is delivered, but also who is included in shaping and guiding the practice.

5.1 Sensory and communication adaptations

In practice, inclusive meditation often involves replacing or supplementing auditory elements with visual or tactile alternatives. Adaptations may include:

- Visual cues – such as visual timers, on-screen text, or gradual light changes to signal transitions

- Auslan or signed guidance – where meditation instructions are delivered via sign language rather than spoken word [46]

- Written scripts – including captions, subtitles, or pre-session transcripts for guided meditations

- Tactile signals or vibration devices used as transitions for meditation stages or breathing rhythms – such as feather gestures, or gentle shoulder taps [44, 47]

These adaptations not only make meditation more accessible for Deaf, deaf, and hard of hearing participants, but also reflect the values of embodied presence, visual engagement, and relational communication that are central to Deaf culture [44]. Research by Goodrich et al. [34] demonstrated that mindfulness can be adapted successfully for adults with severe speech and physical impairments, emphasising the importance of flexible, multi-sensory approaches in inclusive meditation.

5.2 Facilitator communication, posture, and positioning

In group settings, inclusive meditation design also involves attention to facilitator posture and communication style. Consistent and natural eye contact, a measured pace of signing or speech, and open body posture are essential for maintaining a welcoming and visually oriented environment. In Auslan and other signed languages, non-manual markers—such as facial expressions and body movement—carry significant meaning. Facilitators should be mindful of these features, ensuring they are both expressive and culturally attuned.

Facilitation strategies may include the use of Deaf or Deaf-led instructors, co-facilitation with interpreters, or visual demonstration methods that emphasise kinaesthetic and spatial awareness. For example, some meditation leaders use hand gestures to cue breath pacing, or stand in open, visible spaces to maintain visual flow. These methods are not only inclusive but can deepen engagement for all participants by grounding the meditative experience in embodied presence.

5.3 Cultural values, connection, and storytelling

Inclusive meditation supports relational connection and group cohesion by encouraging open-ended sharing, encouraging personal storytelling, and validating individual experience. These culturally aligned strategies foster a sense of safety, respect, and support among participants.

When designed with cultural and sensory responsiveness, inclusive meditation can become a powerful tool for healing, self-awareness, and community connection—especially for those whose experiences have historically been excluded from mainstream wellness and therapeutic programmes.

6. Foundations for inclusive and sustainable practice

Building meditation spaces and practices that are truly inclusive of Deaf, deaf, and hard of hearing individuals requires deliberate design choices and ongoing reflection. This section outlines key foundations for sustainable inclusion, including proactive planning, visual and tactile adaptations, participant feedback mechanisms, and Deaf-led co-design. Inclusion is not a one-off adjustment; it is a foundational commitment that informs every aspect of how meditation experiences are structured, delivered, and sustained [44, 63].

6.1 Planning for inclusion

Inclusive meditation begins with thoughtful planning. Facilitators and program developers must consider the communication needs of participants from the outset. This includes booking qualified interpreters when spoken instruction will be used, ensuring captioning is available for video materials, and preparing written guides or visual supports in advance [74, 75]. Meditation spaces should be arranged to allow clear sightlines between participants, instructors, and interpreters, supporting visual access for all [76, 77].

Facilitators should also be aware of lighting, seating arrangements, and the positioning of visual anchors such as projected text or signed guidance. These details enhance comfort, clarity, and connection within the practice space.

Facilitators benefit from training in Deaf culture, visual communication, and the use of interpreters or Deaf collaborators. Such preparation fosters cultural safety, reduces unintentional exclusion, and strengthens facilitator confidence. Incorporating Deaf cultural knowledge is consistent with principles of inclusive practice and linguistic justice [75–77].

6.2 Visual, tactile, and movement adaptations

Adaptations are central to inclusive practice. Deaf-accessible meditation often includes:

- Visual anchors such as slow-paced signing, captioned videos, or projected text instructions [45, 46]
- Tactile cues such as feather touches, light vibrations, or shoulder taps to signal transitions [44, 47]
- Movement-based techniques including mindful walking, yoga, or hand gestures aligned with breath [31]

These adaptations not only increase accessibility, they also align with Deaf cultural values of embodiment, visual rhythm, and spatial engagement. Programmes such as Auslan Soul Yoga demonstrate the potential for culturally aligned, movement-based meditation options in Australia [39]. Signing affirmations, rather than silently reciting them, may enhance embodied engagement and reinforce linguistic and cultural identity for Deaf participants [44, 46]. These practices align meditation with visual communication norms and support spiritual self-expression. They are not simply substitutes for sound but affirm different sensory ways of being.

6.3 Verifying understanding through teach-back

Inclusive practice includes verifying comprehension in respectful and culturally aware ways. Implementing "teach-back" methods—where participants rephrase or demonstrate instructions—helps facilitators confirm understanding, especially across different language structures [44, 76, 77].

This is especially important with Deaf participants, as eye contact or nodding may be intended to signal continued attention, but can be misinterpreted as full understanding when confusion remains. Auslan and other signed languages differ structurally from English, and clarity must be confirmed through interactive, embodied feedback.

6.4 Community consultation and co-design

Effective inclusion requires collaboration, not assumption. Meditation offerings should be shaped through consultation with Deaf community members and practitioners [44]. Co-design means inviting Deaf people to actively contribute to the structure, content, and delivery of programmes.

Deaf-led meditation sessions or co-facilitated formats model accessibility while fostering cultural alignment and authenticity. Some Deaf individuals have integrated meditative approaches into both secular and faith-based practices, including visual prayer, tactile rhythm, and narrative-based reflection. These culturally resonant methods—whether grounded in Christian spiritual traditions or secular mindfulness—highlight the diversity of Deaf contemplative experience and the potential for meaningful adaptation beyond formal programmes [44, 76, 77]. Such approaches enhance relevance and increase participant trust and sustainability over time [75].

6.5 Sustaining inclusion over time

For accessibility to endure, it must be embedded in systems—not treated as an optional feature. Organisations and facilitators should:

- Plan for ongoing interpreter funding and captioning
- Include accessibility goals in strategic planning
- Provide professional development on inclusive design
- Build feedback loops with Deaf participants
- Prioritise continuity of accessible formats in apps, workshops, and retreats [44, 74]

Sustainable practice honours accessibility as a core value, not an afterthought. It reflects a deeper ethical commitment to equity, respect, and the belief that meditation should be available to all. An essential element of sustainable inclusion—particularly in spoken-guidance settings—is the use of qualified interpreters, which is explored in Section 7 The Importance of Interpreters.

6.6 Sustaining practice in everyday life

Inclusive and sustainable meditation practice extends beyond structured sessions. For many Deaf, deaf, and hard of hearing individuals, integrating mindfulness into everyday life is essential—not only for continuity, but for ensuring accessibility in personal routines and fluctuating environments.

Small, consistent practices—such as brief breathing pauses or tactile grounding techniques—can be especially effective. Short periods of breath awareness, visual focus, or gentle body scans can be embedded in daily transitions such as waking, commuting, or preparing meals [67, 78]. Tactile or visual reminders—such as a subtle hand gesture, a vibration timer, or a visual breathing app—can help prompt mindful pauses without relying on sound [44].

Because Deaf individuals often manage heightened visual attention throughout the day, it is important that mindfulness practices do not add to sensory fatigue. Facilitators can offer participants strategies to engage with meditation in ways that are restorative rather than overstimulating—such as lying down with the eyes open, using natural movement, or focusing on grounding through touch or stillness [34, 47].

Encouraging participants to adapt practices to their own rhythms and communication preferences helps build autonomy and sustainability. This may involve journaling in Auslan via video, using tactile objects such as beads or textured stones to anchor attention, or setting visual intentions in the morning.

Ultimately, integrating meditation into daily life affirms it as a flexible, embodied, and culturally relevant practice—one that supports wellbeing without relying on rigid formats or inaccessible expectations.

7. The importance of interpreters

Among the most essential components of putting inclusive design into practice is ensuring communication access for Deaf, deaf, and hard of hearing participants. In settings where meditation relies on spoken instruction, the use of qualified interpreters becomes essential to inclusion. Ensuring effective communication is a cornerstone of inclusive meditation for Deaf, deaf, and hard of hearing individuals. In settings where meditation is guided verbally, qualified interpreters are often essential to ensure Deaf participants can engage with the full experience [44, 75–77].

Interpreters bridge communication gaps by translating spoken instructions into sign language or, where appropriate, into other visual communication methods. However, simply having an interpreter present is not enough. Interpreters working in meditation settings must be familiar with meditation-specific terminology and practices to convey instructions with the appropriate pacing, tone, and conceptual accuracy [44, 76, 77, 79, 80]. For example, an interpreter translating instructions for mindful breathing, visualisation, or body scans must be able to reflect the slow, deliberate pace and the contemplative tone of the original guidance. Where possible, interpreters should be briefed in advance on meditation terminology, session structure, and tone. This preparation supports accurate pacing and emotional tone. Facilitators should also be mindful of lighting and positioning so participants can clearly see both the interpreter and any visual aids. In some programmes, dual-mode communication—such as combining Auslan guidance with on-screen text—further improves clarity and accessibility [75–77].

When meditation is conducted in group settings, interpreters also support full social inclusion by facilitating communication during group discussions, question and answer sessions, and reflections on practice. Without interpreters, Deaf participants may be excluded from key learning moments, shared insights, and the communal aspects that often enhance meditation experiences.

Family members or unqualified individuals should not be used as interpreters in formal settings, as they may lack the neutrality or linguistic skill required for effective communication. Family members may not have the necessary linguistic proficiency or neutrality required to ensure accurate, confidential interpretation. Professional interpreters, by contrast, are trained to maintain the integrity of communication while preserving participants' privacy and autonomy [74]. Communication access is essential for ethical and effective therapeutic practice, and their recommendations are equally relevant in meditation contexts, where accessibility and inclusion rely on qualified, culturally aware interpreters [81, 82].

Depending on the context, meditation sessions may use either in-person interpreters or video remote interpreting (VRI) services. In-person interpreters are generally preferred for meditation, as they can adjust more intuitively to the atmosphere, physical positioning, and group dynamics of a meditation space. However, if in-person interpreters are unavailable, VRI may provide a viable alternative—provided the technology is reliable and the visual setup does not disrupt the meditative environment.

Interpreter fatigue is another important consideration, especially in longer or emotionally intense practices. Auslan interpreters must process and translate nuanced content in real time while attending to group dynamics and speaker variability. As a result, interpreters may benefit from briefings prior to sessions and opportunities to clarify terminology or spiritual language ahead of time.

Facilitators should be mindful of how their own communication habits affect interpreter flow and participant understanding. Avoiding unnecessary metaphors, pausing for interpretation, and maintaining visual contact with participants (rather than solely with the interpreter) helps ensure clarity and connection. Ethical collaboration with interpreters includes not only respecting their professional role but also recognising when Deaf participants may prefer alternatives such as visual-only guidance or pre-recorded, signed meditation material [63, 75].

In addition to collaboration with interpreters, facilitators should consider the visual needs of Deaf participants. Line of sight should be maintained at all times, and speakers should address participants directly—not just the interpreter. Practitioners should also avoid visually distracting clothing or backlighting that may affect visual communication. Where possible, interpreters should receive content briefings ahead of sessions to clarify terminology or spiritual language. Some programmes combine multiple modes of communication, such as signed guidance with on-screen text or Auslan-led instruction, which can offer additional clarity and cultural alignment [75–77].

Ultimately, the presence of interpreters should be part of a broader strategy for accessible design—not the sole solution. Incorporating Deaf-led facilitation, co-creating content with Deaf practitioners, and offering multiple communication modalities enhances both autonomy and cultural safety. Skilled and culturally aware interpreters are vital partners in creating accessible meditation spaces. Their presence enables Deaf, deaf, and hard of hearing participants to fully engage, reflect, and benefit from meditation without facing unnecessary communication barriers. Communication accessibility must be planned thoughtfully—not as an afterthought.

8. Conclusion

Meditation offers well-established psychological, emotional, and physical benefits. However, traditional meditation practices have often relied heavily on auditory cues, inadvertently excluding Deaf, deaf, and hard of hearing individuals. By examining the purposes and techniques of meditation, the variations across traditions, and the specific challenges posed by sound-reliant practices, this chapter has outlined pathways toward greater inclusivity.

Adapting meditation for Deaf communities requires more than simply translating words—it involves fundamentally rethinking the sensory modalities through which meditation can be taught and experienced. Visual, tactile, and movement-based adaptations provide meaningful alternatives that align with Deaf cultural and linguistic norms. Inclusive practice also demands careful attention to Deaf-aware communication, respect for sign languages such as Auslan, and the thoughtful use of interpreters.

Accessible meditation spaces, culturally aligned delivery methods, and the ongoing development of Deaf-informed resources are essential to ensuring that meditation becomes a welcoming, empowering experience for all participants. Despite progress, barriers persist—such as inconsistent interpreter access, a shortage of mental health professionals fluent in Auslan, and limited availability of culturally accessible wellness resources in Australia [59, 74].

Practitioners are encouraged to reflect with humility on their own assumptions and habits—recognising, as illustrated in the author's own experience with inclusive recording (see Notes), that even well-meaning professionals can overlook accessibility unless deliberate care is taken.

A recent pilot project conducted by the author, titled Accessible Contemplation: A Deaf-Inclusive Pilot of Christian and Secular Visual Meditation, explored culturally responsive meditation using visual contemplative practices. The project, developed by a hard of hearing practitioner in consultation with a Deaf advisor, is currently under review for publication and offers an applied example of how meditation can be meaningfully adapted in partnership with Deaf communities [83]. It highlights the importance of inclusive design, culturally aligned delivery, and the integration of spiritual as well as secular options in broadening access to meditative wellbeing.

Looking ahead, inclusive meditation practice must continue evolving in step with both technological advancements and the insights of Deaf communities themselves. Emerging tools—such as haptic feedback devices, captioned meditation apps, and AI-supported Auslan translation—offer promising avenues for expanding access. However, technology alone is not a substitute for cultural understanding or ethical engagement. Ongoing research, practitioner training, and Deaf-led resource development are essential to ensure that accessibility is not treated as a one-off innovation but as a sustained commitment to equity. As the field of contemplative practice grows, so too must our collective efforts to ensure that every body—and every way of being—has a place within it. As awareness grows, and as practitioners and researchers continue to innovate in respectful collaboration with Deaf communities, meditation can truly fulfil its promise as a universally accessible path to inner peace, resilience, and wellbeing.

Acknowledgements

The author acknowledges that portions of the material presented in this book chapter are adapted from manuscripts developed as part of the requirements for the Graduate Certificate in Teaching Meditation at the University of Divinity.

This chapter was inspired by the author's engagement in the University of Divinity's Graduate Certificate in Teaching Meditation program. The insights gained through this course, particularly during the practicum component, significantly shaped both the direction and content of the work presented here.

The author would especially like to thank Dr. Donovan Cresdee—a proud Deaf man with a PhD in Applied Linguistics—for his generous support and guidance in the development and delivery of meditation offerings tailored for Deaf, deaf, and hard of hearing communities in Adelaide, South Australia, during the year 2024. His collaboration was instrumental in the author's practicum, where a Deaf-focused meditation program was delivered in partial fulfilment of the Graduate Certificate requirements.

Conflict of interest

The author declares no conflict of interest.

Notes

Dr. Nadine Pelling is a clinical psychologist who works across both academia and private practice in Adelaide, Australia. She has been at the University of South

Australia since 2003, which is scheduled to merge with the University of Adelaide in 2026 to form the new Adelaide University. She and her daughter, Jasmine, are both hard of hearing and study Auslan, which they identify as their chosen second language. Jasmine is the model in **Figures 1–4** as follows. Originally from Canada, Dr. Pelling trained as a counselling psychologist at Western Michigan University before relocating to Australia in 2000.

Nadine strongly advocates for the use of interpreters when communicating with members of the Deaf community. She also encourages the learning of Auslan as a way of fostering respectful, inclusive communication and deeper engagement with Deaf culture. Nadine believes that Deaf individuals should lead the teaching of sign language and Deaf Awareness, as part of resisting audism—the belief that hearing people and ways of communicating are inherently superior [55]. As someone who is hard of hearing, Nadine is generally reluctant to be positioned as a 'representative' of the Deaf community. However, she actively advocates for Deaf recognition, inclusion, and access.

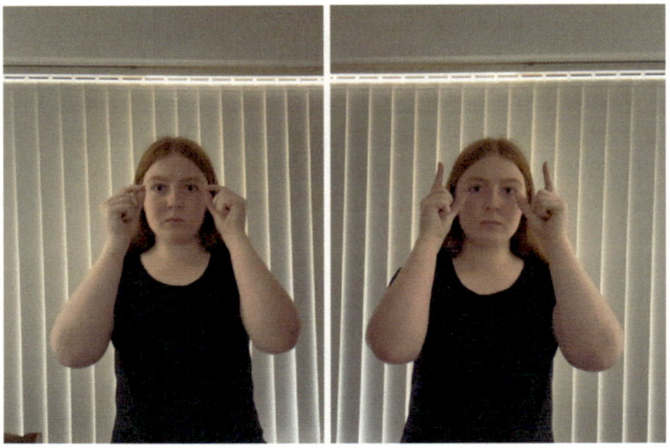

Figure 1.
Aware (one sign using finger movement, fingers move from closed to open).

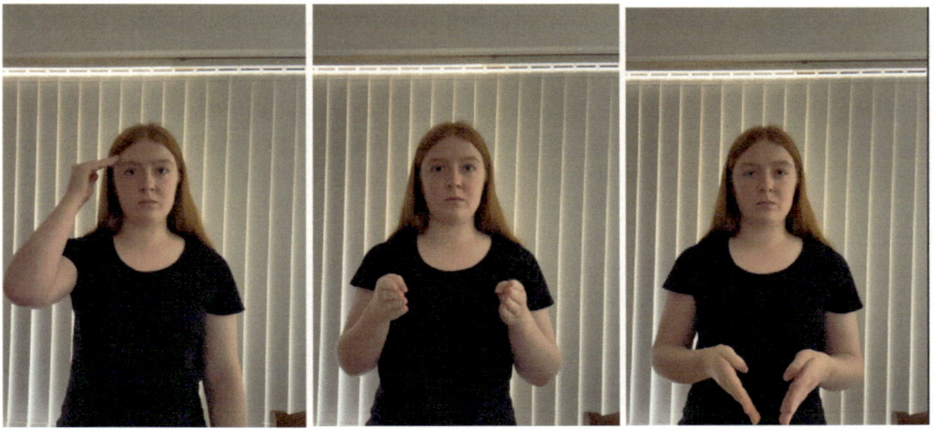

Figure 2.
Mind-focus (two signs, sign for mind and then sign for focus which involves the movment of two hands).

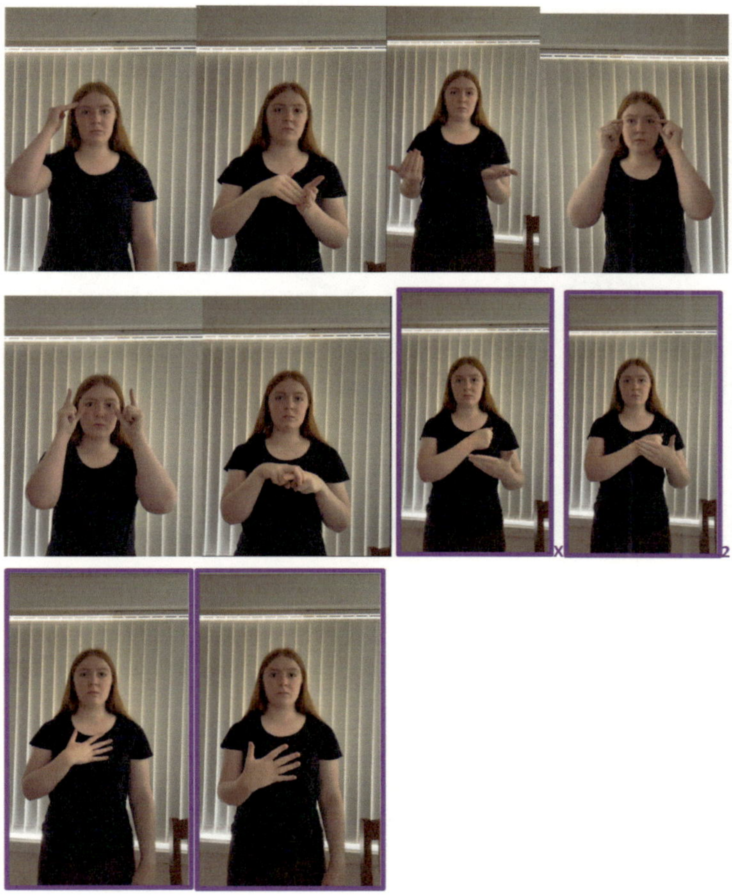

Figure 3.
Mindfulness (10 pictures indicating signs for mind, now, aware, sitting posture, heartbeat, breathing ... x2 indicates a repeated motion such as a heartbeat or breathing).

This chapter cites a videorecorded mini lecture created by Nadine and presented in a conversational style with a university colleague, discussing communication with Deaf individuals and the importance of interpreters. The following is how Nadine states this videorecorded conversation came about:

> *Our university program developers had requested content on the topic of communicating with the Deaf for an undergraduate communication course, and I was invited to participate by a colleague—given my Auslan studies and lived experience as a hard of hearing person. The following is the short conversation that led to a video rather than audio recording being created:*
>
> *Pressed for time (as we so often are in academe), my colleague and thoughtful partner in conversation suggested: "Maybe we just do a quick audio recording instead of video..."*
>
> *I replied, with wry humour, "I don't think so."*
>
> *Then silence.*

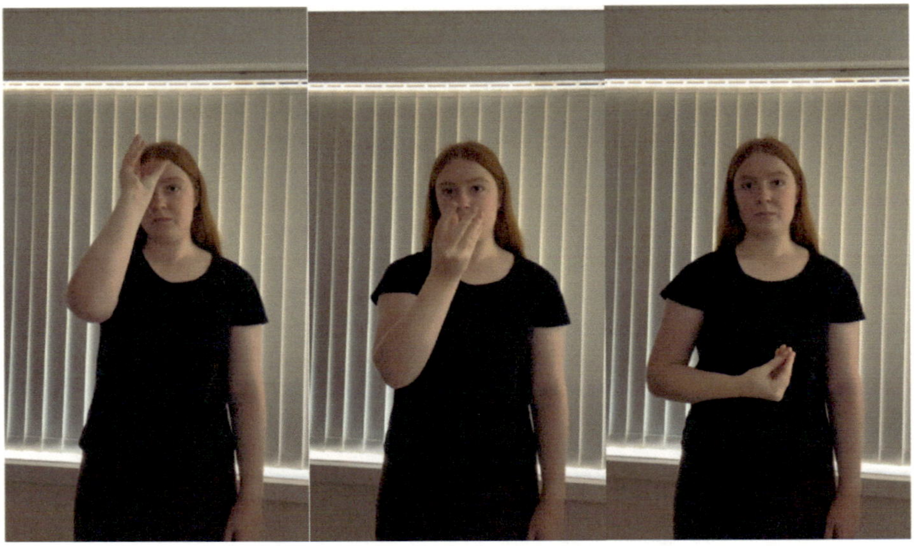

Figure 4.
Meditation (one sign composed of movement from forehead to chest/heart).

> *Then more silence—punctuated only by my blank and expectant expression, held with steady eye contact.*
>
> *It was a classic moment in academia — a reminder that even when discussing inclusive communication, we may forget to practise it unless we pause and reflect. I appreciated that my colleague did pause, did reflect, and then simply said, "Of course. We'll do video." His openness to learning in that moment strengthened both the collaboration and the message we were hoping to convey.*

Example Auslan meditation translation

See **Figures 1–4**.

DOI: http://dx.doi.org/10.5772/intechopen.1011002

Author details

Nadine J. Pelling
University of South Australia (Merging in 2026 with the University of Adelaide to Form Adelaide University), Magill, South Australia, Australia

*Address all correspondence to: nadine.pelling@adelaide.edu.au

References

[1] Jamil A, Gutlapalli SD, Ali M, Oble MJP, Sonia SN, George S, et al. Meditation and its mental and physical health benefits in 2023. Cureus. 2023;**15**(6):e40650. DOI: 10.7759/cureus.40650

[2] Spadaro R, Provident I. Health benefits of mindful meditation. In: Seaward BL, editor. Essentials of Managing Stress. Cham (CH): Springer; 2020. pp. 159-176. DOI: 10.1007/978-3-030-30892-6_11

[3] Korecki JR, Schwebel FJ, Votaw VR, Witkiewitz K. Mindfulness-based programs for substance use disorders: A systematic review of manualized treatments. Substance Abuse Treatment, Prevention, and Policy. 2020;**15**(1):51. DOI: 10.1186/s13011-020-00293-3

[4] McClintock AS, Marcus M. Mindfulness-based approaches in addiction treatment. In: El-Guebaly N, Carrà G, Galanter M, Baldacchino AM, editors. Textbook of Addiction Treatment. Cham (CH): Springer; 2021. DOI: 10.1007/978-3-030-36391-8_27

[5] Ramadas E, Lima MP, Caetano T, Lopes J, Dixe MDA. Effectiveness of mindfulness-based relapse prevention in individuals with substance use disorders: A systematic review. Behavioral Sciences (Basel). 2021;**11**(10):133. DOI: 10.3390/bs11100133

[6] Maloney S, Montero-Marin J, Kuyken W. Mindfulness-based cognitive therapy—Taking it further (MBCT-TiF) compared to ongoing mindfulness practice (OMP) in the promotion of well-being and mental health: A randomised controlled trial with graduates of MBCT and MBSR. Behaviour Research and Therapy. 2024;**173**:104478. DOI: 10.1016/j.brat.2024.104478

[7] Sparby T, Sacchet MD. Defining meditation: Foundations for an activity-based phenomenological classification system. Frontiers in Psychology. 2022;**12**:795077. DOI: 10.3389/fpsyg.2021.795077

[8] Eifring H. Asian traditions of meditation: What is meditation and types of meditation. In: Eifring H, editor. Asian Traditions of Meditation. Honolulu (HI): University of Hawai'i Press; 2016. pp. 1-35

[9] Chang VY, Palesh O, Caldwell R, Glasgow N, Abramson M, Luskin F, et al. The effects of a mindfulness-based stress reduction program on stress, mindfulness self-efficacy, and positive states of mind. Stress and Health. 2004;**20**(3):141-147. DOI: 10.1002/smi.1011

[10] Kabat-Zinn J. Mindfulness-based interventions in context: Past, present, and future. Clinical Psychology: Science and Practice. 2003;**10**(2):144-156. DOI: 10.1037/a0022062

[11] Sangma D, Bharani M. Spiritual values in Buddhism and Christianity: A philosophical study. Journal of Asian Zoroastrianism. 2024;**45**:788-800. DOI: 10.53555/jaz.v45i2.3917

[12] Flarey D. Meditation instructor and eastern and western purposes in meditation. AIHCP Health Care. 2023:11. Available from: https://aihcp.net/2019/09/27/meditation-instructor-and-eastern-and-western-purposes-in-meditation/

[13] Timbers VL, Hollenberger JC. Christian mindfulness and mental

health: Coping through sacred traditions and embodied awareness. Religions. 2022;**13**(1):62. DOI: 10.3390/rel13010062

[14] Garzon F, Benitez-DeVilbiss A, Turbessi V, Offei Darko YT, Berberena N, Jens A, et al. Christian accommodative mindfulness: Definition, current research, and group protocol. Religions. 2022;**13**(1):63. DOI: 10.3390/rel13010063

[15] Gill J. To Call on his Name: Perspectives on the Jesus Prayer. Durham (UK): Sacristy Press; 2019

[16] Johnston W. The Inner Eye of Love: Mysticism and Religion. San Francisco (CA): HarperOne; 1995

[17] Chen B, Yang T, Xiao L, Xu C, Zhu C. Effects of mobile mindfulness meditation on the mental health of university students: Systematic review and meta-analysis. Journal of Medical Internet Research. 2023;**25**:e39128. DOI: 10.2196/39128

[18] Costa A, Barnhofer T. Turning towards or turning away: A comparison of mindfulness meditation and guided imagery relaxation in patients with acute depression. Behavioural and Cognitive Psychotherapy. 2016;**44**(4):410-419. DOI: 10.1017/S1352465815000387

[19] Yamabe N. Concentration and visualization techniques in Buddhist meditation. In: Farias M, Brazier D, Lalljee M, editors. The Oxford Handbook of Meditation. Oxford: Oxford University Press; 2021. DOI: 10.1093/oxfordhb/9780198808640.013.19

[20] Huyser-Honig J. Visio Divina: Sacred Seeing to Encounter God. Grand Rapids, MI, USA: Calvin Institute of Christian Worship; 2021. Available from: https://worship.calvin.edu/resources/articles/visio-divina-sacred-seeing-encounter-god

[21] Manneh E. Praying with Your Eyes: How to Get Started with Visio Divina. Busted Halo; 2023. Available from: https://bustedhalo.com/ministry-resources/praying-with-your-eyes-how-to-get-started-with-visio-divina

[22] Efthimiadis-Keith H, Lindegger G. The subjective experience of using Ignatian meditation by male and female south African university students: An exploratory study. Journal of Religion and Health. 2014;**53**(5):1456-1471. DOI: 10.1007/s10943-013-9764-4

[23] Nicotera A. The circle of insight: A process for deepening Ignatian imagination and inviting Hope. Jesuit Higher Education: A Journal. 2023;**12**(2):3-14. DOI: 10.53309/2164-7666.1457. Available from: https://epublications.regis.edu/jhe/vol12/iss2/2/

[24] Tran T, Donnelly C, Nalder E, et al. Occupational therapist-led mindfulness-based stress reduction for older adults living with subjective cognitive decline or mild cognitive impairment in primary care: A feasibility randomised control trial protocol. BMJ Open. 2020;**10**(6):e035299. DOI: 10.1136/bmjopen-2019-035299

[25] Dudeja J. Analysis and benefits of chant-less Sohum/Humsa mantra meditation. Sports Engineering. 2018;**3**:198-203

[26] Guleria A, Kumar U, Kishan SSK, Khetrapal CL. Effect of "SOHAM" meditation on the human brain: An fMRI study. Psychiatry Research: Neuroimaging. 2013;**214**(3):462-465. DOI: 10.1016/j.pscychresns.2013.06.012

[27] Joshi N, Godiyal P. Effectiveness of so hum meditation in reducing the level of academic stress among first semester B.Sc. Nursing students. International Journal of Advanced Research. 2024;**12**:583-587

[28] Elstad T, Ulleberg P, Klonteig S, Hisdal J, Dyrdal GM, Bjorndal A. The effects of yoga on student mental health: A randomised controlled trial. Health Psychology and Behavioral Medicine. 2020;**8**(1):573-586. DOI: 10.1080/21642850.2020.1843466

[29] Keating T. Open Mind, Open Heart: The Contemplative Dimension of the Gospel. 20th Anniversary ed. New York: Continuum; 2002

[30] Banushi B, Brendle M, Ragnhildstveit A, Murphy T. Breathwork interventions for adults with clinically diagnosed anxiety disorders: A scoping review. Brain Sciences. 2023;**13**(2):256. Available from: https://www.mdpi.com/2076-3425/13/2/256

[31] Schmalzl L, Crane-Godreau MA, Payne P. Movement-based embodied contemplative practices: Definitions and paradigms. Frontiers in Human Neuroscience. 2014;**8**:205. DOI: 10.3389/fnhum.2014.00205

[32] Barcaccia B, Baiocco R, Pozza A, Pallini S, Mancini F, Salvati M. The more you judge the worse you feel: A judgemental attitude towards one's inner experience predicts depression and anxiety. Personality and Individual Differences. 2019;**138**:33-39. DOI: 10.1016/j.paid.2018.09.012

[33] Hytman L, Amestoy ME, Ueberholz RY, Fiocco AJ. Cultural adaptations of mindfulness-based interventions for psychosocial well-being in ethno-racial minority populations: A systematic narrative review. Mindfulness. 2025;**16**:21-41. DOI: 10.1007/s12671-024-02501-8

[34] Goodrich E, Wahbeh H, Mooney A. Teaching mindfulness meditation to adults with severe speech and physical impairments: An exploratory study. Neuropsychological Rehabilitation. 2015;**25**(1):112-135. DOI: 10.1080/09602011.2014.970201

[35] Kropp A, Sedlmeier P. What makes mindfulness-based interventions effective? An examination of common components. Mindfulness. 2019;**10**(10):2060-2072. DOI: 10.1007/s12671-019-01167-x

[36] Valluri J, Gorton KL, Smith RA. Effectiveness of loving-kindness micro-practices on chronic pain and stress outcomes in nurses: An online, double-blind, randomized-controlled pilot study. International Journal of Caring Sciences. 2024;**17**(1):45-56

[37] Farias M, Brazier D, Lalljee M, editors. The Oxford Handbook of Meditation. Oxford: Oxford University Press; 2021. DOI: 10.1093/oxfordhb/9780198808640.001.0001

[38] Pope Francis. General Audience: Catechesis on Prayer – 31. The Meditation. Vatican.va; 2021. Available from: https://www.vatican.va/content/francesco/en/audiences/2021/documents/papa-francesco_20210428_udienza-generale.html

[39] Holub I. Yoga. Available from: https://auslansoulyoga.com.au [Accessed: June 23, 2025]

[40] Knabb J, Johnson E, Garzon F. Introduction to the special issue: Meditation, prayer, and contemplation in the Christian tradition: Towards the operationalization and clinical application of Christian practices in psychotherapy and counseling. Journal of Psychology and Christianity. 2020;**39**(1):5-11

[41] Finley J. Christian Meditation: Experiencing the Presence of God – A Guide to Contemplation. New York: HarperCollins; 2002

[42] Bennett JM. Blessed silence: Explorations in Christian contemplation and hearing loss. Journal of Moral Theology. 2017;**6**(2):138-157

[43] Rosellini B. Exploring mindfulness as a culturally sensitive intervention for the deaf community [Dissertation]. Denver: Graduate School of Professional Psychology; 2015

[44] Ruiz R. Why Your Meditation Lesson Must Be More Accessible. Mashable; 29 Mar 2022. Available from: https://mashable.com/article/mindfulness-meditation-meditating-with-disability

[45] Carers Australia. Mindfulness: Session One – AUSLAN Translation. YouTube; 19 Aug 2021. Available from: https://youtu.be/fbmguszK94Q?si=_E1pYcXa2Owsr8SL

[46] Deaf Websites. Mindfulness and Meditation for Deaf Individuals. Available from: https://deafwebsites.com/mindfulness/ [Accessed: June 23, 2025]

[47] Vincent C, Wittich W, Bergeron F, Hotton M, Achou B. Shopping when you are deafblind: A pre-technology test of new methods for face-to-face communication. Societies. 2021;**11**(4):131. DOI: 10.3390/soc11040131

[48] Karimi H, Ghasemipour M, Dehghan F. The relationship between mindfulness and psychological well-being: The mediating role of emotion regulation. Journal of Contextual Behavioral Science. 2019;**13**:1-6

[49] Aussie Deaf Kids. Terminology for Deafness. Available from: https://www.aussiedeafkids.org.au/about-communication/australian-sign-language/terminology-for-deafness/ [Accessed: June 23, 2025]

[50] National Deaf Children's Society. Glossary: D. Available from: https://www.ndcs.org.uk/information-and-support/glossary/glossary-d/ [Accessed: June 23, 2025]

[51] Educational Audiology Association. Recommended Terminology When Referring to Hearing Differences. 2023. Available from: https://edaud.org/wordpress/wp-content/uploads/2023/10/RecommendedTerminology2023.pdf

[52] Australian Government Style Manual. Use Respectful Language. Available from: https://www.stylemanual.gov.au/accessible-and-inclusive-content/inclusive-language/people-disability [Accessed: June 23, 2025]

[53] Deafblind Information Australia. Terminology. Available from: https://www.deafblindinformation.org.au/about-deafblindness/sensory-impairment/deafness-and-hearing-impairment/terminology/

[54] Bauman HDL, Murray JJ. Deaf Gain: Raising the Stakes for Human Diversity. Minneapolis: University of Minnesota Press; 2014

[55] Bauman HDL. Audism: Exploring the metaphysics of oppression. Journal of Deaf Studies and Deaf Education. 2004;**9**(2):239-246. DOI: 10.1093/deafed/enh025

[56] Vago DR, Silbersweig DA. Self-awareness, self-regulation, and self-transcendence (S-ART): A framework for understanding the neurobiological mechanisms of mindfulness. Frontiers in Human Neuroscience. 2012;**6**:296. DOI: 10.3389/fnhum.2012.00296

[57] Haidar H, Bathelt J, Baker E. Meditation for well-being in the deaf

community: A visual adaptation framework. Journal of Disability Studies. 2023;**33**(2):150-161. DOI: 10.1177/17446295231129213

[58] Meditation Australia. Code of Ethics and Conduct. Available from: https://meditationaustralia.org.au/membership/code-ethics-conduct-rules-association/ [Accessed: June 23, 2025]

[59] Brown PM, Cornes A. Mental health of deaf and hard-of-hearing adolescents: What the students say. Journal of Deaf Studies and Deaf Education. 2014;**20**(1):75-81. DOI: 10.1093/deafed/enu031

[60] Aldalur A, Pick LH. Acculturative stress, mental health, and well-being among deaf adults. Journal of Deaf Studies and Deaf Education. 2023;**28**(4):387-398. DOI: 10.1093/deafed/enad015

[61] O'Connell N. Opportunity Blocked: Deaf People, Employment and the Sociology of Audism. 2021. Available from: https://www.researchgate.net/publication/348886121_Opportunity_Blocked_Deaf_People_Employment_and_the_Sociology_of_Audism

[62] Australian Psychological Society. Code of Ethics. Melbourne (AU): Australian Psychological Society; 2007

[63] Pelling NJ. General ethical principles. In: Pelling NJ, Burton LJ, editors. The Elements of Ethical Practice: Applied Psychology Ethics in Australia. Abingdon (UK): Routledge/Taylor & Francis; 2019

[64] Ludwig DS, Kabat-Zinn J. Mindfulness in medicine. Journal of the American Medical Association. 2008;**300**(11):1350-1352. DOI: 10.1001/jama.300.11.1350

[65] Boxall A-M. Accessible Services for Deaf People Who Use Auslan in the Hospitals and Health Services (v.6). Deaf Australia; 2021. Available from: https://deafau.org.au/wp-content/uploads/2020/12/Hospitals-and-Health-Services-Auslan-v6.pdf [Accessed: April 14, 2025]

[66] Amundsen R, Riby LM, Hamilton C, Hope M, McGann D. Mindfulness in primary school children as a route to enhanced life satisfaction, positive outlook and effective emotion regulation. BMC Psychology. 2020;**8**(1):71. DOI: 10.1186/s40359-020-00428-y

[67] Davis DM, Hayes JA. What are the benefits of mindfulness? A practice review of psychotherapy-related research. Psychotherapy. 2011;**48**:198-208. DOI: 10.1037/a0022062

[68] Goldsby TL, Goldsby ME, McWalters M, Mills PJ. Effects of singing bowl sound meditation on mood, tension, and well-being: An observational study. Evidence-Based Complementary and Alternative Medicine. 2017;**22**(3):401-406. DOI: 10.1177/2156587216668109. Epub 2016 Sep 30

[69] Parmentier FBR, García-Toro M, García-Campayo J, Yañez AM, Andrés P, Gili M. Mindfulness and symptoms of depression and anxiety in the general population: The mediating roles of worry, rumination, Reappraisal and Suppression. Frontiers in Psychology. 2019;**10**:506. DOI: 10.3389/fpsyg.2019.00506

[70] Germer C, Neff K. Teaching the Mindful Self-Compassion Program: A Guide for Professionals. New York: Guilford Press; 2019

[71] Zeidan F, Johnson SK, Diamond BJ, David Z, Goolkasian P. Mindfulness meditation improves cognition: Evidence

of brief mental training. Consciousness and Cognition. 2010;**19**(2):597-605. DOI: 10.1016/j.concog.2010.03.014. Epub 2010 Apr 3

[72] Frederick TV, Muldoon TP. Ignatian spirituality and psychotherapy. Journal of Psychology and Christianity. 2020;**39**(1):12-23

[73] Wernik U. The use of prayer beads in psychotherapy. Journal of Religion and Health. 2009;**48**(3):308-316. DOI: 10.1007/s10943-008-9201-1

[74] Department of Social Services. Auslan Interpreter Support. Available from: https://www.dss.gov.au/auslan-interpreter-support [Accessed: June 23, 2025]

[75] Pelling NJ, Lushington K. Communicating with Deaf and Hard of Hearing Populations [Video Lecture]. Magill, South Australia: University of South Australia; 2025

[76] Bontempo K. Signed language interpreting. In: Mikkelson H, Jourdenais R, editors. The Routledge Handbook of Interpreting. Abingdon (UK): Routledge; 2015. pp. 112-124

[77] Bot H. Interpreting in mental health care. In: Pöchhacker F, editor. The Routledge Handbook of Interpreting. Abingdon (UK): Routledge; 2015. pp. 364-379

[78] Bodian S. Meditation for Dummies. 4th ed. Hoboken (NJ): John Wiley & Sons; 2016

[79] Orozco E. Working with interpreters while delivering trauma therapy. In: Pelling NJ, Burton L, editors. The Elements of Ethical Practice: Applied Psychology Ethics in Australia. London: Routledge; 2019. pp. 4-12. DOI: 10.4324/9780429259319

[80] Pelling NJ. The use of interpreters in psychotherapy. Psychotherapy in Australia. 2005;**12**(1):68-73

[81] Anderson ML, Glickman NS, Mistler LA, Gonzalez M. Working therapeutically with deaf people recovering from trauma and addiction. Psychiatric Rehabilitation Journal. 2015;**39**(1):27-32. DOI: 10.1037/prj0000146

[82] Vernon M, Miller KR. Interpreting in mental health settings. American Annals of the Deaf. 2002;**146**(5):429-434. DOI: 10.1353/aad.2012.0200

[83] Pelling NJ. Accessible Contemplation: A Deaf-Inclusive Pilot of Christian and Secular Visual Meditation [Unpublished Manuscript]. Under Review.

Section 2

Clinical Outcomes

Chapter 6

Exploring the Relationship between Resilience and Self-Realisation as Understood by Young Adults Practicing Sahaja Yoga

Shivani Patil

Abstract

Resilience, defined as adaptive behaviour in the face of adversity, is influenced by spirituality, with self-realisation playing a pivotal role in identity development, particularly during life transitions. There is an Eastern and Western understanding of self-realisation. Unlike other spiritual systems, Sahaja Yoga offers a unique perspective as its practice commences with self-realisation. This chapter presents research which investigates the relationship between resilience and self-realisation among young adults practising Sahaja Yoga. Findings suggest that self-realisation contributes to resilience by fostering meaning, purpose, and identity. This study provides insights into self-realisation as a mechanism for enhancing resilience, with implications for resilience-based interventions targeting young adults.

Keywords: resilience, self-realisation, Sahaja yoga, meditation, yoga, spirituality

1. Introduction

The world today is rapidly changing and full of conflicts. People express resilience to navigate these situations. For young people and the generation of tomorrow, it is notably complex, as they search their identity—their 'self'—in these uncertain times. However, manifesting resilience is associated with individuals who have a sense of meaning and purpose [1, 2], which is asserted as they express self-realisation [3, 4]. Yet, the relationship between resilience and self-realisation is yet to be examined.

Philosophies from around the world articulate a desire for self-realisation that can be summarised as a Western and Eastern understandings. The first focuses on an outward approach—the manifestation of the self through one's work—and the second emphasises an inward approach—the comprehension of consciousness. The practice presented here—Sahaja Yoga (SY)—is a yoga-based meditation related to the last approach.

This chapter introduces a research project examining the relationship between resilience and self-realisation as understood by young adult practicing SY. First, theoretical frameworks within this research are established, followed by the methodologies used in the research. Then findings are presented. Lastly, the chapter discusses the newfound perspectives of self-realisation and their significance for understanding resilience. The findings contribute to the ongoing debate around resilience being either a trait, an outcome or a process and the search for the best wellbeing interventions for young people in distress.

2. Theoretical framework

2.1 Resilience

Resilience has become an important topic for promoting mental health and wellbeing [5]. Overall, resilience refers to successful adaptive behaviour in the face of adversity [6, 7]. However, it is complex, being multidisciplinary and context-specific and, hence, thought of in many ways [8].

The concept of resilience includes a trait, an outcome, and a process [6]. Resilience can be defined as an "adaptive stress-resistant personal quality" [9] or as a personal trait that "helps individuals cope with adversity and achieve good adjustment and development" [10]. Resilience as an outcome occurs as a positive psychological adaptation determined by various factors and can be nurtured through training and interventions [11]. It is most recently defined as a multidimensional, dynamic, and variable process that involves active adaptation and rapid recovery from adversity [12, 13].

Consequently, multiple origins and factors for resilience frequently interact, including biological, psychological and dispositional elements, social support, and other attributes of social systems [14, 15].

2.2 Resilience and spirituality

Among promoting factors, spirituality positively influences resilience [16–21] and was even described by manning as "the path to resilience" [22]. Spirituality involves seeking, finding, and expressing meaning and purpose [21, 23] and experiencing connections with one's deeper self, others, and the environment [24]. It influences coping mechanisms and promotes mental health and wellbeing [25].

Self-realisation is a central concept of existential search in the West [26] and spirituality in the East [27, 28].

Understandings of self-realisation in relation to resilience are scarce, and only [3] has precisely attempted to link those domains. Other authors, such as Liu [29], show the connection between self-realisation and resilience (without defining the terms) as the realisation of the self through self-achievement at work in adverse and difficult conditions.

Extensive discussion has been given to self-realisation or self-actualisation (synonymous in this paper), a concept studied in both Western and Eastern traditions. Both interpretations of self-realisation emphasise individuals' overall wellbeing and contribution to resilience [30, 31].

2.3 Self-realisation in the west

The Western understanding of self-realisation stems from the Greek philosophers' idea of eudaimonic happiness and wellbeing [3, 32, 33]. Aristotle connected self-realisation with the "activity of the soul in accord with virtue", a form of "personal excellence; that is, achieving the best that is within us" [30]. Similarly, eudaimonic wellbeing suggests that happiness and self-realisation are attained when individuals fulfil and manifest their full potential or are "fully functioning" [34]. Based on these concepts, contemporary psychologists and human scientists have formulated various frameworks of self-realisation (e.g. see [35–37]).

2.4 Self-realisation in the east - Indian philosophy

Eastern understanding presents self-realisation as the gaining of enlightenment and as life's main objective [38]. For the sake of simplicity, this paper will focus on the view rooted in Indian philosophy. It considers self-realisation as the aim of spiritual practice, allowing one to experience something larger, a state beyond suffering and the mind, an expansion of consciousness. It takes primarily the form of self-knowledge [28, 39], understanding one's identity as the Atman—"spirit" [40, 41]. Self-realisation is the aim of Yoga [42, 43]. Yoga is "the science of self-realisation" [27]. Self-realisation was the final goal of this practice, which is the same as Yoga, meaning the union with a higher consciousness.

2.5 Sahaja yoga

In contrast, Sahaja Yoga (SY) takes self-realisation as the first step in its spiritual practice [44]. SY emphasises mental silence as meditation, unlike some other systems [45]. It was inaugurated by Nirmala Srivastava, known as Shri Mataji Nirmala Devi, in the 1970s, first in India, then in the UK, and many countries worldwide (ibid). SY follows the ancient yogic traditions of awakening the Kundalini and activating the Chakras.

Menon and colleagues [46] showed that SY practice significantly improves self-esteem, resilience, and mental wellbeing through descriptive and correlation analysis of three scales: the Rosenberg self-esteem scale, brief resilience scale and The Warwick–Edinburgh mental well-being scale. The practice of SY has been qualified with health improvements in different domains, including heart, liver, pain, brain-related diseases as well as stress and resilience [46–52].

3. Aim and objectives

This research explores the relationship between resilience and self-realisation in the understanding and living experience of young adults practising SY, since this specific relationship has yet to be examined.

There are three objectives for this research:

- To explore young adults' understanding of resilience and self-realisation within the framework of SY,
- To examine the perceived relationship between self-realisation and resilience among young adults practising SY,
- To identify the perceived mechanisms through which self-realisation may influence resilience among young adults practising SY.

The study may offer new insights into promoting resilience and mental health and could have implications for developing interventions aimed at enhancing resilience among young adults.

4. Methodologies

4.1 Research design

The paper used primary data, which gave comprehensive insights into the connection between self-realisation and resilience, making this project an exploratory research endeavour. To study perceptions, a qualitative research method was necessary, as it focuses on understanding the participants' behaviours, beliefs, and assumptions [53]. Thus, qualitative data was collected with semi-structured interviews as they provided the most thorough understanding of people's perspectives. The interview guide was constructed using the researcher's knowledge of SY and of the literature.

A pilot interview helped make the researcher aware of their biases and adjust questions accordingly.

4.2 Research participants

Convenient and purposeful sampling methods were chosen to recruit participants, which allowed the study of a specific but diverse population [54, 55]. The criteria were:

- Practitioners of at least 5 years and continuous SY practice to date.

- Between 20 and 35 years old.

Participants came from different countries—France, the United Kingdom, Australia, India, China, and Lithuania—and came into contact with SY at different stages in life—some started practicing in adulthood, some started in their childhood, and others had their parents practising when they were born.

This sample was selected because people at this age are still discovering their identity while experiencing new life stages (e.g. higher education, marriage, parenthood, etc.). The research included twelve participants (n = 12).

4.3 Data collection

Participants acquainted with the lead researcher were recruited via social media. Individuals received an information sheet summarising the study's purpose and role and the opportunity to read the work when finished.

To mitigate any participant bias, the lead researcher established clear boundaries and maintained reflexivity throughout the interview period, as Noble & Smith [56] recommend.

Semi-structured online interviews were employed to gather the data as they offer researchers flexibility in guiding the interviews and the ability to reach participants worldwide [57]. Since the interviews were semi-structured, responses did not always align directly with the topics of inquiry, but they did reveal relevant areas of interest.

In such cases, every attempt was made to steer the responses back to the original question. Interviews revolved around three main topics: self-realisation, resilience, and the relationship between the two. Interviews lasted between 30 and 60 minutes.

4.4 Data analysis

The recorded interviews, conducted with Google Meet, were transcribed verbatim, and the data was thematically analysed using an inductive process. The objective was to identify shared themes across the replies. The transcripts were reworked for accuracy to the recording, relevant information was highlighted, and finally, the data was refined into subthemes and themes. An analytical method called axial coding was used, involving creating line-by-line codes and comparing data to form categories [58, 59]. Then the codes were grouped into sub-themes based on similarities and, lastly, grouped under themes, representing aspects of the answers to the research questions.

Associations were measured by occurrences in interviews and how participants used them to describe their experiences, pertaining to thematic co-occurrence analysis [60].

4.5 Ethical consideration

Participants received information about the study's nature and goals. They consented by signing a form and verbally before the interview. They were informed that they were free not to answer any questions and could withdraw their data until a specified deadline indicated on the form. After this deadline, the data was anonymised, and the original recordings were deleted.

Participants' confidentiality was strictly maintained to ensure their anonymity. The research data was only accessible to the researcher and their mentor. All participants' data was securely stored according to the 2018 General Data Protection Regulation.

5. Findings

Data analysis revealed three themes—principles, outcomes, and comparative Insights—for understanding self-realisation (**Figure 1**; **Table 1**) and three themes—principles, mechanisms, and characteristics—for understanding resilience (**Figure 2**; **Tables 2** and **3**). Self-realisation and resilience seem to be related as shown in **Figure 3** and **Table 4**.

5.1 Understanding of self-realisation

5.1.1 Principles

5.1.1.1 Nature

Participants were asked about their views on the nature of self-realisation, whether it was a state, a happening that fluctuated or was constant, or anything else. Equal numbers of participants defined self-realisation as a happening, a process, and a state. Some said that the state of self-realisation is a later stage of the initial happening:

> *"I would say self-realisation is a happening...You can establish it as a state within you, but then I would call that probably something else" (P8).*

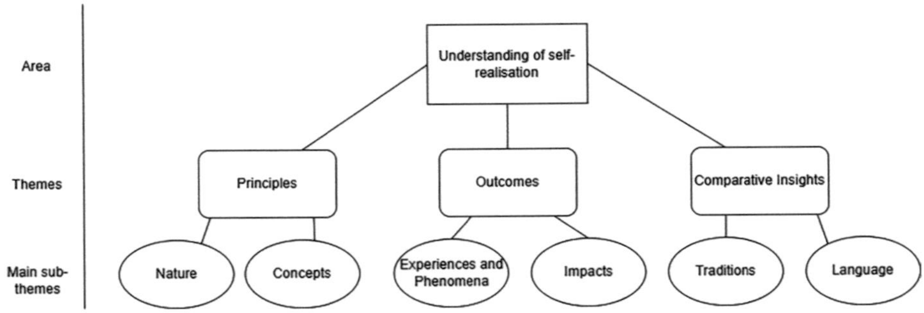

Figure 1.
Understanding of self-realisation.

Themes	Main sub-themes	Sub-themes	Occurrences
Theme 1: Principles of self-realisation—participants' definitions of self-realisation	Sub-theme A—Nature	A state	9
		A happening	8
		A process	8
		A mix/diverse	5
	Sub-theme B—Concepts	SR as a connection to a higher-power/Kundalini awakening and becoming unlimited	12
		SR as knowing the truth, beyond the ego	10
		SR as clarity through awareness	10
		SR as spontaneous but conditioned	9
		SR depends on people and circumstances Born in it/received during childhood/later in life make the path to SR unique	12
		SR with gradient	3
		SR is obtained once but is very subtle so it needs efforts to reinforce the experience	5
Theme 2: Outcomes of self-realisations—participants' experiences and self-realisation impacts	Sub-theme C—Experiences and phenomena	The cold breeze	12
		Above the head	12
		Sensations, hot and cold	12
		Lost concept of time	3

Themes	Main sub-themes	Sub-themes	Occurrences
		Exceptional occurrence	2
		Bliss, joy, and inner peace	5
	Sub-theme D—Impacts	A priceless impact	12
		Be in balance	9
		Living in the moment/be in the present	7
		Thoughtless awareness	12
		Ability to let it go/surrender/ comfort in the process	12
		Decode a situation so make better decision	7
		Unaffected/witness state as the ultimate freedom	7
		Ability to feel it and give self-realisation to others	6
		Personality qualities that others can recognise, even non-practitioners	5
Theme 3: Comparative insights of self-realisation—participants' comparisons of self-realisation in various areas	Sub-theme E—Comparative insights in traditions	Comparison with different cultures	N/A
		Having the same goal	8
		SY simplest and most straightforward	5
		Ancient vs. modern	10
	Sub-theme E—Comparative insights in language	Hard to answer	10
		Interchangeable words	3
		Code-switching	1

Table 1.
Understanding of self-realisation with themes, sub-themes, and occurrences.

Other participants considered it primarily as a state that we "initially... dip in and out of" (P6). Establishing self-realisation as a constant state, agreed by all participants to be the goal, is what people call the "living" (P9) or "ever-evolving" (P2) process.

Sometimes, participants returned to their words to describe a slightly different aspect of self-realisation. For example, P9 said, "I would say it's a happening, is not a process," but later took the opposite view: "It's a process, maybe also." This shows how complex self-realisation is, which can be viewed through several concepts.

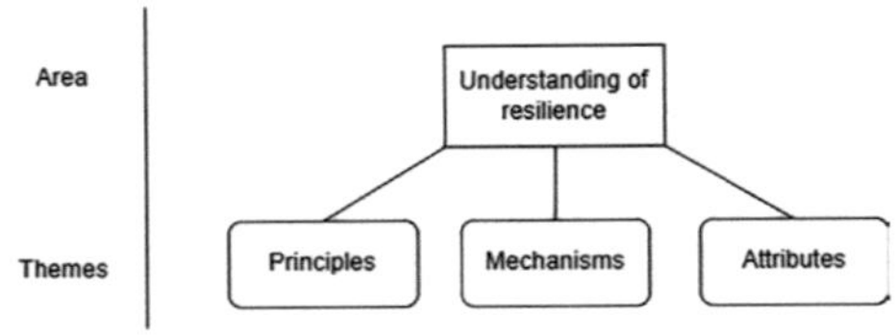

Figure 2.
Understanding of resilience.

Themes	Sub-themes	Occurrences
Theme 1: Principles—Participants' definition of resilience	As overcoming situations	8
	As learning and growing from experience	3
	Unaffected/being in balance	7
	Doing something with consistency	3
	Complete acceptance and stoicism	8
	Resilience exists with vulnerability	2
Theme 2: Mechanisms of resilience	SY practice, especially balancing/clearing techniques	12
	Meditation which allows to be in the present and remove negative feelings like guilt and anger	12
	Stay calm	12
	Faith, acceptance, and surrender	12
	Ability to put into perspective/reframe a situation	6
	Detachment	10
	Finding solution within capabilities	2
	Go into silence, which allows for lucidity	5
	Being with the collective	3
Theme 3: Attributes (Characteristics) of resilience	Being authentic	5
	Being the witness/ability to be unaffected	10
	Courage	2
	Determination	3
	Ability to recover	3
	Being creative	2
	Being flexible	1
	Other attributes	1

Table 2.
Understanding of resilience with themes and sub-themes.

5.1.1.2 Concepts

Self-realisation was described as a connection to a higher power—"Self-realisation is something for me that connects you to God" (P10)—knowing the truth—"So in short, it's the truth" (P2)—and recognising our true identity. In that sense, P2 talked

Subject of the resilience experience told	Occurrences
Job - nanny	2
Job	3
Studies - Law	2
Studies	2
Family issues	5
Note: Some people narrated more than one story	

Table 3.
Subject of the resilience experience told.

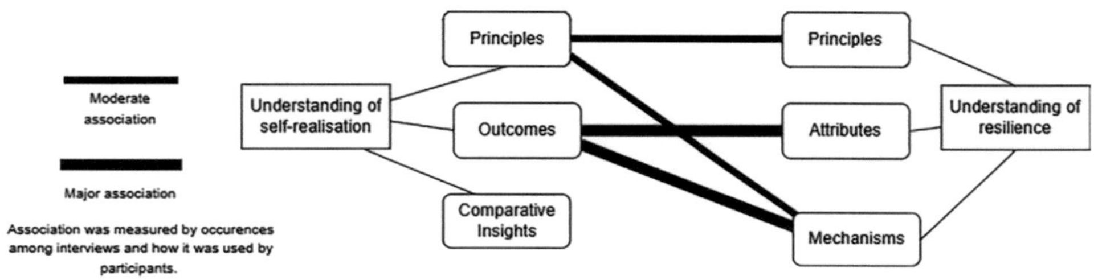

Figure 3.
Relationship between self-realisation and resilience.

Self-realisation themes—Resilience themes	Sub-themes
Principle - Principle	Being balance
Principle - Mechanisms	SY practice (nurturing self-realisation through meditation) leads to resilience
Principle - Mechanisms	By knowing the truth (about world and identity), one can reframe situations
Outcomes - Attributes	Personal qualities developed with self-realisation echoes resilience attributes
Outcomes - Mechanisms	SY practice allows vibrations interpretations which gives indication for the best choice to do
Outcomes - Mechanisms	SY practice (specifically balancing techniques) is completely embedded as a resilience mechanism, meaning that developing self-realisation is priority for resilience
Outcomes - Mechanisms	Going into silence (thoughtless awareness), stay calm, detachment, being the witness and surrender are advantages of self-realisation put into use for resilience
	Lack of clarity

Table 4.
Relationship between self-realisation and resilience with themes, sub-themes, and occurrences.

about "[the] consciousness experiencing meeting itself again", and P1 talked about the removal of "artificial things" to let the expression of the "authentic self".

It involves "Kundalini awakening" and this energy going through the top of the head to the "seventh chakra" called "Sahasrara", and the removal of influences such as "the ego and super-ego" (P2; P5).

Participants believed self-realisation allows one to go "beyond human limitations" and reach their "full potential" (P2; P6; P8), leading to "balance in your chakras, in your being" (P8). By balance, participants refer to a state where "the things that happen to you don't affect you negatively or positively, but you live in a state of balance and hence of wellbeing" (P6).

It is described as a "subtle", "spontaneous" process that cannot be comprehended through mental work, be forced or "controlled", and happens at the right time (P10; P1).

While it is spontaneous, some conditions must be met to experience it, such as "seeking the truth" and "surrendering] to God" (P11). P2, P8, and P10 also described the "more mundane process of actually trying to express that desire through a meditation (P8)". P3 reported that self-realisation depends on people and their circumstances.

Additionally, there are "gradations" of self-realisation, and it is something that needs nurturing to become fully established (P8; P3; P11). Indeed, if one does not "entertain the process, it could fade away" (P3), "like when a plant is growing" (P10).

Some participants believed one can be born with self-realisation (P4), while others needed to discover it through "penance" or "sufferings" (P6; P12).

5.1.2 Comparative insights

5.1.2.1 Traditions

Participants discussed how self-realisation can be linked to different philosophies and cultures, with some noting distinctions between "East" and "West" (P8) or specifying philosophies like "Christianity, Islam, Hinduism, Western psychology (Jung) and Chinese philosophy" (P5). Only P9 expressed that there was a difference with other cultures since they were not talking about Kundalini awakening and could not "give self-realisation".

Most agreed that religions and spiritual movements share the goal of self-realisation (P1; P8): "Every single spiritual movement talks about the ascent of humanity, the movement towards sainthood, towards being the best possible version of yourself, to being at one with God and one with everything."

According to participants, achieving self-realisation through SY practice is simple, in contrast to the harder methods used in ancient times: "It's been going on for thousands of years back in India, but it was taught from one guru to the students and so on. And the student had to prove he was worthy" (P7).

SY practice allowed for giving self-realisation "without efforts" to "anyone", "anywhere", and "at any time" (P3; P5; P7; P8), which was not possible before.

Additionally, the time of establishment of SY influenced practitioners' understanding. For instance, P12 recalled:

> *"Here, means out of China, because every other country starts Sahaja Yoga very early. But us was... Like this year is only the 30th year. So for us, the understanding of Sahaja was different."*

5.1.2.2 Language and communication

Most participants found it hard to answer some questions, especially the ones dealing with self-realisation and its nature. This was expressed through sentences such as "This is hard to answer" (P7), "This is a tricky question to answer" (P8), long pauses, phrases like "I don't know" (P2) and even "my brain froze" (P12).

Some participants used the words meditation, self-realisation, and Sahaja Yoga interchangeably. For instance, P8 said that the state of self-realisation is the state of meditation. Other participants also seemed to have the same understanding, and since that state is achieved by Sahaja Yoga practice, participants would often use those terms synonymously.

There were also signs of code-switching, the clearest one being P7's statement: "I don't know how to explain it in non-Sahaja words".

5.1.3 Outcomes

5.1.3.1 Experience and phenomena

When participants talked about self-realisation, they all said they experienced it at the top of and above the head:

> *"That seems to be the point of integration. And when you go above that and beyond that, and reach a point sort of above yourself. That seems to be where you can go without analysing or thinking or feeling anything but just this pure joy of existing and being aware, and that's it." (P2).*

All participants said that they could experience a "cool breeze" when they were in a state of self-realisation, usually when they meditate. These sensations are called "vibrations". Generally, the cool sensations/vibrations are taken as good signs, and heat is a sign of an unbalanced subtle system (conf. **Table 1**). With this, participants are able to decode the "subtleties" of a situation, which gives them an indication of the best choices to make (P1; P8).

Some participants said that they lost the concept of time when they were in the state of self-realisation as they experienced "bliss" and "joy" (P2; P4; P6). Additionally, when participants had self-realised moments, they experienced exceptional occurrences. For example, P7 recalled: "And the fact that I got it, like my results of the exams, there was some stuff that was like 'Oh, my God, how can that be?'".

5.1.3.2 Impacts

All participants highlighted the "priceless" impacts of self-realisation, such as "be completely present" (P2). Self-realisation also allowed to "be in balance", in a relaxed state and in "thoughtless awareness", which means the absence of thoughts or complete inner silence (all participants).

Self-realisation also allowed participants to be their authentic selves, let go, and accept:

> *"But there is a whole universe out there, of other solutions and other ways of living, of doing things, of just existing, that we're able to access once we just let go of this idea. Of these ideas of who we are and what we do and what we, you know... This kind of limited identification with this sense of limited self. So I feel like this moment of meditation, of self-realisation and of self-awareness is a way to just like access so, so much more of who we truly are." (P6)*

It also enabled participants to reframe situations and make decisions based on vibrational indications: "To me, it's like one more tool in your senses and if it's able to help you make better decisions then, that's it" (P1). As P5 said:

> *"[self-realisation] 's supposed to get you to the state of thoughtless and witness state where you don't want to impose anymore. You are just wise, by knowing yourself, your own capabilities. And you just move forward with that".*

In doing that, participants can access "the real freedom [which] is when you're just untouched. But not untouched because you choose, but just because really you just are unaffected. You're able to completely be, and it's not like through an action, it's just a state. The things that happen to you don't affect you negatively or positively, but you live in a state of balance and hence of wellbeing" (P6).

Furthermore, it provided the ability to sense self-realisation in others, give self-realisation to others, and develop qualities such as intelligence, kindness, compassion, creativity, and humility (see **Table 1**).

5.2 Understanding of resilience

5.2.1 Principles

Participants defined resilience in different ways. Some participants described resilience as the act of overcoming fears or difficult situations: "I understand resilience as being able to, maybe, overcome something that would be maybe unpleasant, traumatic" (P3). "You get into an accident and you overcome the fear of going, of doing whatever happened, that's resilience as well" (P7).

Others said that resilience is about learning and growing from mistakes and experiences: "Resilience comes from experiencing things that are not so pleasant but are necessary, almost, for growth" (P2).

Alternatively, participants established that resilience is about being unaffected by extremes and situations, to be in balance under any circumstances: "I would understand resilience as the ability to face both adversity and great fortune without being unduly deterred from, you could say, one's core traits and core personality and core level of joy and happiness" (P8). This gives a state of balance that equals to resilience according to P3.

P11 described resilience as "the consistency of doing something, even if you don't see the results".

P5 went further as to say that Stoicism, as explained by Greek philosophers, was resilience's ultimate expression:

> *"That philosophy of Stoicism is... That's the definition by itself of resilience. It means that you really accept things to a radical level; that everything is a gift, like everything is a message from the universe, from God".*

5.2.2 Attributes

Participants described attributes and features when resilience was experienced or manifested.

Being the witness, or having this ability to be unaffected, was acknowledged to be resilient: "it's just to witness the events without projecting things on it" (P5). This composure is very often associated with being detached and be able "to see the drama playing" (P11).

Additionally, the ability to recover was mentioned by participants. For example P1 said: "How quickly you come back and how much you deviate from your normal self, these two are features of resilience I feel".

Moreover, participants mentioned that to have resilience one needs "creativity", "confidence", "courage", "determination", the ability to be "flexible", the ability to let go—"You need to get to this position of control-free, in opposition of control-freak" (P5) (conf. **Table 2**). Most of those qualities can be nurtured as SY "gives you those [qualities] to help you feel more resilient" (P4).

5.2.3 Mechanisms

Participants mentioned different mechanisms of resilience, of which some are intrinsic to others.

Accepting the conditions gave a first step to resilience: "The bottom line, the thing is accepting things, means that you don't hold judgment anymore on things ... That also means that you're not rejecting your own desires and reality, but you accept reality by itself" (P5).

All participants used their SY practice as a mechanism for resilience. For instance, most participants used meditation and "balancing techniques" to remove negative feelings (P7; conf. **Table 2**).

Moreover, the faith of participants was used as a resilience mechanism. All participants cited the ability to detach from the situation, surrender it, and reframe it (conf. **Table 2**).

Most participants also mentioned the ability to "stay calm", "go into silence" or in thoughtless awareness, where participants took a moment to enter that state so they could bring clarity and "become incredibly lucid", which allowed them to think of solutions within their capabilities (P10; P7; P6).

Lastly, some participants mentioned that being with the "collective" helped them overcome situations, thanks to people's support.

5.3 The relation between self-realisation and resilience

Self-realisation and resilience are related in different ways, although not always straightforwardly (see **Table 3**). A first point in common is the balanced state that is associated with both self-realisation and resilience:

> *"being self-realised, it means you're balanced. ... I think these situations only come if you are in these two imbalances. And so that's why being self-realised is great. No more challenges in life" (P3).*

With SY practice, one gains tools to develop and establish self-realisation in life, increasing resilience. One gains a subtle awareness which provides a connection to and understanding of a higher order that involves the "all-pervading power", of "divine" nature, also referred to as Kundalini by participants: "whatever happens, happens for a reason... So it's all part of a bigger plan and so Sahaja Yoga really helps me to understand that" (P7).

The understanding happened through the sensations, "the vibrations" one gets, which give "indications" on best action and move on (P8). It also reveals the subtle truths of reality and identity, through which participants could reframe circumstances: "When I meditate, I'm able to go into that space where I can just be myself... And through that state of being then I can face things" (P10).

Going into inner silence, staying calm, detaching, being the witness, and surrendering are advantages of self-realisation for resilience (see **Table 3**). Indeed, the qualities developed by self-realisation through SY practice are the attributes and mechanisms of resilience:

> *"So feeling more confident in yourself, feeling more independent, feeling more secure in yourself. If you're not secure in yourself, you don't feel like you're able stand on your own two feet, you will naturally be swayed by others. And you start to be affected more and less resilient... you can shape yourself and your future, and based on understanding yourself better. And through these tools and techniques of Sahaja Yoga and self-realisation, that is possible" (P4).*

Lastly, participants were asked to recount a story when they thought self-realisation helped. About half explained how self-realisation helped with their jobs and in daily life, others relayed how it assisted in their studies, and some narrated how it comforted them during a time when they had family issues. As P6 said, "it's something that kind of infuses your life".

6. Discussion

The study's participants described different aspects of self-realisation—a happening, a process, and a state. These dimensions are associated with the concepts of self-realisation and resilience.

When self-realisation is associated with Kundalini awakening, then it is a happening. This is consistent with the Indian sacred texts about Kundalini and D. Frawley in his book Ayurveda and Yoga [27]. The certainty of connection with a higher power and the ensuing faith provided participants with the resilience to move forward, which is also suggested in the literature [16, 18].

When self-realisation relates to its establishment and the becoming of the authentic and unlimited self, then self-realisation is a process. Here, two points can be examined: Self-realisation in the manifestation process of identity and self-realisation gradients.

Findings reflect Eastern philosophies, which focused on the internal process of identity, the I and non-I, harnessed through self-cultivation and self-knowledge [28]. In contrast, from a Western perspective, Caruso [26] argued that the search for and understanding of self-knowledge served for the task of becoming oneself. The emphasis was on an outward manifestation, found in the literature as scholars [61, 62] linked self-realisation with external achievements—"I am self-realised because I do". This expression of identity is mainly asserted through professional life (ibid).

Participants mentioned gradients of self-realisation manifesting several ascending spiritual states. This also echoes the aims of spirituality, especially in Indian philosophy [40], but also the ecological self-model put forward by Naess [63] and Wang [37].

In this process, belief in being looked after and guided in the search and experience of the self generates resilience through the acceptance of events.

Participants related self-realisation to a constant balanced state, to thoughtless awareness of the present moment and the subtle world. According to them, this is achieved through the practice of meditation. The balanced state, where one is detached and unaffected by stimulus, gives resilience as the perception of adversity and challenges changes, finding purpose and meaning in the circumstances. This echoes Ryff's study [3], which associates self-realisation with eudaimonic wellbeing. However, Crawford and colleagues [18] also warned that spirituality can negatively affect resilience. For instance, when trauma or hardship destroys faith in a higher power or leads to a negative relationship with this higher authority, it may reduce the likelihood of resilience following adversity (ibid). Likewise, although all participants embraced self-realisation, their experiences were not always relatable to the narrative of the practice. Because of these incongruences, some participants stopped practising SY then started anew. This difference between narrative and experience is called the theory-practice gap or research-practice gap [64, 65]. In the spiritual academic field, this narrative is called the "storyworld", which relates directly to identity and how one sees the world [66]. In constructing or discovering our identity, our storyworld can change to align with our understanding of our living experiences, creating eudaimonic wellbeing.

According to the findings, various outcomes can manifest from the different dimensions of self-realisation, including new experiences and personal changes. These mirror previous SY research [45, 46, 50, 51, 67]. Brain studies involving SY showed positive improvement, like the expansion of white and grey matter [52, 67, 68], which may lead to better regulation. Hendriks and colleagues' research [50] showed that engaging in SY meditation might be connected to a distinct group of positive character traits, including forgiveness, gratitude and self-regulation, also mentioned by participants.

Findings showed that all participants used meditation as a mechanism for resilience. Robust literature supports practices like meditation and mindfulness to increase and maintain wellbeing [69]. Good and colleagues [70] suggested that mindfulness contributes to the development of resilience in various ways. These include aiding in recovery from harmful events, promoting growth in the face of adversity, and facilitating recovery with positive emotion [70, 71]. These elements are also found in participants' experiences. Looking at employee resilience, Buranapin et al. [71] emphasise two understandings of mindfulness: Eastern and Western. The former feeds into the latter, meaning that the passive mind (e.g. awareness and attention) can change into an active mind, encouraging creativity, inquisitiveness, receptiveness to the surroundings, and active engagement with them. Participants' experiences also contain these components.

The findings highlighted different concepts of resilience, which were also mentioned in previous studies. Resilience as overcoming aligns with the common definition of resilience [6]. As such, it echoes with resilience viewed as a process. Moreover, participants' understandings of resilience resonated with Lecomte's description [72]—the ability to grow from experiences or to reframe situations, transforming them from negative to positive—which allows the capacity to develop and nurture resilience through interventions [73, 74]. This resonated with participants' accounts that it is possible to develop resilience, either through personal qualities or with specific techniques developed through SY.

Nevertheless, participants' understanding questions the nature and manifestation of resilience. Participants' accounts suggest that it could be a trait, a process or an outcome—a long-running debate in the literature [75]. Some scholars argue that resilience is a mix of both outcomes and processes [7], viewing it as "the success of the coping process involved given the circumstances" [76]. Both views acknowledge the roles of various factors—life events, challenges, personal attributes, and systems [75, 77]. In this case, scholars talk about protective/risk factors, coping mechanisms, and other developmental constructs such as hardiness and a sense of coherence [6, 14].

However, it is less common to associate resilience with complete acceptance and remaining unaffected to maintain balance, as presented by participants. Moreover, findings showed that attributes and mechanisms of resilience were the same (i.e.

detachment, being the witness). This may be because participants mixed their SY understanding with that of resilience. In fact, Facco [78] argued that the "epistemologically sound, non-dualistic paradigm" of Eastern philosophies allowed having a metaphysical understanding of resilience, "enabling one to live well, die well, and remain in a state of unshakable resilience". More broadly, scholars [79, 80] showed that resilience was culture-specific, which may have implications in interpreting what resilience is and its manifestations.

7. Limitations

The design and methodology impose limitations on the study, which was narrowed to the research's acquaintances, restricting the generalisability of the findings. There was also a risk of bias since the researcher is a SY practitioner, which may have transmuted in the methodology. To mitigate any bias, the researcher established clear boundaries, maintained reflexivity, and sought external supervision. Additionally, questions around resilience could be framed differently, such as querying about its nature by SY practitioners. Moreover, SY is a dynamic practice that is developing with its practitioners. Thus, the findings are also limited in time.

8. Conclusion

Nowadays, resilience is regarded as an important component of wellbeing when coping with a stressful life. This study showed that SY practitioners developed resilience through their spiritual self-realisation. Self-realisation was associated with different concepts. Implications for resilience were discussed.

Yet, this opens for further research to look into SY practitioners' demographics such as gender, age, or practice duration. It also invites comparison with other meditation practices. Additionally, researchers could conceptualise resilience within SY practice for resilience and wellbeing interventions.

Acknowledgements

I would like to extend my sincere thanks to Mia Vulovic and Marcelo Saad foe finding me and giving me the opportunity to publish my research.

Special thanks to my research supervisor, Justin Haroun, and to the University of Westminster which is the institution that allowed me to this research.

I express gratitude to all the individuals who contributed to the success of this research by dedicating their time and sharing their experiences. In a broader sense, I appreciate the support of the Sahaja Yoga community, which has enabled me to connect with the study's participants.

Lastly, I am deeply thankful to my spiritual mother, Shri Mataji Nirmala Devi, for her nurturing guidance and for ensuring the smooth progression of everything.

Conflict of interest

The authors declare no conflict of interest.

Additional materials

The additional materials mentioned in this chapter can be downloaded at: https://cdn.intechopen.com/public/docs/supplemental/Themes_and_codes.xlsx.

Author details

Shivani Patil
University of Westminster, London, United Kingdom

*Address all correspondence to: luciepatil@gmail.com

References

[1] Wexler LM, DiFluvio G, Burke TK. Resilience and marginalized youth: Making a case for personal and collective meaning-making as part of resilience research in public health. Social Science & Medicine. 2009;**69**:565-570

[2] Rutten BPF, Hammels C, Geschwind N, Menne-Lothmann C, Pishva E, Schruers K, et al. Resilience in mental health: Linking psychological and neurobiological perspectives. Acta Psychiatrica Scandinavica. 2013;**128**:3-20. DOI: 10.1111/acps.12095

[3] Ryff CD. Self-realisation and meaning making in the face of adversity: A eudaimonic approach to human resilience. Journal of Psychology in Africa. 2014;**24**:1-12. DOI: 10.1080/14330237.2014.904098

[4] Lewis NA, Hill PL. Sense of purpose promotes resilience to cognitive deficits attributable to depressive symptoms. Frontiers in Psychology. 2021;**12**:698109

[5] Davydov DM, Stewart R, Ritchie K, Chaudieu I. Resilience and mental health. Clinical Psychology Review. 2010;**30**:479-495. DOI: 10.1016/j.cpr.2010.03.003

[6] McCubbin L. Challenges to the Definition of Resilience. San Francisco: ERIC; 2001

[7] Pooley JA, Cohen L. Resilience: A definition in context. Australian Community Psychologist. 2010;**22**:30-37

[8] Southwick SM, Bonanno GA, Masten AS, Panter-Brick C, Yehuda R. Resilience definitions, theory, and challenges: Interdisciplinary perspectives. European Journal of Psychotraumatology. 2014;**5**:25338. DOI: 10.3402/ejpt.v5.25338

[9] Ahern NR, Ark P, Byers J. Resilience and coping strategies in adolescents. Paediatric Nurse. 2008;**20**:32-36. DOI: 10.7748/paed2008.12.20.10.32.c6903

[10] Hu T, Zhang D, Wang J. A meta-analysis of the trait resilience and mental health. Personality and Individual Differences. 2015;**76**:18-27. DOI: 10.1016/j.paid.2014.11.039

[11] Kalisch R, Müller MB, Tüscher O. A conceptual framework for the neurobiological study of resilience. The Behavioral and Brain Sciences. 2015;**38**:e92. DOI: 10.1017/S0140525X1400082X

[12] Fergus S, Zimmerman M, Fergus S, Zimmerman MA. Adolescent resilience: A framework for understanding healthy development in the face of risk. Annual Review of Public Health. 2005;**26**:399-419. DOI: 10.1146/annurev.publhealth.26.021304.144357

[13] Luthar SS, Cicchetti D, Becker B. Research on resilience: Response to commentaries. Child Development. 2000;**71**:573-575. DOI: 10.1111/1467-8624.00168

[14] Luthar SS, Cicchetti D. The construct of resilience: Implications for interventions and social policies. Development and Psychopathology. 2000;**12**:857-885

[15] Friborg O, Hjemdal O, Rosenvinge JH, Martinussen M. A new rating scale for adult resilience: What are the central protective resources behind healthy adjustment? International Journal of Methods in Psychiatric Research. 2006;**12**:65-76. DOI: 10.1002/mpr.143

[16] Schwalm FD, Zandavalli RB, de Castro Filho ED, Lucchetti G. Is there a relationship between spirituality/religiosity and resilience? A systematic review and meta-analysis of observational studies. Journal of Health Psychology. 2022;**27**:1218-1232. DOI: 10.1177/1359105320984537

[17] Vanistendael S. Resilience and spirituality. In: Monroe, B, Oliviere, D. editors. Resilience in Palliative Care: Achievement in Adversity. Vol. 2007. New York: Oxford University Press; 2007. pp. 115-135

[18] Crawford E, Wright MO, Masten AS. Resilience and spirituality in youth. In: Roehlkepartain EC, editor. The Handbook of Spiritual Development in Childhood and Adolescence. London: SAGE Publication; 2006. pp. 355-370

[19] Kim S, Esquivel GB. Adolescent spirituality and resilience: Theory, research, and educational practices. Psychology in the Schools. 2011;**48**:755-765. DOI: 10.1002/pits.20582

[20] Helmreich I, Kunzler A, Chmitorz A, König J, Binder H, Wessa M, et al. Psychological interventions for resilience enhancement in adults. Cochrane Database of Systematic Reviews. 2017;**2017**:CD012527. DOI: 10.1002/14651858.CD012527

[21] Gnanaprakash C. Spirituality and resilience among post-graduate university students. Journal of Health Management. 2013;**15**:383-396. DOI: 10.1177/0972063413492046

[22] Manning LK. Navigating hardships in old age: Exploring the relationship between spirituality and resilience in later life. Qualitative Health Research. 2013;**23**:568-575. DOI: 10.1177/1049732312471730

[23] Lepherd L. Spirituality: Everyone has it, but what is it? International Journal of Nursing Practice. 2015;**21**:566-574. DOI: 10.1111/ijn.12285

[24] Naor L, Mayseless O. The therapeutic value of experiencing spirituality in nature. Spirituality in Clinical Practice. 2020;**7**:114

[25] Cotton S, Larkin E, Hoopes A, Cromer BA, Rosenthal SL. The impact of adolescent spirituality on depressive symptoms and health risk behaviors. Journal of Adolescent Health. 2005;**36**:529. DOI: 10.1016/j.jadohealth.2004.07.017

[26] Caruso G. The meaning of life between the self and the normative process of self-realisation. Human Affairs. 2019;**29**:489-496. DOI: 10.1515/humaff-2019-0044

[27] Frawley D. Yoga and Ayuryeda: Self-Healing and Self-Realization. Twin Lakes, Wis: Lotus Light Pub; 1999

[28] Peters MA. Educational philosophies of self-cultivation: Chinese humanism. Educational Philosophy and Theory. 2022;**54**:1720-1726. DOI: 10.1080/00131857.2020.1811679

[29] Liu R. In the face of instability and marginalisation in a gendered craft industry: Self-realisation and resilience of the self-employed craftswomen in Jingdezhen, China. International Journal of Business Anthropology. 2022;**12**:67-77

[30] Ryff CD, Boylan JM, Kirsch JA. Eudaimonic and hedonic well-being: An integrative perspective with linkages to sociodemographic factors and health. In: Lee MT, Kubzansky LD, VanderWeele TJ, editors. Measuring Well-Being. 1st ed. New York: Oxford University Press; 2021. pp. 92-135. DOI: 10.1093/oso/9780197512531.003.0005

[31] Brooks S, Reynolds S. The exploration of *becoming* as a yoga practitioner and its impact on identity formation, health, and well-being. Journal of Occupational Science. 2024;**31**:354-370. DOI: 10.1080/14427591.2023.2253802

[32] Ryff CD. Eudaimonic Well-Being and Health: Mapping Consequences of Self-Realization. In: Waterman AS, editor. The best within us: Positive psychology perspectives on eudaimonia. Washington: American Psychological Association; 2013. pp. 77-98. DOI: 10.1037/14092-005

[33] Taylor AE. Self-realization—A criticism. International Journal of Ethics. 1896;**6**:356-371

[34] Ryan RM, Deci EL. On happiness and human potentials: A review of research on hedonic and eudaimonic well-being. Annual Review of Psychology. 2001;**52**:141-166. DOI: 10.1146/annurev.psych.52.1.141

[35] Maslow AH. Motivation Personality. New York: Harper & Row; 1970

[36] Tønnesvang J. The structure of self-realisation. Journal of Theoretical and Philosophical Psychology. 2006;**26**:51

[37] Wang C-L. Towards self-realisation: Exploring the ecological self for education. In: Hung RA, editor. Kaleidoscopic View of Chinese Philosophy of Education. New York: Routledge. 2018. pp. 60-70

[38] Cottingham JM. From the self to the Self: An exploration of the process of Self-realisation in the context of Indian psychology [PhD thesis]. Auckland University of Technology; 2015

[39] Wilson M. Encounters with nature as a path of self-realisation: A meaning-making framework. Journal of Transpersonal Research. 2011;**3**:11-29

[40] Tripathi RC, Ghildyal P. Selfhood in search of godhood. Psychology and Developing Societies. 2013;**25**:43-76. DOI: 10.1177/0971333613477319

[41] Durga TK, Sridhar MK, Nagendra HR. Consciousness in upanishads. International Journal of Sanskrit Research. 2018;**4**:66-69

[42] Michelis ED. A History of Modern Yoga: Patanjali and Western Esotericism. London: Continuum. 2005

[43] Singh S, Bhaskar R, Hartwig M. The emotions, thought and self-realisation. In: Singh S, Bhaskar R, Hartwig M, editors. Reality and its Depths: A Conversation between Savita Singh and Roy Bhaskar. Singapore: Springer; 2020. pp. 133-152. DOI: 10.1007/978-981-15-4214-5_7

[44] Coney J. Sahaja Yoga: Socializing Processes in a South Asian New Religious Movement. New York: Routledge. 1999

[45] Manocha R, Noyce J, Rohowyj A, Turek G. Sahaja yoga. Australian Journal of Clinical Hypnotherapy and Hypnosis. 2005;**26**:22

[46] Menon S, Singh S, Kaur M. The effect of Sahaja yoga meditation on self-esteem, resilience and mental well-being among young adults. Mind and Society. 2022;**11**:81-90

[47] Rai UC. Medical Science Enlightened—Nes Insights into Vibratory Awareness for Holistic Health Care. London, New York, Sydney Moscow: Life Eternal Trust; 1993

[48] Rai S, Rai M, Kattimani Y, Agarwal V. Sahaja Yoga for Management of Stress & Life Style Diseases. New Delhi: Beyond Medicine. 2016. pp. 1069-1071

[49] Rai MS, Kattimani YR, Rai SU, Inamdar RS. Heart rate variability changes during Sahaja yoga meditation. International Journal of Physiology. 2019;7:109-113

[50] Hendriks T, Pritikin J, Choudhary R, Danyluck C. Exploring the relationship between character strengths and meditation: A cross-sectional study among long-term practitioners of Sahaja yoga meditation. International Journal of Applied Positive Psychology. 2022;7:31-45. DOI: 10.1007/s41042-021-00052-0

[51] Hendriks T. The effects of Sahaja yoga meditation on mental health: A systematic review. Journal of Complementary and Integrative Medicine. 2018;**15**(3):20160163. DOI: 10.1515/jcim-2016-0163

[52] Dodich A, Zollo M, Crespi C, Cappa SF, Laureiro Martinez D, Falini A, et al. Short-term Sahaja yoga meditation training modulates brain structure and spontaneous activity in the executive control network. Brain and Behavior. 2019;**9**:e01159. DOI: 10.1002/brb3.1159

[53] Choy LT. The strengths and weaknesses of research methodology: Comparison and complimentary between qualitative and quantitative approaches. IOSR Journal of Humanities and Social Science. 2014;**19**:99-104

[54] Andrade C. The inconvenient truth about convenience and purposive samples. Indian Journal of Psychological Medicine. 2021;**43**:86-88. DOI: 10.1177/0253717620977000

[55] Jager J, Putnick DL, Bornstein MH. More than just convenient: The scientific merits of homogeneous convenience samples. Monographs Society Res Child. 2017;**82**:13-30. DOI: 10.1111/mono.12296

[56] Noble H, Smith J. Ensuring validity and reliability in qualitative research. Evidence-Based Nursing. 2025;**0**:ebnurs-2024-104232. DOI: 10.1136/ebnurs-2024-104232

[57] Opdenakker RJG. Advantages and disadvantages of four interview techniques in qualitative research. Forum Qualitative Sozialforschung= Forum: Qualitative Social Research. 2006;**7**:art-11

[58] Punch KF. Introduction to Social Research: Quantitative and Qualitative Approaches. 2nd ed. London: Sage; 2005

[59] Allen M. The SAGE Encyclopedia of Communication Research Methods. Thousand Oaks, London, New Delhi, Singapore: SAGE publications. 2017

[60] Scharp KM. Thematic co-occurrence analysis: Advancing a theory and qualitative method to illuminate ambivalent experiences. The Journal of Communication. 2021;**71**:545-571. DOI: 10.1093/joc/jqab015

[61] de Dieu RJ, Andrianarizaka MT, Randriamiharisoa MA, Rasoamparany JMH. Effect of an Individual's self-realisation on work performance. Modern Economy. 2022;**13**:116-129

[62] Thunman E, Persson M. Self-realisation through work and its failure. In: Neckel S, Schaffner AK, Wagner G, editors. Burnout, Fatigue, Exhaustion. Cham: Springer International Publishing; 2017. pp. 173-194. DOI: 10.1007/978-3-319-52887-8_8

[63] Naess A. Self-realization: An ecological approach to being in the world. The Trumpeter. 1987;**4**(3):35-42

[64] McIntyre D. Bridging the gap between research and

practice. Cambridge Journal of Education. 2005;**35**:357-382. DOI: 10.1080/03057640500319065

[65] Bansal T, Bertels S, Ewart T, MacConnachie P, O'Brien J. Bridging the research-practice gap. Academy of Management Perspectives. 2012;**26**:73-92. DOI: 10.5465/amp.2011.0140

[66] Baldwin C, Furlotte C, Liu Q. Spirituality and narrative identity: Three case studies. Religions. 2023;**14**:1287

[67] Hernández SE, Suero J, Barros A, González-Mora JL, Rubia K. Increased grey matter associated with long-term Sahaja yoga meditation: A voxel-based morphometry study. PLoS One. 2016;**11**:e0150757

[68] Perez-Diaz O, Góngora D, González-Mora JL, Rubia K, Barrós-Loscertales A, Hernández SE. Enhanced amygdala–anterior cingulate white matter structural connectivity in Sahaja yoga meditators. PLoS One. 2024;**19**:e0301283

[69] Joyce S, Shand F, Tighe J, Laurent SJ, Bryant RA, Harvey SB. Road to resilience: A systematic review and meta-analysis of resilience training programmes and interventions. BMJ Open. 2018;**8**:e017858

[70] Good DJ, Lyddy CJ, Glomb TM, Bono JE, Brown KW, Duffy MK, et al. Contemplating mindfulness at work: An integrative review. Journal of Management. 2016;**42**:114-142. DOI: 10.1177/0149206315617003

[71] Buranapin S, Limphaibool W, Jariangprasert N, Chaiprasit K. Enhancing employee resilience through eastern spirituality and western scientific mindfulness. Cogent Business & Management. 2024;**11**:2377766. DOI: 10.1080/23311975.2024.2377766

[72] Lecomte J. Guérir de son enfance. Paris: Odile Jacob. 2004

[73] Connor KM, Zhang W. Resilience: Determinants, measurement, and treatment responsiveness. CNS Spectrums. 2006;**11**:5-12. DOI: 10.1017/S1092852900025797

[74] Southwick S, Pietzrak R, White G. Interventions to enhance resilience and resilience-related constructs in adults. In: Southwick SM, Litz BT, Charney DS, Friedman MJ, editors. Resilience and Mental Health: Challenges across the Lifespan. Cambridge: Cambridge University Press; 2011. pp. 289-306

[75] Herrman H, Stewart DE, Diaz-Granados N, Berger EL, Jackson B, Yuen T. What is resilience? Canadian Journal of Psychiatry. 2011;**56**:258-265. DOI: 10.1177/070674371105600504

[76] Leipold B, Greve W. Resilience: A conceptual bridge between coping and development. European Psychologist. 2009;**14**:40-50. DOI: 10.1027/1016-9040.14.1.40

[77] Ungar M. Resilience, trauma, context, and culture. Trauma, Violence, & Abuse. 2013;**14**:255-266. DOI: 10.1177/1524838013487805

[78] Facco E. Hypnosis for resilience. OBM Integrative and Complementary Medicine. 2020;**5**:1-20

[79] Ungar M. Resilience across cultures. British Journal of Social Work. 2008;**38**:218-235

[80] Blessin M, Lehmann S, Kunzler AM, van Dick R, Lieb K. Resilience interventions conducted in western and eastern countries—A systematic review. International Journal of Environmental Research and Public Health. 2022;**19**:6913

Chapter 7

Taking a Breath: Evidence-Based Techniques for Stress Reduction in Children and Adolescents in Prolonged Stress Situations

Asaf Gitler, Yosef Kula, Carmit Katz and Yori Gidron

Abstract

This chapter focuses on the application of mind–body practices to support the emotional and physical well-being of children and adolescents in healthcare and therapeutic settings. Emphasizing the critical role of self-regulation techniques in fostering resilience, the chapter explores a range of accessible and evidence-based interventions, including diaphragmatic breathing, autogenic training, progressive muscle relaxation, guided imagery, mindfulness-based relaxation, and cognitive strategies. The discussion highlights the unique challenges faced by young individuals dealing with stress, anxiety, and psychosomatic symptoms, offering practical guidance for clinicians and caregivers to implement these techniques effectively. Through age-appropriate adaptations and interactive methods, the chapter aims to equip children and adolescents with lifelong tools for emotional regulation and stress management. By integrating theoretical insights and practical applications, this work contributes to a growing body of knowledge on the importance of fostering mind–body harmony in younger populations.

Keywords: children and adolescent stress, stress management, emotional regulation, evidence-based techniques, body mind interventions

1. Introduction

Recent global challenges, such as the COVID-19 pandemic, natural disasters, economic crises, security-related incidents, wars, and various other health-related events worldwide, highlight the urgent need for accessible, evidence-based tools to promote mental and physical well-being. This document responds to this growing demand, offering a practical resource for therapists, counselors, educators, and other professionals working with individuals and families.

Recognizing the unique stressors faced by children, adolescents, and their families, this document provides a narrative, non-systematic review of effective, evidence-based stress management techniques tailored to younger populations. These techniques have demonstrated efficacy in reducing stress levels, enhancing mental and physical health, and addressing various psychosocial challenges.

The stress management practices discussed in this document, such as diaphragmatic breathing, mindfulness, and progressive muscle relaxation, have demonstrated potential benefits in relieving stress and anxiety. Additionally, these techniques can improve social skills, lessen stress-related physical pain, and enhance performance in educational settings. While these methods have been thoroughly validated for adults, this document specifically addresses the necessary adaptations for using them with children and adolescents, ensuring they are delivered age-appropriate for maximum effectiveness.

Professionals utilizing these techniques with younger populations are encouraged to understand the nuances and adaptations detailed in this resource. Conversely, therapists intending to apply these practices with adults should seek updated guidelines tailored to adult care. This document aims to empower professionals to foster resilience and well-being in diverse populations during these challenging times by bridging evidence-based methods with practical applications. Stress is an inevitable part of life, yet evidence-based methods exist to effectively manage and reduce its impact. This chapter focuses on providing practical, research-supported tools for managing stress, particularly among children and adolescents, emphasizing the role of adults as key facilitators in the process. By equipping young individuals with accessible and effective strategies, we can contribute to their immediate well-being, long-term resilience, and overall health.

The foundation of this document rests on the following principles:

1. *Acknowledging the universal truth*: Although stress is a universal unavoidable experience, well-established, evidence-based approaches to mitigate its effects and improve coping mechanisms are exists.

2. *The importance of stress reduction techniques*: Effective stress management goes beyond promoting relaxation and personal well-being. It also enhances focus, concentration, academic performance, and social skills. Furthermore, unmitigated stress, particularly in war or crisis situations, is linked to medium to severe physical illnesses. Conversely, learning to manage stress can significantly reduce these risks.

3. *The critical role of adults in implementation:* This document underscores the call to action for adults (whether they are healthcare professionals, educators, or parents) to introduce and model these techniques to both young individuals and their peers.

2. Strategic approach to developing this chapter

The tools and techniques presented in this chapter were chosen based on the following criteria:

1. *Research-based foundation*: Only evidence-based tools with demonstrated efficacy through empirical studies are included.

2. *Simplicity and practicality*: The techniques are simple, easy to learn, implement, and teach, ensuring accessibility to diverse audiences.

3. *Suitability for children and adolescents*: The tools are specifically adapted to the developmental stages and unique needs of younger populations, ensuring they can readily learn and practice these skills.

Our main focus is on equipping children and adolescents with skills rooted in cognitive behavioral principles rather than just imparting theoretical insights.

3. Key concepts in the Core of the document

3.1 Stress

The concept of stress is described in various ways in the literature, including as a trigger, a response, and the physiological consequences of that response [1]. Cohen et al. [2] define stress broadly as a condition where external demands challenge an individual's ability to adapt, potentially leading to illness. Even in the absence of extreme events like war, many students in primary and secondary education experience significant stress, with rising rates of stress-related health issues [3]. Common stressors for children and adolescents include lack of supportive caregivers [4], poverty [5], academic pressure [6, 7], bullying [8], and more [9]. Approximately 35% of children face health problems linked to stress [10].

3.2 Acute stress

The stress response is a natural reaction to threatening stimuli. Various external events activate the "stress system" through a series of responses occurring across three dimensions: psychological—emotional expression and cognitive processes; behavioral—fight-or-flight response; and physical/physiological—autonomic nervous system and hormonal system responses [11].

The autonomic nervous system comprises two subsystems: the sympathetic nervous system and the parasympathetic nervous system [12, 13]. The parasympathetic system is predominantly active during rest and routine states, regulating continuous physiological activities such as breathing, heart activity, digestion, secretion, cell regeneration, hormonal activity, blood pressure, and inflammation. On the other hand, the sympathetic system is highly active during emergencies, stress, and threats. It orchestrates the "fight-or-flight" response to manage emergencies, redirecting energy to skeletal muscles for rapid and sudden reactions while halting digestive functions. During sympathetic activation, blood flow changes, blood vessels in the skin constrict, muscle tension increases, and heart and brain activity alters [1, 12, 14].

The hypothalamus-pituitary–adrenal (HPA) axis is the primary hormonal stress system, initiating a hormonal response in the adrenal glands that triggers cortisol production [15]. Additionally, the locus coeruleus-adrenal axis is activated, releasing high levels of adrenaline to accelerate heart rate.

3.3 Chronic stress

Prolonged exposure to chronic stress keeps the body in a state of heightened arousal. The allostatic load model [16, 17] describes the effect of prolonged exposure to stress on an axis that begins with allostasis and ends with allostatic load. To maintain stability, the organism must adapt its internal environment to external demands, which has been termed allostasis [18]. In challenging situations, the body, as two missions, initiates the allostatic system and turns it off when the threat is passed [17]. The most common allostatic reaction of the body includes neural and hormonal activations that produce hormones, catecholamines, and cytokines. This response impacts multiple body systems, including the brain, the immune and cardiovascular systems, and metabolic activity [16, 19]. When an allostatic state persists over time, an allostatic load is created and is associated with the development of chronic morbidities such as increased inflammatory conditions, exhaustion, depression, and diabetes [20–22].

Prolonged exposure to stress is linked to chronic illnesses such as increased inflammation, fatigue, depression, and diabetes [20–22]. Common symptoms of chronic stress include recurrent abdominal pain, affecting 10 to 30% of school-age children [23], as well as headaches [24, 25], chest pain, nausea, and diarrhea. Among these, headaches are the most common somatic complaint, while abdominal pain is the most prevalent gastrointestinal symptom [25]. These symptoms often overlap with anxiety disorders, which affect 9 to 30% of children and adolescents [3].

4. Stress management methods for children and adolescents

The biopsychosocial model posits that illness is not just a physical disorder but affects multiple functional levels, including cellular and organ systems and an individual's role within their family and society. This model highlights the interconnectedness of the body and mind and their interaction with the social environment. The interplay between biological, psychological, and socio-cultural factors significantly influences treatment outcomes [26–28]. Understanding health issues requires considering biological and physical aspects alongside psychological and social influences. For example, research indicates that social support can enhance survival rates in cancer patients [29] and that higher stress levels can lead to increased respiratory infections [30].

Self-regulation methods and psychophysiological tools (mind–body techniques) for reducing stress responses have been used for thousands of years in martial arts and practices such as meditation and yoga. The development of research combined with cultural influences has led to the concept of "stress management" as we know it today. Relaxation techniques encompass a range of behavioral therapeutic interventions aimed at relieving physical tension and fostering positive emotions in stressful situations. Relaxation is a key component of all types of meditation, facilitating a calm and deep state of mind and body [31]. Importantly, relaxation techniques are central to most therapeutic programs addressing stress-related problems [32].

By the 1970s, research began examining the effectiveness of relaxation training for children. Despite challenges like unclear definitions and inconsistent variables, studies suggested that these techniques could help with learning, behavioral, and some physical disorders [33]. By the 1980s, stress management techniques similar to those used today were identified. In 1988, it was reported that 10 to 20% of American children with psychological or physical conditions likely faced issues related to stress [34].

Contemporary literature offers children and adolescents a wide array of evidence-based, non-pharmacological stress management techniques that can be practiced in hospitals, schools, or even at home. These techniques address various issues, from routine pain and disease-related pain (e.g., cancer, irritable bowel syndrome, asthma) to psychiatric disorders [3, 35–38].

Numerous effective stress reduction techniques for children and adolescents are highlighted in the literature. These include breathing exercises, meditation and mindfulness techniques, guided imagery, progressive muscle relaxation, autogenic training, and even digital applications. All are considered effective in supporting and treating stress and related disorders, such as anxiety disorders, headaches, abdominal pain, preoperative anxiety, postoperative pain, and behavioral and attention-deficit disorders [32, 39–52]. These evidence-based techniques have been successfully implemented in various settings, including schools, clinics, and hospitals.

Research evidence underscores that children experiencing significant stress, even in infancy, may suffer long-term consequences [53]. Thus, the ability of children and adolescents to cope with stress is of paramount importance. Acquiring coping skills during childhood aids in regulating their responses to stressful events and is essential for their future physical and psychological well-being [54, 55]. The following sections will present evidence-based techniques for equipping children with stress management tools.

5. Evidence-based, accessible, and practical techniques for working with children and adolescents

5.1 Breathing education and breathing exercises

5.1.1 Theoretical background

Our breathing patterns are closely linked to emotional states [56]. There is a bidirectional relationship between breathing and mental state, breathing is influenced by emotional state and can also influence it [57, 58]. During stressful situations, the body adopts specific breathing patterns, such as chest breathing or hyperventilation (rapid and shallow breaths exceeding 20 breaths per minute). Many individuals live for years without awareness of their breathing. Poor and inefficient breathing habits are often characterized by reduced use of the diaphragm during normal breathing.

Modern society places significant emphasis on flattening and tightening the abdomen, restricting the diaphragm's natural ability to move up and down and perform its function. This leads to losing the natural depth of breathing, resulting in fast and shallow respiration.

Breathing is the only function of the autonomic nervous system that can be consciously controlled. Breathing techniques have been used in practices like yoga and meditation for thousands of years to enhance performance. In Western culture, slow breathing techniques (often using biofeedback) have primarily been developed for therapeutic purposes, independent of spiritual or religious practices [59, 60].

5.1.2 Slow paced breathing (SPB)

This technique involves guiding individuals to reduce their normal breathing rate (12–20 breaths per minute) to approximately six breaths per minute. SPB can also be practiced without biofeedback devices, making it accessible in time- or resource-constrained settings [61]. There are various SPB techniques in which practitioners consciously control one or more respiratory parameters: frequency, depth, or the ratio of exhalation to inhalation [60]. Proper training emphasizes reducing the breathing rate and lengthening the exhalation phase [62]. It focuses on observing abdominal movement, where the abdomen expands due to diaphragm expansion during inhalation. It minimizes reliance on chest breathing, avoiding unnecessary activation of upper body muscles [60, 63, 64].

5.1.3 Benefits of slow breathing techniques

SPB enhances neural and brain activity related to emotional regulation and mental and physical well-being. It has been shown to be effective in treating conditions such as hypertension and heart disease [65–67]. Research [60] has widely supported the efficacy of these techniques, including studies involving children and adolescents [46] and diverse psychopathological conditions [42]. These techniques provide a practical, evidence-based tool for reducing stress and improving overall well-being in children and adolescents, making them an invaluable component of stress management programs in educational and clinical settings.

For a guide to SPB practice, see Appendix 1.

5.2 Progressive muscle relaxation (PMR)

5.2.1 Theoretical background

Progressive muscle relaxation (PMR) is an effective stress reduction technique developed by Edmund Jacobson in the twentieth century. As early as 1905, Jacobson observed that students in deep relaxation exhibited minimal startle responses to sudden noises. This discovery became the focus of his research and therapeutic work [68, 69]. Through his studies, Jacobson explored the relationship between muscle tension and various physical and mental disorders. He concluded that tension and anxiety are closely linked to muscle tension, positing that "mental calmness is a natural result of physical relaxation" [69].

Achieving a complete absence of contractions by relaxing muscle fibers is considered the physiological antithesis of tension, making it an effective tool for managing physical or mental stress. Jacobson found that systematically tensing and releasing different muscle groups and learning to differentiate between feelings of tension and relaxation significantly reduces muscle contractions and promotes a deep sense of relaxation [70].

PMR was introduced in 1934 as a process involving systematically tensing and relaxing 16 muscle groups. It remains one of the most widely used relaxation techniques. The method involves tensing and releasing different muscle groups in a structured sequence while focusing on the contrast between the tensed and relaxed states. Participants are instructed to tense a specific muscle group while inhaling and release the tension while exhaling. This practice cultivates self-awareness of the distinction between stress and relaxation states, eventually enabling relaxation without active muscle engagement [43].

Key objectives of PMR:

1. *Increased skeletal muscle relaxation*: Reducing muscle tone and physical tension through tensing and releasing specific muscle groups.

2. *Enhanced discrimination ability*: Learning to engage only the necessary muscles while avoiding excessive tension in other areas. This is achieved by isolating specific muscle groups and identifying tension and relaxation.

3. *Reduced sympathetic activity*: Lowering physiological arousal through skeletal muscle feedback to the brain, signaling a heightened state of relaxation. This promotes balance and regulation within the body's autonomic systems.

PMR has been extensively validated for managing stress and illness. It has been found effective in reducing headaches, improving insomnia, and serving as an adjunctive treatment for cancer, chronic arthritis pain, and irritable bowel syndrome [41]. Among cardiac patients, PMR combined with medication reduced hospitalizations more effectively than medication alone [71].

5.2.2 Impact on cortisol and the immune system

Research examines how Progressive Muscle Relaxation (PMR) affects salivary cortisol levels and may benefit the immune system. Cortisol, produced by the hypothalamic–pituitary–adrenal (HPA) axis, peaks shortly after waking to aid daily activities, with stress potentially causing sudden spikes. Relaxation practices like PMR can help reverse stress-related hormonal responses and support immune function [72, 73].

5.2.3 Evidence supporting PMR for children and adolescents

PMR is widely recognized among adults, but research on its application for children is less extensive. However, existing studies indicate its potential in reducing stress and associated symptoms in younger populations. For example:

- In a randomized controlled trial, adolescents aged 11–17 practicing PMR for 15–20 minutes daily reported significantly lower perceived stress levels after three weeks compared to a control group [74].

- A study by Jong et al. [75] found that three months of PMR reduced the frequency and intensity of headaches—one of the most common stress symptoms in children—by more than 50% for nearly half of the participants aged 9–18. This reduction persisted for six months after practice ended.

- Tsai et al. [76] compared stress reduction training with and without PMR in high school students and found that adding PMR led to greater cortisol reductions in the intervention group.

PMR has also been shown to be effective in treating various anxiety disorders in children [77].

5.2.4 Conclusion

PMR is an accessible and evidence-based technique with broad applicability, from reducing physical tension to improving emotional regulation. Its efficacy in children and adolescents highlights its value as a key component in stress management and mental health interventions.

For a guide to PMR practice, see Appendix 2.

5.3 Autogenic training

5.3.1 Theoretical background

The term *autogenic training* was coined nearly a century ago by German psychiatrist Johannes Heinrich Schultz [78]. Schultz found that simple verbal statements encouraging passive focus could influence body perception and significantly calm autonomic nervous system activity [78]. In this technique, individuals use verbal statements to address their psychological and physiological experiences with guidance from a therapist. This approach is based on psychological and biological principles, focusing on body awareness to promote control and relaxation. AT is a simple, safe, and accessible approach that helps participants develop a sense of control and calm, as well as internal body awareness, enabling them to manage stress-related physical symptoms in a relatively short time. Research has shown that autogenic training is effective for children and adolescents [79].

The basic training lasts between 10 and 20 minutes and is relatively short. It involves a series of mental exercises that promote self-regulation through self-suggestion. The three fundamental principles of self-suggestion are:

1. Repeating verbal statements that focus on different parts of the body.

2. Passively attending to sensations of warmth and heaviness in the body without making any active effort.

3. Reducing attention to both internal and external sensory distractions [80].

During the sessions, the trainer guides the participant to focus on physical sensations in various parts of the body, which can be consciously perceived with mindfulness. For example, when focusing on the hands, one might feel them becoming increasingly heavy during relaxation (due to decreased muscle tension in the arms and shoulders). As relaxation deepens, a sense of warmth may follow, reflecting increased blood flow to the skin in peripheral areas.

5.3.2 Key statements used in AT

The training includes six key statements, each focusing on a specific body region or sensation [81, 82]:

1. *Heaviness in the limbs:* "My arms and legs are heavy." This statement connects the participant to bodily sensations and the training instructions, facilitating relaxation as skeletal muscles release tension.

2. *Warmth in the limbs*: "My hands and feet are warm." This statement reflects increased peripheral blood flow during relaxation, raising the temperature in these areas.

3. *Heart activity:* "My heartbeat is calm and regular." Even if the participant cannot feel their pulse, this statement fosters awareness of cardiac activity, promoting relaxation and a steady heart rate.

4. *Breathing:* "My breathing is slow and calm." This is typically practiced after basic diaphragmatic breathing exercises. Such breathing (often called abdominal breathing) uses the diaphragm to expand lung capacity rather than chest muscles. Slow, regular diaphragmatic breathing (6–8 breaths per minute) optimizes oxygen and carbon dioxide balance, inducing physical and mental relaxation.

5. *Warmth in the upper abdomen*: "My solar plexus is warm and calm." Relaxation enhances blood flow to the abdominal region and digestive system, resulting in a sensation of warmth. Conversely, stress reduces blood flow to these areas.

6. *Coolness in the forehead*: "My forehead is cool." This focus promotes awareness of physical sensations, leading to vasoconstriction in the head area and relaxation of the frontal muscle.

5.3.3 AT learning and application

The six statements are introduced gradually during training, beginning with foundational motivational engagement and initial exercises in body awareness and diaphragmatic breathing [83].

Structured progression is essential to fostering skill acquisition. For instance, early sessions might focus on the heaviness and warmth of the limbs, dedicating more time to these sensations. As skills develop, participants move on to other areas, integrating previously mastered statements into each session.

By repeating these statements, participants enter a stress-free state of relaxation and enhance their ability to focus attention. Once basic proficiency in focusing on specific areas is achieved, sessions can expand to address additional aspects. Training usually includes around ten sessions, after which participants can practice independently or use therapist-provided audio recordings customized to their needs. Independent practice between sessions generalizes relaxation and self-regulation skills to daily life, often yielding significant results within two weeks [82].

5.3.4 Evidence of efficacy

AT has been shown to reduce stress and anxiety in adults, with numerous systematic reviews supporting its effectiveness (e.g., [84, 85]). Evidence in children, though more limited, also indicates its potential:

- *Group AT sessions*: In a study of 50 children aged 5–13, eight weeks of 30-minute group AT sessions significantly reduced stress in children with emotional and behavioral issues [79].

- *Randomized controlled trial:* A study of 70 children found that 12 weekly AT sessions improved attention, reduced anxiety symptoms, and enhanced well-being compared to a control group [86].

- *Physiological effects:* In a study without a control group, AT reduced cortisol levels, blood pressure, and heart rate in adolescents with adjustment disorders [87].

5.3.5 Conclusion

Autogenic training is a flexible, evidence-based method that can be taught individually or in small groups for various age groups. PMR therapeutic advantages include stress reduction, anxiety management, and improved emotional and physical well-being.

For a guide to AT practice, see Appendix 3.

6. Basic meditation and mindfulness techniques

6.1 Theoretical background

Meditation and mindfulness encompass a "family of techniques that share the deliberate focus of attention on the present experience, avoiding engagement with the content or meanings of arising thoughts or sensations". Meditation techniques typically include four general components: a quiet environment, a visual or auditory focal point (e.g., a mantra), a passive attitude, and a comfortable posture. The literature details a wealth of specific meditation practices [88].

Mind–body interventions can prevent the activation of the stress response system. Moreover, meditation has been shown to enhance brain activity in the medial prefrontal cortex in adults, indicating improved emotional regulation [89]. Mindfulness, a related practice, is defined as the intentional, nonjudgmental moment-to-moment awareness of one's experiences, fostering a connection between thoughts, emotions, and behaviors.

Mindfulness involves cultivating an open awareness of the present moment without attachment to outcomes or judgments. The central component of mindfulness practice is focused attention on the breath. Additional key elements include distinguishing between bodily and mental experiences and recognizing one's personal reactions.

One of the most well-known and extensively studied mindfulness interventions is the Mindfulness-Based Stress Reduction (MBSR) program developed by Jon Kabat-Zinn at the University of Massachusetts Medical School. This eight-week program includes weekly 2–2.5-hour group sessions led by a trained instructor, daily guided home practice, and a full-day mindfulness retreat [88, 90].

6.2 Goals of mindfulness training

Formal mindfulness training aims to teach individuals multiple aspects of attention, such as:

1. Recognizing when the mind wanders and repeatedly redirecting attention to a focused area (e.g., the breath).

2. Developing sustained attention.

3. Cultivating open awareness without being swept away by thoughts, emotions, or bodily sensations.

Mindful breathing regulates the autonomic nervous system, focuses the mind, and enhances self-awareness [91].

6.3 Efficacy of mindfulness

Mindfulness-based reduction (MBSR) has been studied in various populations and settings, including schools and hospitals:

- A meta-analysis of the efficacy of MBSR in clinical and non-clinical settings with children and adolescents found it effective for stress reduction (effect size 0.33) and anxiety and depression [92].

- A review of 24 school-based MBSR programs found the highest efficacy in reducing stress (effect size 0.3) and improving cognitive performance [93].
- A recent review of MBSR interventions for school students highlighted their efficacy specifically for stress reduction (effect size 0.55) [94].

Body Scan Meditation is particularly beneficial for children and adolescents among the various mindfulness practices. This mindfulness exercise involves systematically directing attention to different parts of the body, from toes to head, helping participants become more aware of their physical sensations, reducing stress, and enhancing emotional regulation.

For a guide to Body Scan Meditation, see Appendix 4.

7. Guided imagery/visualization

7.1 Theoretical background

Guided imagery, or visualization, is a process in which individuals create mental images that engage physical-sensory, visual, and auditory elements. This technique is commonly used in interventions ranging from sports psychology and performance enhancement to behavioral therapy [95]. Imagination is a uniquely human ability, allowing individuals to step away from the "here and now" and create alternative realities. It provides a magical glimpse into other possibilities. The method is simple to learn, accessible, and versatile, making it suitable for professionals across fields—including non-clinical roles—working with children facing various challenges [96]. The effectiveness of visualization has been demonstrated across therapeutic, educational, and healthcare professions. It is particularly effective with children, adolescents, and adults [96]. Imagination is a basic psychological function, enabling individuals to conceive of scenarios and ideas that are not directly perceived through the physical senses. It supports planning, flexible reflection on past events, out-of-the-box thinking, and emotional regulation—either by amplifying or suppressing emotions.

Applications of Imagination in Guided Imagery:

- *Memory rehabilitation and learning*: Guided imagery helps restore memory and enhance learning capabilities.
- *Strategic problem-solving*: It fosters creative solutions by enabling individuals to manage emotions differently and discover new strategies.
- *Stress management*: Particularly in extreme life circumstances, imaginative coping reframes meanings, providing emotional relief and adaptability.

Both children and adults use imaginative reframing, leveraging spontaneous expressions of creativity, such as play, humor, narratives, or metaphors, to construct new meanings in their lives [95, 97]. These non-verbal mental activities tap into the human ability to think in "as-if" scenarios, fostering emotional release, flexibility, and a sense of meaning.

7.2 Structure of guided imagery practice

Guided imagery combines behavioral techniques like physical relaxation with cognitive interventions, including:

1. *Physical relaxation*: Encouraging bodily relaxation through systematic muscle release or deep breathing exercises.

2. *Cognitive engagement*: Directing attention to positive imagery, drawing on memory recall, and generating new sensory experiences.

3. *Self-regulation*: Offering a non-invasive way to achieve emotional balance and self-awareness.

This blend makes guided imagery particularly well-suited for children and adolescents [98].

7.3 Guided imagery: Process, benefits, and evidence

Three active steps in guided imagery:

1. *Body relaxation*: Begin by relaxing the body to help the child focus on physical sensations. Gradually release muscle tension starting from the feet and moving upward to the head, accompanied by deep breathing.

2. *Spontaneous or directed mental reconstruction*: Encourage the child to visualize a favorite place or cherished experience, either real or imagined. This involves vividly imagining sights, sounds, smells, tastes, and sensations as if they are being experienced in the present moment. Use personalized language for each participant.

3. *Returning to reality*: After spending time in the imagined safe space, guide the child to return gradually to their surroundings. Reassure them that they can mentally revisit this positive experience anytime they wish.

7.4 Adaptive benefits of guided imagery

Embracing flexible imagination and playful strategies through guided imagery builds resilience and a sense of control. This adaptability enhances psychological endurance, fosters a more positive outlook, and improves self-confidence [99].

The vivid imagery created during guided visualization helps individuals relax, prepare for stressful situations, and reduce symptoms like performance anxiety, back pain, headaches, high blood pressure, and gastrointestinal sensitivity.

7.5 Integration with other relaxation techniques

Guided imagery is often combined with other methods, such as progressive muscle relaxation (PMR). This multimodal approach amplifies its therapeutic effectiveness [100].

Research evidence on guided imagery:

1. *Guided imagery and PMR for abdominal pain*: A study comparing guided imagery combined with PMR to breathing exercises in children with abdominal pain (a common stress symptom) found that the guided imagery group reported fewer days with pain and reduced absences from daily activities like school and extra-curricular activities [24].

2. *Health behavior and stress reduction*: In a study of 111 adolescent girls participating in a four-week intervention to improve health behaviors related to obesity, combining guided imagery with healthy lifestyle education significantly reduced physiological (cortisol levels) and psychological stress compared to the control group, which received lifestyle education alone [101].

3. *Preoperative anxiety and postoperative pain*: Research on children aged 6–12 undergoing minor surgery found that combining guided imagery and relaxation exercises significantly reduced preoperative anxiety and postoperative pain compared to standard care ($p < .001$ for both measures). This study highlights guided imagery as a non-pharmacological, effective method to reduce anxiety and pain, with the potential to decrease reliance on anesthetics and pain medications [51].

7.6 Conclusion

Guided imagery is a powerful, evidence-based relaxation technique that is easy to implement and effective for reducing stress, anxiety, and pain. Its flexibility and adaptability make it particularly suitable for children and adolescents, enabling them to develop emotional resilience and self-regulation skills.

For a guide to guided imagery safe place training, see Appendix 5.

8. Cognitive emotional regulation: Reframing

8.1 Theoretical background

8.1.1 Emotional regulation through cognitive reframing: Mechanisms and implications

8.1.1.1 Introduction

Emotions are among the most challenging aspects of human experience to navigate. Research highlights significant interactions between thoughts, emotions, and behaviors, which collectively form core areas of focus in psychological research and therapy. Emotional regulation refers to an individual's ability to influence the type, intensity, and expression of their emotions. Various emotional regulation strategies exist, but cognitive approaches have been shown to be particularly effective in mitigating distress.

8.1.1.2 Cognitive reframing and minimization

One of the most comprehensive meta-analyses in psychology demonstrated that cognitive emotional regulation, specifically through *reframing* and *minimization*, exerts the most significant positive effects on emotional well-being, surpassing the impact of emotional expression alone [102].

- *Reframing*: Reframing involves altering one's perception of a stressful situation from catastrophic to neutral or even positive. For example, after a car accident, an individual might say, "Car accidents are common in densely populated countries" (neutral reframing) or "The accident made me more mindful and cautious while driving" (positive reframing).
- *Minimization*: This strategy reduces the perceived severity of an event. Following a car accident, for instance, one might say, "The airbag saved me, and I only sustained minor injuries".

8.1.1.3 Empirical evidence supporting reframing

Recent research underscores the physiological and emotional benefits of reframing:

1. *Trauma and inflammation*: A recent study found that reframing mitigated and, in some cases, entirely neutralized the link between childhood trauma and inflammatory markers in adulthood [103].
2. *Childhood anxiety*: A study focused on children found that anxious children who employed reframing strategies successfully reduced their negative emotions [104].

8.1.1.4 Teaching reframing to children and adolescents

Reframing is not only effective but also relatively easy to teach, especially to adolescents. Cognitive strategies like reframing complement relaxation techniques in managing stress responses, making them essential tools for emotional regulation.

8.1.1.5 Neurobiological mechanisms of reframing

Advances in neuroimaging have illuminated the mechanisms underlying cognitive reframing. A meta-analysis of 48 studies revealed that reframing activates brain regions critical for cognitive and linguistic control of meaning, such as the prefrontal cortex, while simultaneously reducing activity in the amygdala region associated with emotional responses [105].

These findings have profound implications for treating stress-related conditions, including post-traumatic stress disorder (PTSD), highlighting reframing as a powerful tool for improving emotional resilience.

8.1.1.6 Conclusion

The ability to teach cognitive reframing to children and adolescents is vital. It equips them with practical skills to manage stress effectively, fostering resilience and emotional well-being. As research continues to demonstrate its effectiveness, reframing should be integrated into therapeutic practices and educational frameworks, ensuring young individuals are well-equipped to navigate life's emotional challenges.

DOI: http://dx.doi.org/10.5772/intechopen.1008771

Cognitive reframing, combined with relaxation techniques, provides a holistic approach to emotional regulation and stress management, benefiting individuals across developmental stages.

For a guide to cognitive appraisal practice, see Appendix 6.

9. Relaxation-induced anxiety, causes, and management

9.1 Overview

It should be noted that relaxation techniques are generally effective in reducing stress, subjective anxiety, and physiological arousal. However, some evidence suggests that these methods may induce or exacerbate anxiety in certain individuals, a phenomenon known as Relaxation-Induced Anxiety (RIA). Symptoms of RIA include restlessness, excessive sweating, trembling, palpitations, or rapid breathing experienced during relaxation [106].

9.2 Theoretical explanations

The mechanisms underlying RIA are categorized into five related but distinct theories [107]:

1. *Unexpected reactions*: The practitioner may become alarmed by physiological, behavioral, or emotional responses that emerge automatically during relaxation.

2. *Fear of losing control*: The practitioner may fear losing control or overexerting effort to achieve relaxation, paradoxically increasing tension.

3. *Attention to anxiety*: Relaxation may direct attention to their anxiety, intensifying the experience.

4. *Internal focus*: Fear of engaging with internal experiences may heighten anxiety.

5. *Intrusive thoughts or memories*: Relaxation might bring up distressing thoughts, memories, or concerns unrelated to the relaxation practice.

9.3 Recommendations for managing RIA

1. *Alternate techniques*: If one relaxation method (e.g., PMR) induces anxiety, switching to an alternative technique, such as mindful breathing or guided imagery with pleasant content, may produce an effective relaxation response.

2. *Gradual exposure*: Anxiety during relaxation may result from a heightened awareness of previously unnoticed tension-related cues. Consistent practice and repeated exposure to these cues can help reduce their associated tension over time.

3. *Structured practice*: To improve the learning process, relaxation training should follow a graded approach:

- Start with short sessions, incorporate breaks, and gradually increase session duration.
- Use a well-lit room and introduce conversations between relaxation attempts.
- Begin with seated relaxation before transitioning to lying-down exercises.

9.4 Additional tools for stress reduction

1. *Physical activity*: Encourage regular exercise, whether through sports, dancing, yoga, or simple activities. Physical activity releases endorphins and natural stress relievers.
2. *Creative outlets*: Promote creative activities such as drawing, music, or writing to allow children and adolescents to express emotions safely and non-verbally.
3. *Consistent routine*: A stable daily routine provides a sense of security and reduces stress.
4. *Time in nature*: Outdoor activities, such as hiking or playing outside, are highly calming and improve mood.
5. *Social support*: Fostering open communication and a supportive environment where children feel heard and understood is vital.
6. *Hobbies and interests*: Encouraging hobbies and enjoyable activities can significantly alleviate stress.
7. *Adequate sleep*: Ensuring sufficient sleep is critical for effective stress management. Establishing a consistent bedtime routine can help.

It is important to emphasize that:

- *Professional intervention plays a crucial role in maintaining the mental health of children and adolescents*, especially when regular relaxation techniques or self-managed stress reduction methods are insufficient. Similar to relaxation methods, professional therapy offers evidence-based approaches tailored to the unique psychological needs of young children and adolescents.
- *Therapists can utilize a variety of techniques*, including cognitive behavioral therapy (CBT), which is highly effective in altering thought and behavior patterns [108, 109].
- *Play therapy is particularly beneficial for younger children to express emotions non-verbally* [110, 111].
- *Parental guidance and family therapy can help address issues in family dynamics that contribute to stress* [112].

Additionally, *group therapy* provides a supportive environment where peers facing similar challenges can share experiences and coping strategies.

These therapeutic approaches, administered by skilled professionals, are an integral part of fostering the supportive and healing environment essential for the psychological, physical, and social development of children and adolescents.

10. Conclusions and summary

> *"You cannot prevent the birds of sorrow from flying over your head, but you can prevent them from building nests in your hair – ."Chinese Proverb*

Stress is an inevitable part of life but is not always negative. It is a natural physiological response that alerts the body to potential danger, activating the fight-or-flight response for survival. Stress can also enhance awareness and mobilize resources in challenging situations. Ancient wisdom and modern science agree that stress cannot be eliminated from human life. However, research consistently shows that specific techniques can alleviate stress and promote mental health in both children and adults. Relaxation methods are simple to learn and use, effectively reducing stress levels.

Each individual responds differently to stress, making it essential to identify personal stressors. While some sources of stress are obvious, such as strained relationships or academic struggles, uncovering the root cause of anxiety can sometimes be challenging. Relaxation techniques empower children to manage everyday stressors and enhance coping mechanisms.

Integrating relaxation techniques into daily life, supported by digital tools like mobile apps and smartwatches, can facilitate stress tracking and management. These tools measure metrics such as heart rate, oxygen levels, and physical activity, making stress monitoring accessible.

By modeling these techniques and encouraging their use, adults can guide children and adolescents toward better stress management. Tailoring interventions to the child's needs ensures their effectiveness.

This document provides a comprehensive overview of evidence-based stress management techniques for children and adolescents, offering valuable insights for academics, health and education professionals, parents, and caregivers. Integrating these techniques into daily life fosters resilience, improves mental and physical well-being, and equips the younger generation to navigate life's challenges.

A. Appendices – Relaxation and stress management practice protocols

A.1 Appendix 1 – Diaphragmatic breathing

1. *Breathe from the belly instead of the chest:* Relax the chest and shoulder muscles, allowing the abdomen to expand as you inhale. This technique uses the diaphragm effectively, increasing lung capacity.

2. *Inhale through the nose*: Breathing through the nose cleans and warms the air before it enters the lungs, improving the respiratory process. Hold the breath for one or two seconds after inhaling, then exhale slowly.

3. *Extend the exhalation phase*: Lengthen the exhalation to better activate the parasympathetic nervous system, which is responsible for relaxation and recovery.

4. *Slow your breathing rate:* The breathing rate acts as an internal clock regulating various bodily systems, including the heart and vascular systems. Aim to gradually reduce your breathing rate to 6–8 breaths per minute.

5. *Practice effortlessly*: Avoid over-focusing on perfection. Let yourself breathe freely while following these guidelines gently.

A.2 Appendix 2 – Progressive muscle relaxation (PMR)

Preparation and execution instructions:

- Sit comfortably in a chair or recliner. Relax your shoulders, arms, and legs.
- Begin with diaphragmatic breathing: Inhale through the nose and exhale through the mouth slowly, expanding the diaphragm fully.
- Close your eyes if comfortable.
- Sequentially tense and relax specific muscle groups as described below. Hold each contraction for 4–5 seconds and release slowly while exhaling.

Recommended sequence:

1. Hands:
    - Clench both fists.
    - Tighten forearm muscles.
    - Tense upper arm muscles.
2. Legs:
    - Point toes forward (straight line with shins).
    - Flex toes upward (toward shins).
    - Tighten calf muscles.
    - Tighten thigh muscles.
3. Torso:
    - Tighten pelvic muscles (e.g., glutes).
    - Contract lower abdominal muscles.

- Tighten diaphragm with a deep breath.
- Squeeze chest and shoulder muscles inward.

4. Head and neck:
   - Lower head toward the chest.
   - Move head backward, facing upward.
   - Rotate head slowly from side to side.
   - Tighten facial muscles ("sour face").
   - Stretch mouth into a wide smile.

A.3 Appendix 3 – Autogenic training

Guided instructions:

1. Preparation:
   - Sit or lie down comfortably. Ensure your body is fully supported.
   - Take several diaphragmatic breaths, focusing on the rhythm and depth of your breathing.
2. Verbal statements:

Repeat the following affirmations slowly, 5–7 times each:

- *Breathing*: "My breathing is calm and steady."
- *Heartbeat*: "My heartbeat is calm and regular."
- *Body warmth*: "My body is warm and relaxed".
- *Heavy limbs*: "My arms and legs feel heavy."
- *Forehead coolness*: "My forehead feels cool".

3. Conclusion:

   When ready to end the practice, take a deep breath, stretch your arms, and slowly return to your surroundings.

A.4 Appendix 4 – Body scan exercise

1. Begin in a comfortable position:
   - Sit or lie down, close your eyes, and take a few deep breaths.

2. Focus on body parts sequentially:
    - Start with your toes, then move to the soles, heels, ankles, calves, knees, and thighs.
    - Progress to the pelvis, lower back, abdomen, chest, and upper back.
    - Continue with shoulders, arms, hands, neck, and head.
    - Pay attention to sensations such as tension, relaxation, or pressure.
3. Conclude:
    - Finish with a deep breath and gently stretch before returning to the present moment.

A.5 Appendix 5 – Guided imagery: Safe place

1. Preparation:
    - Begin with diaphragmatic breathing and body relaxation exercises.
2. Visualization:
    - Imagine yourself in a safe and peaceful place (e.g., a beach, forest, or familiar location).
    - Focus on sensory details: the feel of the ground, the sounds around you, the temperature, and any smells or sights.
3. Anchor the experience:
    - Stay in this imagined place for a few minutes, absorbing its calming influence.
    - When ready, return gradually to the present moment.

A.6 Appendix 6 – Cognitive reframing with children

1. *Explain the connection between thoughts and feelings*: Discuss how thoughts influence emotions and behaviors.
2. *Identify negative thoughts*: Encourage children to verbalize their thoughts in challenging situations.
3. *Teach reframing*: Explain how to view situations differently, like changing a picture's frame.
4. *Practice together*: Use real-life or hypothetical scenarios to model and practice reframing.

5. *Encourage positive self-talk*: Replace negative internal statements with affirming alternatives (e.g., "I'll try my best" instead of "I can't do this").

6. *Reinforce with examples*: Share your personal experiences with reframing to inspire them.

7. *Praise and journal*: Encourage keeping a journal to track negative thoughts and reframed alternatives, praising their efforts and progress.

Note: These exercises are designed to support stress reduction and emotional regulation. Regular practice and appropriate adaptations can enhance their effectiveness for individuals of all ages.

Author details

Asaf Gitler[1,2*], Yosef Kula[2,3], Carmit Katz[3,4] and Yori Gidron[2]

1 The International Community Stress Prevention Center ICSPC (NGO), Israel

2 The Neurocognitive Regulation Laboratory of Health and Illness, Faculty of Health and Welfare Sciences, Department of Nursing, University of Haifa, Israel

3 The Haruv Chair for the Study of Child Maltreatment, Hebrew University of Jerusalem, Israel

4 The Paul Baerwald School of Social Work and Social Welfare, Hebrew University of Jerusalem, Israel

*Address all correspondence to: asafgitler@gmail.com

References

[1] Kemeny ME. The psychobiology of stress. Current Directions in Psychological Science. 2003;**12**(4):124-129

[2] Cohen S, Gianaros PJ, Manuck SB. A stage model of stress and disease. Perspectives on Psychological Science: A journal of the Association for Psychological Science. 2016;**11**(4):456-463

[3] Saps M, Seshadri R, Sztainberg M, Schaffer G, Marshall BM, Di Lorenzo C. A prospective school-based study of abdominal pain and other common somatic complaints in children. The Journal of Pediatrics. 2009;**154**(3):322-326

[4] Chrousos GP. Stress and disorders of the stress system. Nature Reviews. Endocrinology. 2009;**5**(7):374-381

[5] Loman MM, Gunnar MR. Early experience and the development of stress reactivity and regulation in children. Neuroscience and Biobehavioral Reviews. 2010;**34**(6):867-876

[6] Evans GW, Schamberg MA. Childhood poverty, chronic stress, and adult working memory. Proceedings of the National Academy of Sciences of the United States of America. 2009;**106**(16):6545-6549

[7] Napoli M, Krech PR, Holley LC. Mindfulness training for elementary school students: The attention academy. Journal of Applied School Psychology. 2005;**21**(1):99-125

[8] Duckworth AL, Quinn PD, Tsukayama E. What no child left behind leaves behind: The roles of IQ and self-control in predicting standardized achievement test scores and report card grades. Journal of Educational Psychology. 2012;**104**(2):439-451

[9] Kena G, Hussar W, McFarland J, de Brey C, Musu-Gillette L, Wang X, et al. The condition of education. United States Department of Education. 2016;**2016**:347

[10] Kassymova K, Kosherbayeva N, Sangilbayev S, Schachl H. Stress management techniques for students. In: Proceedings of the International Conference on the Theory and Practice of Personality Formation in Modern Society (ICTP-PFMS 2018). Amsterdam, Netherlands: Atlantis Press; 2018

[11] Lynch T, Davis SL, Johnson AH, Gray L, Coleman E, Phillips SR, et al. Definitions, theories, and measurement of stress in children. Journal of Pediatric Nursing. 2022;**66**:202-212

[12] Glick DB, Glick G, Stein EJ. The autonomic nervous system. Basics of Anesthesia. 2019;**6**:70-82

[13] McCorry LK. Physiology of the autonomic nervous system. American Journal of Pharmaceutical Education. 2007;**71**(4):1-11

[14] Wehrwein, EA., Orer, HS., Barman, SM. Overview of the Anatomy, Physiology, and Pharmacology of the Autonomic Nervous System. 2016. DOI: 10.1152/physrev.00041.2006

[15] Frodl T, O'Keane V. How does the brain deal with cumulative stress? A review with focus on developmental stress, HPA axis function and hippocampal structure in humans. Neurobiology of Disease. 2013;**52**:24-37

[16] McEwen BS, Stellar E. Stress and the individual: Mechanisms leading to

disease. Archives of Internal Medicine. 1993;**153**(18):2093-2101. DOI: 10.1001/archinte.1993.00410180039004

[17] McEwen BS. Protective and damaging effects of stress mediators. New England Journal of Medicine. 1998;**338**(3):171-179

[18] Sterling P, Eyer J. Allostasis: A new paradigm to explain arousal pathology. In: Fisher S, Reason J, editors. Handbook of Life Stress, Cognition and Health. New York: John Wiley; 1988. pp. 629-649

[19] McEwen BS. Physiology and neurobiology of stress and adaptation: Central role of the brain. Physiological Reviews. 2007;**87**(3):873-904. DOI: 10.1152/physrev.00041.2006

[20] Guidi J, Lucente M, Sonino N, Fava GA. Allostatic load and its impact on health: A systematic review. Psychotherapy and Psychosomatics. 2021;**90**(1):11-27

[21] McEwen BS, Wingfield JC. The concept of allostasis in biology and biomedicine. Hormones and Behavior. 2003;**43**(1):2-15

[22] Thayer JF, Yamamoto SS, Brosschot JF. The relationship of autonomic imbalance, heart rate variability and cardiovascular disease risk factors. International Journal of Cardiology. 2010;**141**(2):122-131. DOI: 10.1016/j.ijcard.2009.09.543

[23] Valizadeh L, Farnam A, Farshi MR. Investigation of stress symptoms among primary school children. Journal of Caring Sciences. 2012;**1**(1):25

[24] Weydert JA, Shapiro DE, Acra SA, Monheim CJ, Chambers AS, Ball TM. Evaluation of guided imagery as treatment for recurrent abdominal pain in children: A randomized controlled trial. BMC Pediatrics. 2006;**6**(1):29

[25] Zwart J-A, Dyb G, Holmen TL, Stovner LJ, Sand T. The prevalence of migraine and tension-type headaches among adolescents in Norway. The Nord-Trøndelag health study (head-HUNT-youth), a large population-based epidemiological study. Cephalalgia: An International Journal of Headache. 2004;**24**(5):373-379. DOI: 10.1111/j.1468-2982.2004.00680.x

[26] Engel GL. The need for a new medical model: A challenge for biomedicine. Science. 1977;**196**(4286):129-136

[27] Engel GL. Sounding board. The biopsychosocial model and medical education. Who are to be the teachers? The New England Journal of Medicine. 1982;**306**(13):802-805

[28] George E, Engel L. The clinical application of the biopsychosocial model. The American Journal of Psychiatry. 1980;**137**(5):535-544

[29] Nausheen B, Gidron Y, Peveler R, Moss-Morris R. Social support and cancer progression: A systematic review. Journal of Psychosomatic Research. 2009;**67**(5):403-415

[30] Cohen S. The Pittsburgh common cold studies: Psychosocial predictors of susceptibility to respiratory infectious illness. [keynote presentation at the 8th international congress of Behavioral medicine; Mainz, Germany, august 25-28, 2004]. International Journal of Behavioral Medicine. 2005;**12**(3):123-131

[31] Hussain D, Bhushan B. Psychology of meditation and health: Present status and future directions. International Journal of Psychology and Psychological Therapy. 2010;**10**(3):439-451

[32] Benson H, Greenwood MM, Klemchuk H. The relaxation response: Psychophysiologic aspects and clinical applications. International Journal of Psychiatric in Medicine. 1975;**6**(1-2):87-98

[33] Richter NC. The efficacy of relaxation training with children. Journal of Abnormal Child Psychology. 1984;**12**(2):319-344

[34] Perrin JM, MacLean WE Jr. Children with chronic illness: The prevention of dysfunction. Pediatric Clinics of North America. 1988;**35**(6):1325-1337

[35] Ball TM, Shapiro DE, Monheim CJ, Weydert JA. A pilot study of the use of guided imagery for the treatment of recurrent abdominal pain in children. Clinical Pediatrics. 2003;**42**(6):527-532

[36] Beauchemin J, Hutchins TL, Patterson F. Mindfulness meditation may lessen anxiety, promote social skills, and improve academic performance among adolescents with learning disabilities. Complementary Health Practice Review. 2008;**13**(1):34-45

[37] Christensen J, Fatchett D. Promoting parental use of distraction and relaxation in pediatric oncology patients during invasive procedures. Journal of Pediatric Oncology Nursing: Official Journal of the Association of Pediatric Oncology Nurses. 2002;**19**(4):127-132

[38] Higa-McMillan CK, Francis SE, Rith-Najarian L, Chorpita BF. Evidence base update: 50 years of research on treatment for child and adolescent anxiety. Journal of Clinical Child and Adolescent Psychology: The Official Journal for the Society of Clinical Child and Adolescent Psychology, American Psychological Association, Division 53. 2016;**45**(2):91-113

[39] Alexander AB, Miklich DR, Hershkoff H. The immediate effects of systematic relaxation training on peak expiratory flow rates in asthmatic children. Psychosomatic Medicine. 1972;**34**(5):388-394

[40] Birnie KA, Noel M, Chambers CT, Uman LS, Parker JA. Psychological interventions for needle-related procedural pain and distress in children and adolescents. The. Cochrane Database of Systematic Reviews. 2018;**10**(10):CD005179

[41] Bougea A, Spantideas N, Chrousos GP. Stress management for headaches in children and adolescents: A review and practical recommendations for health promotion programs and well-being. Journal of Child Health Care: For Professionals Working with Children in the Hospital and Community. 2018;**22**(1):19-33

[42] Brown RP, Gerbarg PL, Muench F. Breathing practices for treatment of psychiatric and stress-related medical conditions. The Psychiatric Clinics of North America. 2013;**36**(1):121-140

[43] Charalambous A, Giannakopoulou M, Bozas E, Marcou Y, Kitsios P, Paikousis L. Guided imagery and progressive muscle relaxation as a cluster of symptoms management intervention in patients receiving chemotherapy: A randomized control trial. PLoS One. 2016;**11**(6):e0156911

[44] Hock RA, Bramble J, Kennard DW. A comparison between relaxation and assertive training with asthmatic male children. Biological Psychiatry. 1997;**12**(4):593-596

[45] Hölzel BK, Carmody J, Vangel M, Congleton C, Yerramsetti SM, Gard T, et al. Mindfulness practice leads to increases in regional brain gray

matter density. Psychiatry Research: Neuroimaging. 2011;**191**(1):36-43

[46] Kurth L, Engelniederhammer A, Sasse H, Papastefanou G. Effects of a short mindful-breathing intervention on the psychophysiological stress reactions of German elementary school children. School Psychology International. 2020;**41**(3):218-238

[47] Petosa R, Oldfield D. A pilot study of the impact of stress management techniques on the classroom behavior of elementary school students. The Journal of School Health. 1985;**55**(2):69-71

[48] Shapiro DH. Meditation: Self-Regulation Strategy and Altered State of Consciousness. New York: Aldine; 1980

[49] Sridhar S, Suprabha BS, Shenoy R, Shwetha KT, Rao A. Effect of a relaxation training exercise on behavior, anxiety, and pain during buccal infiltration anesthesia in children: Randomized clinical trial. International Journal of Paediatric Dentistry. 2019;**29**(5):596-602

[50] Thabrew H, Stasiak K, Hetrick SE, Wong S, Huss JH, Merry SN. E-health interventions for anxiety and depression in children and adolescents with long-term physical conditions. The Cochrane Database of Systematic Reviews. 2018;**2018**(8):6-23

[51] Vagnoli L, Bettini A, Amore E, De Masi S, Messeri A. Relaxation-guided imagery reduces perioperative anxiety and pain in children: A randomized study. European Journal of Pediatrics. 2019;**178**(6):913-921

[52] Yates A. Stress management in childhood. La Clinica Pediatrica. 1983;**22**(2):131-135

[53] Atkinson L, Jamieson B, Khoury J, Ludmer J, Gonzalez A. Stress physiology in infancy and early childhood: Cortisol flexibility, Attunement and coordination. Journal of Neuroendocrinology. 2016;**28**(8):1-12

[54] Dubow EF, Tisak J. The relation between stressful life events and adjustment in elementary school children: The role of social support and social problem-solving skills. Child Development. 1989;**60**(6):1412-1423

[55] Rutter M, Bailey A, Bolton P, Le Couteur A. Autism and known medical conditions: Myth and substance. Journal of Child Psychology and Psychiatry. 1994;**35**(2):311-322

[56] Homma I, Masaoka Y. Breathing rhythms and emotions. Experimental Physiology. 2008;**93**(9):1011-1021

[57] Ashhad S, Kam K, Del Negro CA, Feldman JL. Breathing rhythm and pattern and their influence on emotion. Annual Review of Neuroscience. 2022;**45**:223-247

[58] Grassmann M, Vlemincx E, Von Leupoldt A, Mittelstädt JM, Van den Bergh O. Respiratory changes in response to cognitive load: A systematic review. Neural Plasticity. 2016;**2016**:1-16

[59] Lauria MJ, Gallo IA, Rush S, Brooks J, Spiegel R, Weingart SD. Psychological skills to improve emergency care providers' performance under stress. Annals of Emergency Medicine. 2017;**70**(6):884-890

[60] Zaccaro A, Piarulli A, Laurino M, Garbella E, Menicucci D, Neri B, et al. How breath-control can change your life: A systematic review on psycho-physiological correlates of slow breathing. Frontiers in Human Neuroscience. 2018;**12**:353

[61] You M, Laborde S, Zammit N, Iskra M, Borges U, Dosseville F, et al.

Emotional intelligence training: Influence of a brief slow-paced breathing exercise on psychophysiological variables linked to emotion regulation. International Journal of Environmental Research and Public Health. 2021;**18**(12):6630. DOI: 10.3390/ijerph18126630

[62] Russo MA, Santarelli DM, O'Rourke D. The physiological effects of slow breathing in the healthy human. Breathe (Sheffield, England). 2017;**13**(4):298-309. DOI: 10.1183/20734735.009817

[63] Hamasaki H. Effects of diaphragmatic breathing on health: A narrative review. Medicine. 2020;**7**(10):65

[64] Liu H, Wiedman CM, Lovelace-Chandler V, Gong S, Salem Y. Deep diaphragmatic breathing-anatomical and biomechanical consideration. Journal of Holistic Nursing. 2024;**42**(1):90-103

[65] Gitler A, Vanacker L, De Couck M, De Leeuw I, Gidron Y. Neuromodulation applied to diseases: The case of HRV biofeedback. Journal of Clinical Medicine. 2022;**11**(19):5927 MDPI AG

[66] Kramer AC, Neubauer AB, Schmiedek F. The effectiveness of a slow-paced diaphragmatic breathing exercise in Children's daily life: A micro-randomized trial. Journal of Clinical Child and Adolescent Psychology. 2023;**52**(6):797-810

[67] Miri S, Hosseini SJ, Takasi P, Mollaei A, Firooz M, Falakdami A, et al. Effects of breathing exercise techniques on the pain and anxiety of burn patients: A systematic review and meta-analysis. International Wound Journal. 2023;**20**(6):2360-2375

[68] Harris GE. Progressive muscle relaxation: Highly effective but often neglected. Guidance and Counseling. 2003;**18**(4):142-148

[69] Jacobson E. The origins and development of progressive relaxation. Journal of Behavior Therapy and Experimental Psychiatry. 1977;**8**(2):119-123

[70] Bernstein D, Borkovec T. Progressive Muscular Relaxation Training. Champaign, IL: Research Press; 1973

[71] van Dixhoorn JJ, Duivenvoorden HJ. Effect of relaxation therapy on cardiac events after myocardial infarction: A 5-year followup study. Journal of Cardiopulmonary Rehabilitation and Prevention. 1999;**19**(3):178-185

[72] Krajewski J, Sauerland M, Wieland R. Relaxation-induced cortisol changes within lunch breaks–an experimental longitudinal worksite field study. Journal of Occupational and Organizational Psychology. 2011;**84**(2):382-394

[73] Pawlow LA, Jones GE. The impact of abbreviated progressive muscle relaxation on salivary cortisol. Biological Psychology. 2002;**60**(1):1-16

[74] Manjushambika R, Prasanna B, Vijayaraghavan R, Sushama B. Effectiveness of Jacobson's progressive muscle relaxation (JPMR) on educational stress among school going adolescents. International Journal of Nursing Education. 2017;**9**(4):110-115

[75] Jong MC, Boers I, van Wietmarschen HA, Tromp E, Busari JO, Wennekes R, et al. Hypnotherapy or transcendental meditation versus progressive muscle relaxation exercises in the treatment of children with primary headaches: A multi-Centre, pragmatic, randomized clinical study. European Journal of Pediatrics. 2019;**178**(2):147-154

[76] Tsai ML, Cheng TH, Yang YK, Wang CJ. A school-based progressive muscle relaxation program for female

adolescents: Development and the effectiveness on physiological and psychological evidence. Healthcare. 2021;**9**(10):1319

[77] Manzoni GM et al. Relaxation training for anxiety: A ten-years systematic review with meta-analysis. BMC Psychiatry. 2008;**8**(1):1-12

[78] Linden W. The autogenic training method of JH Schultz. In: Lehrer PM, Woolfolk RL, editors. Principles and Practice of Stress Management. 2nd ed. New York: Guilford Press; 1993

[79] Goldbeck L, Schmid K. Effectiveness of autogenic relaxation training on children and adolescents with behavioral and emotional problems. Journal of the American Academy of Child and Adolescent Psychiatry. 2003;**42**(9):1046-1054

[80] Luthe W, Schultz JH. Autogenic Therapy. Vol. 2. Grune and Stratton: Medical applications; 1969

[81] Davis M, Eshelman ER, McKay M. The Relaxation and Stress Reduction Workbook. 6th ed. New Harbinger Publications; 2008

[82] Luthe W. About the methods of autogenic therapy. In: Mind/Body Integration: Essential Readings in Biofeedback. Boston, MA: Springer US; 1979. pp. 167-186

[83] Zucker TL, Samuelson KW, Muench F, Greenberg MA, Gevirtz RN. The effects of respiratory sinus arrhythmia biofeedback on heart rate variability and posttraumatic stress disorder symptoms: A pilot study. Applied Psychophysiology and Biofeedback. 2009;**34**(2):135-143

[84] Breznoscakova D, Kovanicova M, Sedlakova E, Pallayova M. Autogenic training in mental disorders: What can we expect? International Journal of Environmental Research and Public Health. 2023;**20**(5):4344

[85] Seo E, Kim S. Effect of autogenic training for stress response: A systematic review and meta-analysis. Journal of Korean Academy of Nursing. 2019;**49**(4):361-374

[86] Guiote JM, Lozano V, Vallejo MA, Mas B. Autogenic meditation training in a randomized controlled trial: A framework for promoting mental health and attention regulation in children. Revista de Psicodidáctica (English ed.). 2022;**27**(1):47-55

[87] Jojić BR, Leposavić LM. Autogenic training as a therapy for adjustment disorder in adolescents. Srpski Arhiv za Celokupno Lekarstvo. 2005;**133**(9-10):424-428

[88] Creswell JD. Mindfulness interventions. Annual Review of Psychology. 2017;**68**(1):491-516

[89] Amundsen R, Riby LM, Hamilton C, Hope M, McGann D. Mindfulness in primary school children as a route to enhanced life satisfaction, positive outlook and effective emotion regulation. BMC Psychology. 2020;**8**(1):71

[90] Kabat-Zinn J. Mindfulness-based interventions in context: Past, present, and future. Clinical Psychology: Science and Practice. 2003;**10**(2):144-156

[91] Emerson LM, de Diaz NN, Sherwood A, Waters A, Farrell L. Mindfulness interventions in schools: Integrity and feasibility of implementation. International Journal of Behavioral Development. 2020;**44**(1):62-75

[92] Kallapiran K, Koo S, Kirubakaran R, Hancock K. Review: Effectiveness of

mindfulness in improving mental health symptoms of children and adolescents: A meta-analysis. Child and Adolescent Mental Health. 2015;**20**(4):182-194

[93] Zenner C, Herrnleben-Kurz S, Walach H. Mindfulness-based interventions in schools: A systematic review and meta-analysis. Frontiers in Psychology. 2014;**5**:603

[94] Fulambarkar N, Seo B, Testerman A, Rees M, Bausback K, Bunge E. Review: Meta-analysis on mindfulness-based interventions for adolescents' stress, depression, and anxiety in school settings: A cautionary tale. Child and Adolescent Mental Health. 2023;**28**(2):307-317

[95] Saulsman LM, Ji JL, McEvoy PM. The essential role of mental imagery in cognitive behaviour therapy: What is old is new again. Australian Psychologist. 2019;**54**(4):237-244

[96] Skeens LM. Guided imagery: A technique to benefit youth at risk. National Youth-At-Risk Journal. 2017;**2**(2):92-106

[97] Blackwell SE. Mental imagery in the science and practice of cognitive behavior therapy: Past, present, and future perspectives. International Journal of Cognitive Therapy. 2021;**14**(1):160-181

[98] Pile V, Williamson G, Saunders A, Holmes EA, Lau JYF. Harnessing emotional mental imagery to reduce anxiety and depression in young people: An integrative review of progress and promise. The Lancet Psychiatry. 2021;**8**(9):836-852

[99] Schwarz S, Grasmann D, Schreiber F, Stangier U. Mental imagery and its relevance for psychopathology and psychological treatment in children and adolescents: A systematic review. International Journal of Cognitive Therapy. 2020;**13**(4):303-327

[100] Nilsson S, Forsner M, Finnström B, Mörelius E. Relaxation and guided imagery do not reduce stress, pain, and unpleasantness for 11- to 12-year-old girls during vaccinations. Acta Paediatrica. 2015;**104**(7):724-729

[101] Weigensberg MJ, Wen CKF, Spruijt-Metz D, Lane CJ. Effects of group-delivered stress-reduction guided imagery on salivary cortisol, salivary amylase, and stress mood in urban, predominantly Latino adolescents. Global Advances in Health and Medicine. 2022;**11**:21649561211067443

[102] Webb TL, Miles E, Sheeran P. Dealing with feeling: A meta-analysis of the effectiveness of strategies derived from the process model of emotion regulation. Psychological Bulletin. 2012;**138**(4):775-808. DOI: 10.1037/a0027600

[103] Jones EJ, Marsland AL, Gianaros PJ. Do trait-level emotion regulation strategies moderate associations between retrospective reports of childhood trauma and prospective changes in systemic inflammation? Stress and Health. 2023;**39**(3):525-538. DOI: 10.1002/smi.3205

[104] Carthy A, McCann C, McGilloway S, McGuinness C. Enhancing the academic and social learning of irish undergraduates through emotional and social skills development. The All Ireland Journal of Teaching and Learning in Higher Education. 2013;**5**(3):1231-12311

[105] Buhle JT, Silvers JA, Wager TD, Lopez R, Onyemekwu C, Kober H, et al. Cognitive reappraisal of emotion: A meta-analysis of human neuroimaging studies. Cerebral Cortex. 2014;**24**(11):2981-2990

[106] Carrington P. Freedom in Meditation. Doubleday: Anchor Press; 1977

[107] Heide FJ, Borkovec TD. Relaxation-induced anxiety: Mechanisms and theoretical implications. Behaviour Research and Therapy. 1984;**22**(1):1-12

[108] Banneyer KN, Bonin L, Price K, Goodman WK, Storch EA. Cognitive behavioral therapy for childhood anxiety disorders: A review of recent advances. Current Psychiatry Reports. 2018;**20**(8):65

[109] Leichsenring F, Steinert C. Is cognitive Behavioral therapy the gold standard for psychotherapy?: The need for plurality in treatment and research. JAMA. 2017;**318**(14):1323

[110] Ray D, Bratton S. What the research shows about play therapy: Twenty-frst century update. In: Baggerly J, Ray D, Bratton S, editors. Child-Centered Play Therapy Research: The Evidence Base for Effective Practice. Hoboken, NJ: Wiley; 2010. pp. 3-33

[111] Bratton SC, Ray D, Rhine T, Jones L. The efficacy of play therapy with children: A meta-analytic review of treatment outcomes. Professional Psychology: Research and Practice. 2005;**36**(4):376

[112] Thongseiratch T, Leijten P, Melendez-Torres GJ. Online parent programs for children's behavioral problems: A meta-analytic review. European Child and Adolescent Psychiatry. 2020;**29**:1555-1568

Chapter 8

How to Facilitate Self-Reflection, Personal Development, and Coping with Stress: Yoga and Yogic Breathing for Increasing Health, Healing and Wellbeing

Ingunn Hagen and Ananda Balayogi Bhavanani

Abstract

The aim of this chapter is to reflect on the therapeutic potential of yoga, and especially yogic breathing for health, healing, and wellbeing. We will do this by focusing on how a university course with yoga theory and practice as the central element could contribute to people's ability for Swadhyaya (self-reflection or self-inquiry), awareness about their need for personal development and self-care, as well as offer strategies for coping with stress. Our point of departure will be the yoga as a fourfold awareness model developed by Dr. Swami Gitananda Giri, founder of the Gitananda Rishi-culture Yoga tradition. The model focuses on how yoga can facilitate awareness about the body, emotions, mind, and meta-awareness (meta-cognition) and their interrelationship, in addition to acknowledging lack of awareness. These insights are relevant for coping with stress, personal development, and selfcare and can be used for teaching students in health care professions courses as well as health professionals. In the chapter, we aim to illuminate the overlap between yoga and yoga therapy and to illustrate how even yoga in educational settings can manifest yoga's therapeutic potentials.

Keywords: yoga, yoga therapy, self-reflection, personal development, coping with stress, yogic breathing, health, healing, wellbeing

1. Introduction

Yoga therapy known traditionally as Yoga Chikitsa is about facilitating healing through principles and practices of yoga, and thus yoga and yoga therapy are overlapping categories. In a recent article, the following definition as earlier envisioned by the IAYT (International Association of Yoga Therapists) was suggested as appropriate: "Yoga therapy is the process of empowering individuals to progress towards improved health and well-being through the application of the teachings and practices of yoga" ([1], p. 45). Yoga therapy is often practiced in dyads between the yoga therapist and care-seeker. Teaching yoga, on the other hand, mostly takes place in group settings in classrooms at yoga ashrams or centers, physically or virtually (through webinars). We propose that both yoga and yoga therapeutic elements can contribute to enhanced coping with stress, healing, and personal development in educational settings.

Thus, the purpose of this chapter is to explore how some selected principles of Yoga and Yoga Therapy can be applied in a classroom or group setting. The starting point and source of inspiration for our reflections was a university course on "Self-reflection, Personal Development, and Coping with Stress".[1] The course was coordinated by the author Hagen, in collaboration with a colleague who was a Jungian therapist.[2] Fifteen people participated in the further education course, which was taught intensively for a week, in person, after an introductory webinar 2 weeks before hand. The students also had to submit an essay 5 weeks after the course in order to have the course approved and get credit. Thirteen of the course participants were women, while two of them were men. They were in the age range mid-thirties to early sixties. Most of the course participants were working with people, primarily in health professions, and as consultants, and leaders. Here is an example of how one of the participants experienced the outcome of the course:

> *Learning to live with a better awareness of how the body works and how emotions affect my health are insights that I have gained through participating in the NTNU course (2024). I have decided to learn more about how practicing yoga can contribute to self-development and create my own happiness so that I can flourish as a person and face aging changes with greater peace of mind.*
>
> *Yoga is a way of life that includes all aspects, which I recognize requires training in several phases. I have started a yogic lifestyle, but I have a long way to go before I have learned the way of life. In the future, I will continue to practice yoga, both the physical exercises and the mental perspective, to find the elements that suit me best. These can probably also be developed and changed over time as I learn to live with a yoga practice.*[3]

As demonstrated in this citation, the person expressed that s/he had gained more awareness about how the body and emotions impacted her/his health and were motivated to develop a yogic lifestyle for the purpose of self-development, happiness, and peace of mind.

In the following, we will describe the yogic teachings of the "Self-reflection, personal development, and the ability to cope with stress" course. Thus, in this chapter, we chose to elaborate on the concepts Swadhyaya or self-reflection, Pranayama or Yogic Breath, and yoga for coping with stress. These concepts were related to central themes in the above-mentioned course. We will focus our discussion on the yogic elements of the course, and

[1] The course was offered at Norwegian University of Science and Technology (NTNU), as an NTNU Further Education Course, by Department of Psychology (Available from: https://www.ntnu.no/videre/gen/-/courses/nv24352,https://www.ntnu.edu/studies/courses/PSY6018/2024#tab=omEmnet).

[2] This colleague was Dr. Dorte Odde, a Danish Jungian Analyst who was mainly working as a therapist but also with Coaching and Supervision. She also has a Ph.D. in Cultural Sociology.

[3] This citation is from one of the essays submitted as part of the course assignments. The essays were delivered anonymously.

in the Appendices, we will share the questions for reflection and practices.[4] The point is to illustrate how to facilitate increased awareness in such an educational setting. We also aim to demonstrate the healing and therapeutic impacts on the participants, especially when they tested out the yogic practices in their everyday lives, as well as wrote about their experiences in an essay, describing what was at stake for them.

We think that both yogic and yoga therapeutic insight can be relevant for the chapter. Thus, we take a few of the Principles of Yoga Therapy from the book *Yoga Therapy for Care Seekers* as our starting point ([2], p. 08). Here we chose to cite only the most relevant ones:

- Become aware of your body, emotions, and mind.
- Calm down your mind and focus inwards.
- Slow down your breath by making it quiet and deep.
- Improve the flow of Healing Pranic Life Energy to all parts of your body (...), thus relaxing, regenerating and reinvigorating yourself.
- Relax your body from toes to head.
- Decrease your stress level by fortifying yourself against the omnipotent stressors in your life.
- Health and happiness are your birthright, claim them and develop them to your maximum potential.

A variation of the last citation ("Health and happiness are your birthright") was put forward as a motto for the course on "Self-reflection, Personal development, and Coping with Stress".

2. Background

The perspective in this chapter is based on the Gitananda yoga tradition, which is a holistic yoga tradition with Patanjali's *Yoga Sutras* as its strong basis (see Ref. [3]). We also draw upon the perspective of Salutogenesis and its focus on factors that contribute to health, and in that sense resembles the Gitananda Yoga tradition. The Salutogenesis perspective emphasizes the Sense of Coherence (SoC) model, where comprehensibility, manageability and meaning are important for a healthy life [4, 5]. There are some commonalities with positive psychology, with is focus on health, happiness, flourishing and meaning. However, while health from the yogic and salutogenic perspective can be seen as a continuum, positive psychology is more concerned with the health part of a dichotomy, as a reaction to the earlier focus on (mental) pathology in psychology [6, 7].

---

[4] In the course in question, my co-teacher Dr. Dorte Odde addressed the Jungian concepts Active Imagination and Individuation, with their related practices.

We also addressed how Dr. Swami Gitananda Giri reminds us that even though health and happiness are our birthright, we are ourselves responsible for re-claiming them [3]. Though health and happiness are important and can be achieved or aimed for through yoga; these are to be seen as byproducts, while we are suggested to focus on a more important goal which is Moksha, or liberation from what is limiting us in life [8, 9]. The aim of yoga is also to calm our mind, to become more aware, and become more balanced in our nervous system and life [3]. We will also discuss how learning about and practicing Swadhyaya (self-reflection), Pranayama or yogic breath, and yoga for coping with stress seem to contribute to increased health, happiness, and personal development or growth.

2.1 Central concepts in the course title

Here we will address the everyday understanding of the central concepts in the course that inspired this article, on "Self-reflection, Personal Development, and Coping with Stress." Self-reflection is about realizing who you are, for yourself, in relation to others, and in different roles. It is about being aware of your values, the process that governs decisions you make and your reflections about their consequences for yourself and others. Self-reflection needs to be a daily and continuous process in life. The related concern in this course was how the notion of Swadhyaya, one of the Niyamas in Patanjali's *Yoga Sutras* may inform our understanding of self-reflection [8, 10].

Personal development can be described as an awareness that you are in a positive and reflexive change process, with body, mind, emotions, and competence. In modern times, it is expected that you take responsibility for your health and happiness. Moreover, personal development is emphasized in social media, to the extent that may put pressure on people, especially young people [11, 12]. In work life, constant self- and competence development is expected, something that puts pressure on employees [13]. The norm is to work on yourself, your relations, as well as to practice lifelong learning. Our concern is how yoga can contribute to positive personal development and the ability to cope with pressure and stress.

Coping with stress can also be dealt with by addressing what makes us stressed and how to deal with stress. Since it can be argued that "stress is in the eyes of the beholder" (see Ref. [14]), our perspective is important for how we experience stress. Selye defined stress as a nonspecific or general response of the body to any demand [15].[5] Stress can also be defined as "an exaggerated response to changes in the external or internal environment" [16]. Thus, stress is response to a stimulus that disturbs our mental or physiological equilibrium. Here we will illuminate how yoga and especially yogic breath could contribute positively to our experience of and coping with stress.

2.2 Explaining yoga and the Gitananda tradition

One challenge in the course that inspired this chapter was the diverse background of the students, where most of them had not practiced yoga earlier. However, a few of them had practiced various aspects of yoga, including meditation.[6] Due to

[5] Hans Selye is often given credit for coining the concept of stress.

[6] Some of the course participants were also yoga teachers, both in Ashtanga yoga and yin yoga. The participants were all adults, working in very diverse professions, like in health professions, as leaders, HR-professionals, or other professions working with people.

their diverse background, there was a need to introduce them to yoga, mainly the Gitananda tradition, and provide a few relevant practice experiences. These introductions are shared here.

As is often referred, the word Yoga is derived from the Sanskrit word "yuj," meaning to "join," "to yoke together," "to unify" and "to unite as one" ([3], p. 1). One of the most quoted Sanskrit definitions of yoga is "*yogah chittavritti nirodhah*," the second sutra from the ancient text *Yoga Sutras* by Maharishi Patanjali (see Ref. [8]). According to Bhavanani, this classical definition of yoga can be translated as yoga being "a discipline to control the whirlpools of the subconscious/unconscious mind" (op.cit.: 6). A general understanding is that yoga calms the fluctuations of the mind and thus creates stillness (also see Ref. [10]).

However, yoga is not only what happens on the yoga mat. Gitananda emphasized that he preferred "yoga as a way of life, a way of integrating one's whole nature, so that all aspects of one's life work in harmony, one with another" ([3], p. 1). Similarly, yoga also means "'integration' at all levels of existence" ([17], p. 2). Thus, yoga is about empowerment. Gitananda describes yoga as "skill in action," referring to Krishna in the Bhagavad Gita. With the global popularity of yoga, a proper cultural appreciation of yoga is needed, rather than misappropriation [18]. This includes understanding yoga in its original context in ancient India, and in citing the original sources of your insight.

In this chapter, we emphasize that yoga is a source of conscious development [3]. Practicing yoga on and beyond the mat is about getting to know oneself for the sake of personal growth, and of self-care. The development achieved through yoga can be described as a process of conscious evolution through a fourfold awareness: developing awareness about the body and how it works, awareness of the emotions and how they impact the body, awareness about how the mind can control the emotions and the rest of the body, and awareness about awareness or meta-cognition. A starting point for this fourfold awareness is acknowledging one's lack of awareness, as pointed out by Ammaji Meenakshi Devi Bhavanani ([3], p. 9). We believe that this model of yoga for developing fourfold awareness, and its focus on the interrelationship of the body, emotions, mind, and meta-awareness can illuminate the holistic contributions of yoga to our balance, health, and wellbeing.

Most yoga traditions in India regard Patanjali's *Yoga Sutras* as their stepping-stone and source of inspiration. In line with this Swami Gitananda introduces the term "no-option yoga,"[7] implying that all yoga needs to be based on the Yama and Niyama from Patanjali's Ashtanga Yoga (the eight limbs of yoga). These are: Yama (social restrictions), Niyama (internal disciplines), Asana (physical postures), Pranayama (regulation of prana or life energy through breath), Pratyahara (withdrawal of the senses), Dharana (concentration), Dhyana (meditation), and Samadhi (union or integration) (see Ref. [19]). The notion of Swadhyaya, which we pay attention to here is one of the above-described Niyama. Niyama can also be described as "ethical observances that cultivate humane qualities and prepare us for the higher, conscious life of yoga" ([8], p. 15).

2.3 Swadhyaya or self-reflection

Our emphasis here is on the fourth Niyama, Swadhyaya, which can be described as self-study or self-analysis. The meaning of the Sanskrit word Swadhyaya is "to

[7] Bhavanani [18]. Available from: https://bhavanani.medium.com/some-core-concepts-of-the-rishiculture-gitananda-yoga-tradition-6ae44823d206.

see clearly one's own nature." Thus, Swadhyaya is about our ability and willingness for self-inquiry by asking questions like, who am I? Why did I do what I did? Are my actions right or wrong? Gitananda describes Swadhyaya as "self-knowledge through introspection" ([3], p. 5). Similarly, Bhavanani describes Swadhyaya as "the important task of introspectional self-analysis" ([8], p. 161). Such a task requires courage and honesty as Swadhyaya is about studying your own nature, not only your strengths, but also your faults and weaknesses. This can sometimes be painful.

Reading philosophical or religious books is recommended to get ideas about human nature and the diversity of human experiences, but we must use these scriptures as "sounding board to understand ourselves" ([8], p. 161). Thus, learning from books becomes Swadhyaya only when it enters our consciousness and is applied to every moment of our lives. Gitananda suggests that Swadhyaya is also about our perception and our cognition: "It is awareness of the accuracy of reports of the senses, as well as the factual basis for one's mental conceptions" (op.cit.). Thus, Swadhyaya is reflecting on how we perceive and understand the world, trying to go beyond our preconceptions and stereotypes.

Introspection and self-analysis are important for our spiritual development. As stated by Patanjali (II, p. 44) "through introspectional self-analysis we become one with our inherent divinity" ([8], p. 188). When we realize where we are in life, we can also understand and better choose where we are going. Gitananda suggests that seeking knowledge of the self can free a person from the illusions caused by the ego. However, getting to know yourself takes patience and even self-devotion ([3], p. 5). Ammaji Meenakshi Devi Bhavanani emphasizes the importance of relationships in self-reflection, "as human relationships are the mirror in which we 'see ourselves' (Swadhyaya)." We are all in different relationships; child-parents, husband-wife, siblings, colleagues, and pupil-teacher, where we all develop different self-knowledge. Swadhyaya is about reflecting on your own feelings, thoughts and actions, the way they are expressed in your own reaction patterns, and the responses you get in your interaction with others. Continuous self-reflection needs to be an integral part of yogic life, for the sake of conscious evolution.

2.4 Pranayama or yogic breath

Pranayama is the fourth limb in Patanjali's description of Ashtanga Yoga (eight limbs of yoga). As it is a powerful tool, it is vital that Pranayama is adapted and learnt gradually, as emphasized by Gitananda [20]. Pranayama or yogic breath is about controlling or regulating the breath to become more aware of Prana – the life-force. Gitananda suggests that "Pranayama is the 'Science of Breath,' the control of the Vital Force (Prana) in the air we breathe" ([3], p. 2). Our breathing needs to be deep, slow, and relaxed to have sufficient absorption of Prana for our nervous system. Pranayama or yogic breath can have important consequences for our life and wellbeing, by increasing our energy, freeing our blockages, and calming down our nervous system.

In the "Self-reflection, Personal Development, and the Ability to cope with Stress" course we recommend Vibhaga Pranayama, or sectional breathing, as a starting point for developing awareness about yogic breathing, as it is the ABC of pranayama and the best way to develop good breath control ([3], p. 11). One starts with Adham Pranayama, breath with focus on the lower, abdominal section of the lungs. Secondly, Madhyam Pranayama, breath with focus on the mind, intra-costal area of the lungs. Thirdly, Adhyam Pranayama, breath with focus on the higher, clavicular area of the lungs. Finally, there is Mahat Yoga Pranayama, complete breath, including a sequential focus on all levels of the lungs.

Moreover, it is important to become aware of the four phases of yogic breathing: Puraka—the incoming breath or inspiration phase, Rechaka—the outgoing breath or expiration phase, Kumbhaka or held-in phase, and Shunyaka or the held-out phase ([3], p. 71; [21], p. 34). In the Gitananda tradition the Savitri Pranayama or solar breath is emphasized, with its tala of 2-1-2-1 (e.g., 6 in, hold in 3, 6 out, hold out 3, or 8-4-8-4, etc.). Breathing is of course important, as it makes the difference between life and death. Yogic breath is also regarded the bridge between our internal and external world. Furthermore, Meenakshi Devi Bhavanani suggests that "We must deepen it, lengthen it, control it, expand it, and become conscious of it and its potentiality, to link us with our Highest Nature. That is the real pranayama, the ancient spiritual Science of vital control" ([21], p. ii).

It is also important to have a certain structure for practicing pranayama, often conveyed as regularity, rhythm, and repetition. Dr. Gitananda suggests that pranayama needs to be practiced as Abhyasa "sustained discipline within a repeated structure" ([20], p. 27). Being realistic is also recommended, in the sense that it is better to practice 10 minutes of pranayama in the morning than plan for a longer practice which is not realized. Pranayama can facilitate personal development as practicing it leads to a pure mind, fit for concentration. Practicing pranayama can also lead to energy in the body and freshness in the mind, thus promoting "Yogic skill in action" ([21], p. 41). Moreover, practice of pranayama also facilitates discrimination (Viveka), knowledge, and wisdom (Jnana).

To summarize, pranayama may contribute to our personal development as it creates a greater sensitivity to the subtler aspects of our conscious and existence, connecting the individual with the universe ([21], pp. 38–40). Pranayama is also suggested to calm and control both emotions and mind.[8] First, by creating a better balance between the sympathetic and para-sympathetic limbs of the autonomic nervous system. And secondly, by enhancing our memory, intelligence, and creativity.

2.5 Yoga for coping with stress

For many people, their everyday life is stressful, for example stressing school days for young people, stress at work for many employees, or stress related to attempting to balance between family and work-life [12, 13]. The World Health Organization, WHO describes stress as of the main reasons for current health problems, both physical and mental ones. To be more specific, in work life employees experience stress when the demands or expectations in the workplace are greater than they can cope with.

---

[8] One example is Kapalabhati, often referred to as the "Skull brightener" or skull cleanser, which is one of the eight classical Pranayamas, and one of the Shat Karmas, purging methods [3].

Another example is Pranava AUM, the healing breath. Pranava AUM can also be related to the sectional breath, where we after in-breath in each section, we breathe out A, U, M, and finally AUM. The vibration prolongs outbreath, increasing our para-sympathetic activation, contributing to ease in the body and peace of mind.

A third example is Bhramari, one of the healing breaths, where the point is to make the nasal sound of a female bee on the forced expiration of the breath (Bhavanani, 2008). The vibrations of Bhramari can be very calming.

Stress over time can lead to serious physical or mental health problems, like backache, fatigue, depression, or anxiety.

However, it is worth noticing that it is often your perception of a situation that determines how you react, whether you get stressed or not: "We may place our body on 'stress alert' quite unconsciously because of our psychological and emotional attitude" ([22], p. 13). Thus, if you cannot avoid stress, which most people cannot, you must become aware of your perception of and experience of stress, to cope better with stress. It matters whether you perceive something as a challenge or as a problem, for whether you become very stressed or not. A certain level of activation or eustress may also facilitate your performance. Through yoga you can also achieve deep relaxation, thus reducing the level of stress you experience.

Moreover, there is increasingly research that demonstrates how practicing yoga strongly reduces the experience of stress and facilitates the ability of coping with stress [19]. Psychological mechanisms include a more positive attitude toward stress, self-awareness, a sense of control, calmness, spirituality, and self-compassion. Biological mechanisms emphasize the autonomic nervous system and achieving better balance between the para-sympathetic and the sympathetic limbs. Learning how to relax through yoga allowed young people who were offered yoga at school to become more aware about stress and relaxation, something that can counteract stress levels [11]. Similarly, in a study of occupational stress, the participants who had practiced yoga expressed that yogic breathing, meditation, and positive self-talk made them calmer, more focused, and relaxed rather than stressed [13].

In the course discussed in this chapter, we challenged people to develop a yogic approach to stress. While some amount of stress (eustress) is necessary to bring out the best of us, we need to learn how to manage distress. Our attitude or perspective toward stress matters! As Swami Gitananda jokingly said: "You don't have problems – you are the problem!" ([2], p. 76). In line with this, a positive frame of mind will help us become more cheerful and less stressed. To change our perspective, we might also follow Maharishi Patanjali's advice, to cultivate Pratipaksha Bhavanam (the Opposite or Contrary View), to achieve balance between the emotions and the mind. To develop our prefrontal cortex and let it override the limbic system (the center of our emotions) through yoga will more likely let us be less overwhelmed by the stress in our lives.

In the chapter "A yogic approach to stress" the following actions were recommended to reduce or eliminate stress ([2], pp. 77–79): Develop awareness of stress and try to get rid of it. Practice movements like asana, walking, swimming, etc. to reduce tension. Practice Yogic relaxation like Shava Asana and Yoga Nidra to become aware and relax the body and mind. Hobbies like music, dance, painting, cooking, gardening and having a pet will relieve our tension and provide positive "flow" experiences. Deep breathing is recommended as "one of the easiest ways to relieve stress". An attitude of detachment and "Let things lie" will help to minimize and relieve stressful situations. Visualization may help us to identify pleasant solutions to problems. Mental techniques like Positive self- suggestion can help us replace negative thoughts with a "I can, and I will"-attitude.

3. Discussion and case examples

In our discussion, we aim to focus on the therapeutic potential of yoga in an educational or classroom setting, illustrated through how a few of the course participants expressed the experienced impact from the course on their health and wellbeing. To recapitulate the purpose of the course, which is our source of inspiration; we introduced definitions of yoga, Patanjali's Ashtanga Yoga (eight limbs of yoga), Swadhyaya or yogic self-reflection, Pranayama or yogic breathing, and discussed coping with stress through yoga. The fourfold model of yoga was emphasized, presenting yoga to increase awareness about the body, emotions, mind, and meta-awareness, starting with a recognition of one's lack of awareness [3]. In the course, there was a mixture of offering students theoretical concepts, practices, as well as opportunities for self-reflection, observation and discussions in small groups, and plenary discussions in the class setting.

A challenge in our case or described course was the diverse background of the students, where most of them had not practiced yoga earlier. However, a few of them had practiced various aspects of yoga, including meditation. Three of the course participants were also yoga teachers, both in Ashtanga Yoga and Yin Yoga, while others had related backgrounds like yoga therapist, MBSR and trauma therapist. Due to their diverse experience with yoga, we chose to introduce the course participants to basic yoga philosophy, theory and practice, based on insights from the Gitananda tradition. The course included practice experiences of Pranayama (yogic breath), Yogic Asanas (poses), group discussion topics like Swadhyaya (self-reflection through introspection), as well as experience of stress and strategies for coping with stress.

The 15 participants in this further education university course on were not "care seekers" in the traditional sense. They were working people, in the age range early thirties to mid-sixties who had signed up for the course on "Self-reflection, Personal Development, and Coping with Stress".[9] The course participants seemed eager to reflect on and make some changes in their lives, as many of them expressed when they introduced themselves. The participants also expressed curiosity and enthusiasm about the various themes of the course. Apparently, we were able to create a rather open atmosphere in the course, where people also could talk about challenges that they had faced in their lives, like "meeting the wall", periods of burn-out and related long-term sick-leave. Several of the participants shared that they had experienced degrees of trauma in life, and many reported that they often experienced stress, related to their work life, balancing family and work, and finding time for themselves.

Most of the course participants expressed that they had decided to attend the course to get some new tools for helping clients in their jobs. But they also gradually realized that the course became important for their own self-care; through self-reflection, personal development, coping with stress, and experience more health and wellbeing. Several of the course participants expressed appreciation for the course format, consisting of lectures, with discussion and questions, practices of Hatha Yoga and Pranayama, and group discussions in small groups of two or three people, and then follow-up panel discussions in the whole group/class.[10] The participants also expressed that the course was different from what they had anticipated, with a lot more personal involvement and practical learning than they were accustomed to in their earlier education.

On the last day of the course the participants had to present a topic for their essay or writing assignment (the exam to get credit for the course). The participants

[9] Available from: https://www.ntnu.edu/studies/courses/PSY6018/2024#tab=omEmnet.

[10] As mentioned earlier, the practices and topics for discussion related to the yogic part of the course will be shared in the Appendix.

who were not able to be present, could send a written presentations by email. We encouraged the course participants to write about something that "was at stake" for them, personally, with other people, at home, or in their workplace. They could also try out some of the practices shared in the course, like yoga, yogic breathing, active imagination, strategies for self-care, or for coping with stress, and then write about their experiences and learning. It seemed like the course had provided inspiration and empowered the participants to make changes in their lives, mostly through Pranayama or yogic breathing, Asanas or yogic postures, and Dhyana or meditation. Others seemed to have benefitted a lot from the self-reflections and hearing other people's reflections. Others again wanted to go deeper into their personalities and challenges through focusing on the Jungian concepts of active imagination and individuation, with their related practices and reflections. Several course participants expressed that they appreciated the opportunities to test the introduced practices, and to write about their experiences, both those in the course and during the weeks when they prepared their essay assignments.

We will provide a few more examples from parts of the conclusory remarks from the students' essays, which were submitted about 5 weeks after the course:

> *Starting with pranayama and experiencing the changes that have occurred has led to a greater curiosity and interest in yoga as a whole. First and foremost, in asanas (physical yoga postures) and dhyana (meditation). I find that I have a more open attitude and am not as skeptical as I was a few months ago. I am more able to quiet my mind and be present here and now. I am more concentrated and present in what I am doing or the task in front of me. It has also opened up for other exercises that are about trying to change thought patterns. I also feel that I am able to be more in my thoughts and mind, without it becoming difficult and I need distractions. A greater experience that thoughts are thoughts, they are not facts and thoughts can be controlled. In an attempt to change a lot of negative thinking, I have also started writing daily gratitude before bedtime. I have also become more curious about my dreams and what they can tell me.*
>
> *Through my new experience, I have seen the value of focusing on the breath and that breathing techniques themselves can be a good tool for stress management. Breathing techniques have been and are important to me, especially in work life in general where deadlines and a high workload can often lead to a stressful everyday life. By regulating my breathing, I feel an immediate change inside me. Both when I practice yoga, but also in other contexts where stress can occur. In my collaboration with a psychomotor physiotherapist, I was made aware that I often breathed high in the chest and very fast. Through breathing techniques, you can actively regulate this yourself to lower the stress reactions in the body. To promote breathing techniques and yoga practice at my current workplace, I have established a "break gym", where employees gather every day just before lunch for simple stretching exercises and/or yoga exercises combined with breathing techniques.*
>
> *For me personally, I see that I can reap benefits from using yoga and yogic breathing both as a private person and in a work context. Often these are also connected, one affects the other. I will continue to practice yogic breathing and hope to incorporate this into my daily routine eventually. And not only in relation to sleep, but also to be able to use it in other stressful situations to gain peace and balance. I also have both faith and hope that this will give me fewer health problems and increased well-being.*

> *I think that I have only just started on my own "yoga journey". I have gained a little insight, but there is still a lot to learn. I have learned that yoga can often provide many positive benefits both in terms of physical and mental health. But the most important thing I take with me is to stop and study myself, reflect on my own life, health and mindset. Then I can further use the tools I have now received to create change, development and life mastery.*

The course participants used this opportunity to address some of the problems they had in their lives, in the past and currently. Many of them expressed that they were motivated to change their lives, to heal traumas, cope with stress and find more time for their own self-care. They also reflected about their own attitudes to life, which also contributed to their stress levels. Many of the participants expressed a positive and optimistic perspective toward taking more control of their own life, wishing to improve their health and wellbeing.

These examples of statements from our participants illustrate that even a short weekly intensive course with a mixture of theory, practice, reflection and discussions could contribute to people's ability for Swadhyaya or self-reflections. The course participants seemed to have become more aware about themselves and their health challenges and demonstrated more meta-awareness. Pranayama was said to be experienced as quite impactful and was one of the elements that several course participants wanted to try as a continued practice and topic for their essays. Several of them also demonstrated a willingness for more self-inquiry, and consequently more self-awareness, including awareness about their need for more self-care.

This increased self-awareness demonstrated by the course participants seems to be in line with the Gitananda model of yoga as fourfold awareness [3], where awareness about the body, emotions, mind, and meta-awareness is potentially achieved through practicing yoga. The students seemed empowered by this increased awareness, which apparently enabled them to become more in charge of changes in their life, including the ability to be in the presence, to focus, to be with themselves, and to try to change their negative thought patterns. Several of the course participants expressed that they had taken this increased awareness with them after the course, and many of them were motivated to continue with yoga and to learn more about yoga for making it part of their new way of life or lifestyle.

Course participants also expressed that yoga and especially yogic breathing, or Pranayama were good tools for stress management. Breathing techniques were seemingly an important part of a personal yoga practice, and valuable for the stress that would occur related to work deadlines and responsibilities. As the course participants expressed that they experienced the positive changes in their own bodies and minds when being able to regulate their stress levels, some also decided to take the yoga practices from the course into their workplace as something to share with their colleagues. One of the participants also reported that she gave a small summary lecture of the "Self-reflection, Personal development, and Coping with Stress"-course in her workplace. The cited course participants, as well as several others expressed that they wanted to continue exploring the yogic tools that they had been exposed in the course.

4. Conclusory remarks

The purpose of this chapter is to reflect on the potentials of yoga, yoga therapeutic aspects, and yogic breathing for improved health, better healing, and increased wellbeing. Yoga and yoga therapy are overlapping categories, but while yoga is often taught in classes yoga therapy is mostly seen to happen in sessions with one yoga therapist. However, regardless of context yoga can contribute to healing, and be a preventive and health promotive practice. In our case, a further education course on "Self-reflection, Personal Development, and Coping with Stress" the focus was on Swadhyaya, Pranayama, and Asanas. The aim was increased self-reflection, and the ability to experience calm and relaxation rather than being overly stressed. In this way, yoga and its therapeutic potential can increase wellbeing and be a "whole person approach to health", to borrow a concept from Majewski and Bhavanani [23].

Apparently, the course on contributed to increased optimism and positive health for the course participants. The increased knowledge and practice of self-reflection and being part of other people's self-reflection through group work made course participants more aware of themselves. Thus, this course facilitated more awareness for the participants of their body, emotions, mind and the ability for meta-awareness, in line the Gitananda model of yoga as fourfold awareness. The increased awareness empowered the course participants and motivated them for making positive changes in their lives. As mentioned, many of the course participants shared that they had experienced trauma in their life, some had experienced "burn-out" after long-time stress. Moreover, too much stress and too little self-care was part of everyday life for most of them. The course participants expressed that they realized that the tools of constant self-reflection, yogic breathing and asanas were the starting point for a better life, with more positive health, continued healing, and wellbeing. Several of them characterized this as the beginning of better self-care and personal development through a more yogic life.

In another recent article, Bhavanani suggests that "This concept of positive health is one of Yoga's unique contributions to modern health care as Yoga has both a preventive as well as promotive role in the health care of our masses" ([9], p. 19). It also seemed that Yoga contributed to a Sense of Coherence (SoC) in the course participants' lives, where their world was experienced as meaningful, understandable, and manageable as emphasized in the Salutogenic perspective also shared in the course (see Ref. [5]). It seemed like the new concepts, practices, and reflective discussions, together with the ability to try out and write about their experiences contributed to the SoC experience. Tools like self-reflection, yogic breathing, and yogic asanas provided awareness, motivation, and visions about a better health and life. More tools for self-awareness, personal development, coping with stress, and self-care are needed in educations settings, especially for students who will work with people (as clients, employees, or students), or those who are already in such professions, like most of our course participants were. Then, improved health and happiness/wellbeing are within reach.

Conflict of interest

The authors declare no conflict of interest.

Thanks

Thank you to all the participants of the course used as a case example! We also express our gratitude to the Gitananda Rishi-culture Yoga Tradition, a holistic and humanistic lineage of Classical Indian yoga.

Note

Our translation of the course title into English is slightly different from our translations, to make it more in line with the intentions of the course.

Appendices

Appendix I

Simple Hatha yoga practice.
Sukha Asana with Sukha Pranayama (contemplation).
Jatis.
Tapping.
Rub hands and cover the eyes.
Vajra Asana with Mukha Bhastrika.
Brahma Mudra (Sukha or Vajra Asana).
Chatus Pada.
Trikona Asana.
Vriksha Asana.
Rishikesh Surya Namaskar.
Dwi Pada Uttana Asana with Savitri Pranayama.
Sarvanga Asana and Viparita Karana Mudra.
Hala Asana.
Paschimottanasana.
Baddhakona Asana and Kriya.
Vakra Asana.
Kapalabhati.
Kaya Kriya.
Shava Asana with Savitri Pranayama

Appendix II

Practical exercise in self-reflection.
Swadhyaya: Reflect on our reaction pattern (own thoughts, feelings, and behaviors) and response in interaction with others.

1. Who are you? Why do you behave the way you do, toward yourself and toward others? Are your actions good (ethical) or bad?

2. How are your thoughts; Are they idealistic and positive, or selfish and negative? What about your feelings?

3. What are your lifestyle habits like, in relation to diet, sleep, and what you spend time and energy on?

4. Common: What are your values and goals in life, and do you live in line with these?

Appendix III

Practices of Pranayama or Yogic Breath.
Sukha Asana and Pranayama – slowly, 6 in 6 out, through the nose.
Jathis, Tapping,
Rub hands and cover the eyes.
Vajra Asana with Mukha Bhastrika.
Vibhaga Pranayama – the ABC of Pranayama.
Vibhaga Pranayama – sectional breathing, with Sparsha Mudra.
Adham Pranayama – focus on the lower parts of the lungs.
Madhyam Pranayama – focus on the mid part of the lungs.
Adhyam Pranayama - focus on the upper part of the lungs.
Mahat Yoga Pranayama – complete breath.
Nishpanda – Makara Asana, Bhujanga Asana, Shashankar Asana.
Vibhaga Pranayma with Hasta Mudras and Sound (Nada).
Adhama Pranayama with Chin Mudra, A.
Madhyama Pranayama with Chin Maya Mudra, O.
Adhyama Pranayama with Adhi Mudra, M.
Brahma Mudra with Pranava AOM (OM).
Nishpanda – Makara Asana, Bhujanga Asana, Shashankar Asana.
Brahmari.
Kaya Kriya – Sukha Pranayama.
Shavasana – Savitri Pranayama, 6 x 3 x 6 x 3.
Marmanasthanam Kriya (22 body parts relaxation)

Appendix IV

Reflection exercise linked to the experience of stress

1. What makes you stressed?

2. How do you react when you are stressed?

3. How do you cope with or handle stress?

4. Common: What are fruitful ways to cope with stress?

Author details

Ingunn Hagen[1*] and Ananda Balayogi Bhavanani[2]

1 Department of Psychology, Norwegian University of Science and Technology (NTNU), Trondheim, Norway

2 Institute of Salutogenesis and Complementary Medicine (ISCM), Sri Balaji Vidyapeeth (SBV), Pondicherry, India

*Address all correspondence to: ingunn.hagen@ntnu.no

References

[1] Bhavanani AB, Sullivan M, Taylor MJ, Wheeler A. Shared foundations for practice: The language of yoga therapy. Yoga Therapy Today. 2019:44-48. Available from: www.iayt.org

[2] Bhavanani AB, Ramanathan M, Dayanidy G, Balaji R, editors. Yoga Therapy for Care Seekers. A Monograph Compiled and Published by Institute of Salutogenesis and Complementary Medicine (ISCM), Sri Balaji Vidyapeeth (SBV); 2023

[3] Gitananda S. Yoga: Step-by-Step. Pondicherry, India: Satya Press; 1981

[4] Antonovsky A. Health, Stress and Coping. San Francisco: Josey-Bass; 1979

[5] Mittelmark MB, Bauer GF. Salutogenesis as a theory, as an orientation and as a sense of coherence. In: Mittelmark MB, Bauer GF, Vaandrager L, Pelikan JM, Sagy S, Eriksson M, Lindström B, Magistretti CM, editors. The Handbook of Salutogenesis. 2nd ed. Springer: Open Access; 2022. pp. 11-19. Available from: https://library.oapen.org/handle/20.500.12657/52407

[6] Seligman M. Authentic Happiness: Using the New Positive Psychology to Realize your Full Potential. New York: Atria paperbacks; 2002

[7] Seligman M. Flourish. A New Understanding of Happiness and Well-Being and How to Achieve Them. Boston and London: Nicholas Brealey Publishing; 2011

[8] Bhavanani AB. Understanding the yoga Darshan. In: An Exploration of the Yoga Sutra of Maharishi Patanjali. Puducherry: Dhivyananda Creations; 2011

[9] Bhavanani AB. Exploring yoga Chikitsa and positive health. Yoga Life. 2024;**55**(04):17-27. Available from: www.rishiculture.in

[10] Jnandev Y. The Yoga Sutras of Maharishi Patanjali. Great Britain: Design Marque; 2019

[11] Hagen I, Skjelstad S, Nayar US. Promoting mental health and wellbeing in schools: The impact of yoga on young people's relaxation and stress levels. Frontiers in Psychology. 2023;**14**:1083028. DOI: 10.3389/fpsyg.2023.1083028. Available from: https://www.frontiersin.org/journals/psychology/articles/10.3389/fpsyg.2023.1083028/full

[12] Hagen I. How can social expectations and related stress among adolescents and young adults be better coped with through practicing yoga? In: Herzog S, editor. The Social Contexts of Young People - Engaging Youth and Young Adults. London, UK: IntechOpen; 2024. ISBN 978-0-85014-046-0. Available from: https://www.intechopen.com/chapters/88811

[13] Hagen I, Hagen Ø. The impact of yoga on occupational stress and wellbeing: Exploring practitioners' experiences. Frontiers in Public Health. 2024;**12**:1-16. Available from: https://www.frontiersin.org/journals/publichealth/articles/10.3389/fpubh.2024.1352197/full

[14] Yogendra J. Cyclopaedia yoga Vol. I. In: All about Asanas and 100 More Topics. 1st ed. Santacruz: The Yoga Institute; 2013. p. 1988

[15] Selye H. Perspectives in stress research. Perspectives in Biology and Medicine. 1959;**2**(4):403-416. DOI: 10.1353/pbm.1959.0000

[16] Bhavanani AB. Stress and Relaxation: A Yogic Approach. Integral Yoga Magazine; 2016. Available from: https://integralyogamagazine.org/stress-relaxation-yogic-approach/

[17] Bhogal RS. Yoga and mental health and beyond. In: A Guide to Self-Management. Lonavla: Kaivalyadhama; 2010

[18] Bhavanani AB. Yoga and cultural misappropriation. In: Based on a Scintillating Saturday Talk. Pondicherry: Dhivyananda Creations; 2021

[19] Hagen I. Lykkeverktøy for Fagfolk Som Jobbar Med Menneske (Happiness Tools for Professionals Who Work with Human Beings). Oslo: Cappelen Damm; 2018. Available from: https://utdanning.cappelendamm.no/_lykkeverktoy-ingunn-hagen-9788202567538

[20] Gitananda S. Pranayama. In: Ananda B, Bhavanani MD, editors. The Fourth Limb of Ashtanga Yoga. An Understanding of Pranayama Based on Gitananda Yoga Teachings in the Tradition of Rishiculture Ashtanga Yoga. Pondicherry: Satya Press; 2008

[21] Bhavanani AB, Bhavanani YD. The importance of Pranayama in yogic discipline. In: Gitananda YS, editor. Pranayama. The Fourth Limb of Ashtanga Yoga. (An understanding of Pranayama Based on Gitananda Yoga Teachings in the Tradition of Rishiculture Ashtanga Yoga.) Contributors and Editors: Bhavanani, Ananda B. and M. D. Bhavanani. Pondicherry: Satya Press; 2008. pp. 29-43

[22] Yogendra J. Cyclopedia Yoga Vol. III, (with Information on the Application of Yogic Approach in the Management of Stress, Psychosomatic and Psychogenetic Diseases). The Yoga Institute: Santa Cruz/Bombay; 2010

[23] Majewski L, Bhavanani AB. Yoga Therapy as a Whole-Person Approach to Health. London: Jessica Kingsley Publishers/Singing Dragon; 2020

Chapter 9

Perspective Chapter: Maternally Centered Social Ecosphere – South Slavic Women's Transgenerational Trauma – Female Biology – A Feminist Perspective through the Lens of Kolo-Informed Trauma

Danica Anderson

Abstract

This chapter explores the intersections of female biology, cultural oral memory practices, and transgenerational trauma healing in the context of healthcare and trauma recovery. Drawing on the experiences of South Slavic women war crimes and war survivors, it introduces the Maternally Centered Social Ecosphere (MCSE) as a foundational framework for mental and physical health interventions. The MCSE integrates epigenetics, neurobiology, and social engagement, offering a holistic model for trauma recovery. The chapter advocates for incorporating female-centered knowledge systems into healthcare to create inclusive and effective interventions. By bridging cultural traditions and healthcare sciences, this approach underscores the biopsychosocial impact of female biology and collective healing practices. In this chapter, an exploration on the intricate relationship between female biology, cultural oral memory practices, and transgenerational trauma healing through the experiences of South Slavic women war crimes and war survivors is outlined. By examining the maternal-centered social ecosphere (MCSE) and the South Slavic oral memory practices, this study underscores the transformative potential of integrating biological inheritance into the transmission of cultural continuity across generations.

Keywords: homeostasis, polyvagal, female-biology, epigenetic, oral memory

1. Introduction

This issue is not defined solely by the absence of women, but by the systemic erasure of maternally-centered ecospheres that has long been the foundation of cultural continuity, adaptation-evolving to healing [1]. Current findings highlight the role of female biology, social epigenetics-memory gene [2, 3], and neuroplasticity in shaping individual and collective adaptation and healing. The chapter advocates for the incorporation of female-centered knowledge systems into trauma research to create inclusive and effective interventions and preventions [4].

The devastation of war extends beyond physical destruction; it deeply alters biological and psychological health across generations. In post-war Bosnia and Herzegovina, South Slavic women's oral memory practices and maternal-centered healing traditions play a crucial role in healthcare interventions for trauma recovery. This chapter presents the still viable traditional cultural and social oral memory practices paradigm with adjustments for modern day conflict, wars and violence adaptations to move from survival to flourishing. Healing through the maternally-centered social ecosphere (MCSE) involves integrating female biology, epigenetics, and cultural practices communal healing traditions as critical components of trauma-informed healthcare.

When I first arrived in Bosnia in 1998, the journey from the Sarajevo airport to nearby towns revealed a landscape of profound devastation—homes reduced to rubble, railways dismantled, and entire communities fractured. These targeted structures were not merely physical but also symbolic of the maternallycentered social ecosphere (MCSE), representing cultural continuity and biological harmony [5]. The ruins of Sarajevo and its rural surroundings stood as a testament to the relentless wars that have ravaged the region for a century, undermining the foundations of female biology and its role in sustaining life. The Balkan War rape camps, where the Yugoslav War Crimes Tribunal finally declared rape a war crime, highlighted the systemic violence against women [6]. Despite such declarations, sex trafficking has become a global issue perpetuated by non-state actors in the aftermath of wars [7].

Institutionalized violence against women centers on targeting the maternal ecosphere, since it is an evolutionary homeostasis. Evolutionary homeostasis according to Wheeler is "living totalities in which life of the whole exceeds the sum of the parts; individuals are phenomenologically embodied and embedded in culture and nature which must be seen as inextricably intertwined and co-dependent and co-evolving" ([8, 9], p. 41). However, the legacy of institutionalized violence against women, particularly in the context of the Balkan War, has created unique challenges for the South Slavic women war survivors [8, 10, 11].

My forensic traumatology training, rooted in understanding trauma across psychological, sociocultural, and biological dimensions, felt insufficient against the stark realities of war's impact on women and marginalized groups. In my fieldwork with South Slavic women war crimes and war survivors in the aftermath of the Balkan War (1991–1995), I reconnected with an innate understanding that healing trauma required a nature communal, embodied approach: the maternally centered social ecosphere, deeply embedded in the Slavic concept of Moist Mother Earth [12, 13].

My experiences as a first-generation Serbian immigrant and the daughter of a WWII Jasenovac concentration camp survivor shaped my awareness of transgenerational trauma [4]. While my family lacked a visible maternally centered social ecosphere as 'displaced persons', remnants of this framework were present in Serbian Orthodox Church rituals, including the Slavic Kolo—a round folk-dance or to be socially engaged in a circle-communal collective embodying oral memory and communal solidarity [14, 15]. In the aftermath of violence and war, there is a need for maternally-centered ecospheres and safe spaces for the excluded, females, the gendered, since what is revealing are the limitations imposed by patriarchal structures.

Given the noticeably absent maternally-centered social ecosphere, it is also absent in western genomic and psychology research. However, I witnessed its visible remnants in Bosnia Hercegovina (BiH), where the Muslim women war crimes and war survivors organized oral memory social engagement rituals such as the Slavic kolo—a communal practice of embodied circular movement or folk dance—and food-centered gatherings. These moments provided brief respites from the relentless demand to survive as females confined to specific sanctioned patriarchal roles.

2. Understanding MCSE in healthcare contexts

MCSE is not merely a cultural construct; it is a biological, psychological, and social framework that impacts gene expression, nervous system regulation, and collective trauma healing. Rooted in epigenetics and neurobiology, MCSE offers a non-pathologizing perspective on trauma, positioning it as an intensified learning process rather than a disorder [4, 16].

The overview framework of maternally-centered social ecosphere resides in the following:

- Epigenetics and Trauma Transmission: Research shows that trauma-induced epigenetic changes are inherited across generations, affecting immune response, stress regulation, and neurological health [17].

- Neurobiological Implications: Polyvagal theory underscores social engagement as a key mechanism for trauma healing. MCSE regulates autonomic states through communal and embodied practices [18].

- Psychosomatic Health and Cultural Healing: The integration of oral memory traditions, kolo-informed trauma therapy, and maternal fright healing rituals provides a biocultural blueprint for trauma interventions.

MCSE is not merely a cultural construct; it is a biological, psychological, and social framework that impacts gene expression, nervous system regulation, and collective trauma healing. Rooted in epigenetics and neurobiology, MCSE offers a female cross-cultural position that is a non-pathologizing perspective on trauma, defining trauma as an intensified learning process rather than a disorder [4].

Epigenetics and Trauma Transmission: Research shows that trauma-induced epigenetic changes are inherited across generations, affecting immune response, stress regulation, and neurological health [19]. For example, studies on Holocaust survivors and their descendants indicate that heightened stress responses persist across generations [11]. Similarly, South Slavic women war crimes and war survivors have experienced maternal fright, which has led to increased anxiety disorders and metabolic changes in their offspring [4, 8, 14]. This illustrates how trauma is not just a psychological imprint but is biologically embedded in future generations. The MCSE framework seeks to address these epigenetic imprints by integrating culturally rooted healing practices that work alongside the body's natural regulatory systems [20].

Neurobiological Implications: According to Polyvagal Theory, social engagement is a key mechanism for trauma healing [18]. When trauma disrupts the autonomic nervous system, individuals may become trapped in hyperarousal (fight-or-flight) or shutdown (freeze response). The MCSE supports trauma survivors by restoring their ability to co-regulate through embodied practices specifically through social engagement. South Slavic women engage in the Kolo, a communal round dance that fosters a sense of connection, rhythm, and predictability—signaling safety to the nervous system [4]. This practice aids in transitioning individuals from survival states to states of neurobiological balance. Healthcare interventions that integrate such communal and movement-based therapies could significantly improve outcomes for trauma survivors suffering from PTSD and other stress-related disorders [21].

Psychosomatic Health and Cultural Healing: Trauma is often stored in the body, manifesting in chronic pain, autoimmune disorders, and reproductive health complications [22]. The MCSE framework acknowledges that oral memory traditions, kolo-informed trauma therapy, and maternal fright healing rituals provide a biocultural blueprint for trauma interventions. In Bosnia-Herzegovina, women who experienced war-related sexual violence have reported healing benefits through social engagement rituals such as storytelling and traditional bioculinary practices, which help regulate the nervous system and restore psychosomatic health [4]. Integrating these cultural practices into trauma recovery programs in healthcare settings would create a more all-inclusive and effective model of care, particularly for war survivors and displaced women. By incorporating these perspectives, MCSE advances a healthcare model that moves beyond individual treatment toward collective healing, integrating cultural knowledge with scientific approaches to trauma recovery.

3. Female biology and transgenerational trauma

The intersection of female biology and trauma reveals the pivotal role of the XX chromosome shaping human adaptation and survival [16]. Superior in its ability to give rise to both XX and XY offspring, the XX chromosome drives evolutionary processes and sustains cultural and diversity continuity [23]. Female biology, including the unbroken mitochondrial DNA line passed from mother to daughter, embodies a biological repository of life experiences [24]. This tacit knowledge[1] informs adaptive responses to trauma, fostering a movement from the survival mechanism of resilience toward growth ([4], pp. 28–30, 44). Thus, my tacit knowledge defines trauma not as a mental illness rather it is an intensified learning scape [4]. While no one chooses to endure trauma, the Slavic expression 'in life there is death and in death there is life' emphasizes the necessity to the need of MCSE for adaptations and evolving.

Epigenetics, the study of heritable changes in gene expression influenced by environmental factors, underscores the interconnectedness of biology and lived experiences. For example. Rosalynn A. Vegas research on mitochondrial memory-transgenerational trauma stated, "autoethnographic anecdotes highlighting the struggles of immigrant women of color—women Donna Haraway might refer to as "cyborg entities" (1991, p. 149)—thereby framing mitochondrial memory as formed through "naturecultural" and intersectional "intra-actions" [27].

Epigenetics does not alter the DNA's fundamental code but instead modifies which genes can be activated or silenced based on life experiences and environmental factors. This dynamic biological process enables individuals to adapt by integrating the lived experiences of past generations into present-day survival and adaptation

[1] Tacit Knowledge - Trauma—an event without precedent—lacks immediate vocabulary. Healing emerges through socially engaged practices that construct meaning, neuroplastic narratives over time [25]. For example, the maternal bonding role, influenced by the female-specific oxytocin hormone—which is present in significantly higher amounts in females compared to males—plays a critical part in nurturing infants through to adulthood [26]. This process demonstrates how non-verbal communication evolves into shared understanding, forming the foundation for adaptive behaviors and social connections.

strategies. Essentially, epigenetic changes reflect the capacity to reauthor memory through adaptive mechanisms, moving beyond survival toward transformation. When examining South Slavic women war crimes and war survivors, their tacit knowledge and their oral memory practices reveals an intrinsic understanding of this epigenetic biological process—demonstrating how ancestral life experiences shape present realities and inform future adaptation.

A recent study in the *Journal of Molecular Psychiatry* examined the epigenetic changes in the sperm cells of men who endured severe childhood stress [28]. This study illustrates the interplay of trauma and epigenetic adaptation, shedding light on the profound impact of early life stressors on gene expression. The findings reveal that these epigenetic changes are not only persistent over decades but also transgenerational, influencing subsequent generations.

This aligns with the maternally centered partnership inherent in female biology, which fosters healing and adaptation across generations. Through oral memory practices, South Slavic women have demonstrated the capacity to integrate these epigenetic shifts into their cultural frameworks, transforming trauma into a vehicle for growth and evolution. As Marianne Guenot from *Live Science* notes, "Uncovering any associations between these stressors and epigenetics is absolutely fascinating because the stressors happened early in the men's lives. This suggests that the epigenetic changes persisted over time, despite decades passing since the events that would have initially triggered them" [29]. These findings underscore the enduring transgenerational nature of epigenetic modifications and their critical role in shaping both individual and communal social engagement within a maternal-centered ecosphere.

Social epigenetics extends this framework, exploring how nature cultural practices and societal conditions shape genetic expressions across generations [27]. For South Slavic women, oral memory practices center on the social engagement serving as mechanisms for encoding and transmitting adaptive responses to trauma [4].

Essentially, female biology fosters a partnership with the XY chromosome, ensuring adaptability through the interplay of genetic diversity and maternal ecosystems. Epigenetic mechanisms and tacit knowledge—the unspoken-teleonomy[2], innate understanding derived from life experiences—serve as a collective memory, molding human evolution through transgenerational adaptation thus evolving and transforming [30]. This interconnectedness highlights the role of women as creators of culture, leveraging both biological and social knowledge to guide communities from survival to thriving [31].

4. Oral memory practices and the maternal ecosphere

Mental Health Benefits of Oral Memory Practices utilized with the women who survived war crimes and armed conflict encompass memory gene activation. Recent studies suggest that non-neural cells store trauma memories, supporting oral traditions as a form of somatic healing [5, 19]. In my two decades plus of Kolo informed trauma practices revealed a cognitive pliability in the use of oral memory practices, rituals to traditions such as their storytelling. By engaging in oral memory transmission, it activates neural plasticity, improving cognitive function and emotional regulation [22].

[2] *Teleonomy* success *over* time: close social cooperation, *adaptive*... Teleonomy is also an implicit (though *unspoken*) influence in ... system to respond to variability and *changing* conditions [30].

Since interconnectedness underscores women's role as the architects of culture, drawing from both biological and social knowledge to guide communities beyond mere survival, patriarchal constraints impose severe and often devastating barriers—denying the recognition that females are not an extension of mankind but the essence of humankind [31]. What became evident among the Bosnian women war crimes and war survivors in my field work was their ability to cultivate a sense of safety within their communities through oral memory social engagements, forging spaces of connection and continuity amidst the remnants of war [4]. By participating in the maternal ecosphere via the psychodynamic oral memory embodied practices [32], women reinforce social bonds, process trauma collectively, and create an environment of safety and support [33]. Oral memory practices embedded in the maternal ecosphere integrate cultural and biological knowledge, transforming trauma into a resource for communal recovery [34, 35].

Maternal fright, a phenomenon deeply rooted in South Slavic oral memory traditions, illustrates the neurobiological impact of transgenerational trauma [35]. A young pregnant woman from Bosnia shared her experience of maternal fright, describing the epigenetics involving genocide and her husband's childhood experiencing the war crimes influenced her pregnancy [34]. Unable to find an existing oral memory ritual or possibly to author a more adaptive remedy to protect her unborn child, she created a new practice by drawing a spiral on her belly, symbolizing Slavic thaumaturgy [17, 34]. This act demonstrates the psychodynamic epigenetic spiritual earth-based nature of oral memory traditions, evolving to address contemporary challenges.

While maternal fright cannot change any person's specific DNA blueprint, traumatic stress and experiences award a point where heritable traits may become malleable through trauma-induced alterations in gene expression [36]. Similar to a toggle switch, the brain tangibly identifies the trauma exposure and distinguishes transgenerational trauma susceptibility requiring prevention and intervention [15, 18]. For South Slavic women and women cross culturally enduring violence, conflict to wars, the maternal ecosphere and their wombs have become tombs eradicating their social epigenetic oral memory practices [34]. However, the women's tacit knowledge interconnecting the biological and environment's so-called causal events play a role in shaping female biology thus human not mankind biology.

5. The Kolo-informed trauma (KIT) framework

Through the use of oral memory, what was observed was a community-centered interventions and preventions concerning PTSD & War Trauma [4, 27]. Healthcare models can integrate MCSE practices into PTSD treatments:

- Group healing retreats: Socially engaged, female-centered retreats (modeled after South Slavic communal healing circles-kolo) support emotional recalibration [14, 18].

- Bioculinary interventions: Traditional foods, seed-sharing practices, and nourishment rituals reinforce nutritional epigenetics in trauma recovery [15, 35].

Kolo-Informed Trauma (KIT) provides a model for integrating female-centered biological, social epigenetics, and cultural knowledge into clinical trauma approaches and research [2]. By emphasizing the interconnectedness of nature and nurture, KIT redefines trauma as intensified learning rather than pathology [14]. This perspective shifts the focus from survival to growth, aligning with the polyvagal theory, which highlights the role of social engagement in regulating the nervous system while igniting neural plasticity [18].

Through KIT sessions, South Slavic women war survivors reclaimed their narratives and reconnected with their cultural oral memory roots. For instance, women-only engendered retreats organized in post-war Bosnia offered a space for laughter, storytelling, and communal healing [4, 12, 37]. These gatherings revealed the importance of culturally embedded oral memory practices in addressing the unique needs of trauma survivors.

Building upon this understanding, my research on Kolo-Informed Trauma (KIT), bioculinary, and biosemiotics reveals the profound interconnection between nutrition, epigenetics, and cultural continuity [4, 15]. The maternal ecosphere does not function in isolation and is nourished through the rituals of food agrarian, foraging to preparation, consumption, and the shared oral memory embedded in these practices [4].

The South Slavic women war crimes and war survivors not only preserved the medicinal integrity of their cultural cuisine but understood on an intrinsic level that the epigenome operates as a dynamic neuroplastic system [2], one that records life experiences, environmental exposures, and, critically, the lived memories sustenance that sustains bodies across generations [34].

With my informed trauma research in Bosnia and Herzegovina, I observed how food served as both a medicinal survival necessity and an adaptive epigenetic tool. Nutritional epigenetic programming, including the concept of "epigenetic drift," underscores how daily dietary choices imprint themselves upon the body's metabolic memory, thus the epigenome, influencing long-term health outcomes [38]. Recognizing this, I facilitated therapeutic interventions rooted in cultural foodways—securing donations for seed banks, ensuring access to traditional cuisines such as coffee, and organizing communal trips to the coast where the women could reconnect with the embodied rituals of nourishment [34]. These bioculinary and biosemiotic engagements reinforced the women's adaptive mechanisms, transforming food into a form of healing, one that extends beyond mere sustenance to an active agent of social epigenetic cultural preservation [15].

6. Maternally centered epigenetic cross talk biological sex-XX and XY, gendered

I examine the intersection of biological sex—XX and XY—gendered trauma and cultural healing through the lived experiences of South Slavic women who have survived war crimes and systemic violence. Gender, as imposed by patriarchal systems, defines the societal expectations placed on women, the engendered, and shapes their perceived roles and behaviors. These survivors illustrate how transgenerational trauma could transform and evolve maternal epigenetic inheritance. This highlights how life experiences shape epigenetic memory, highlighting the intrinsic relationship between female biology and culture [2].

Epigenetics, with its transgenerational properties, describes the genomic mechanisms through which environmental and life experiences encode changes in gene expression without altering DNA sequences [28]. The XX chromosome—superior in its ability to give rise to both XX and XY offspring—is pivotal to driving evolutionary processes, ensuring gender-specific diversity and species survival.

Given that epigenetics is the core of a lifelong series of feedback loops linking the environment to the human genome, XX, Xy and gendered [39], epigenetics operates as a dynamic interface between the environment and the human genome, functioning as a series of interconnected feedback loops that enable constant dialog between lived experience and biological inheritance. Within a maternally centered framework, this process is not passive but an active, adaptive mechanism partnership of XX, Xy, and gendered—one that shapes and reshapes gene expression based on the environment's demands [40].

While, the XX genome, as the foundational biological template, carries an unbroken line of mitochondrial DNA, epigenetic transmission, encoding not just survival mechanisms but the necessary adaptations for thriving across generations. The latter requires partnership, diversity inclusive of XX, Xy and gendered [19]. However, the impact of trauma—transgenerational, cultural, environmental—disrupts these adaptive processes, embedding stress, fear, and systemic oppression into the epigenome, influencing not only individual health but communal survival. The strategic targeting of women, gender-diverse individuals and children are strategic targets of conflict and wars represents a transgenerational trauma in the modern world. It is noted that the impact is not on just XX, but Xy and the gendered [22].

7. Kolo-informed trauma (KIT) highlights how the maternal ecosphere

Kolo-Informed Trauma (KIT) highlights how the maternal ecosphere, through gendered, maternally centered social engagements, plays a critical role in regulating epigenetic states. These epigenetic markers are not simply inherited but are influenced by cultural, environmental, and nutritional factors, shaping the biological function and health of both current and future generations. Nutritional epigenetics—integral to bioculinary and biosemiotic oral memory traditions [15], emphasizes how food, a maternal-gendered knowledge system, serves as an epigenetic modulator, reinforcing the stability of the ecosystem within which the genome exists.

Despite its critical role in species survival and adaptation, female biology has long been relegated to the margins, dismissed or erased entirely within male-default sciences [41]. Women's embodied, experiential knowledge, particularly in trauma adaptation, healing, and transgenerational inheritance—has at best been disparaged and, at worst, systematically eliminated through patriarchal misogyny [42]. The unending survival mechanism, resilience narrative demanded in patriarchy [17], often imposed on women within trauma studies, fails to acknowledge the broader systemic violence that necessitates adaptation in the first place [41].

Understanding these mechanisms is crucial in dismantling male-default scientific paradigms [41] that overlook the epigenetic agency of the XX genome in shaping species evolution, adaptation, and the transgenerational inheritance of knowledge. The epigenetic cross-talk and XX requires the gylanic partnership—all in sync—to sustain the survival and evolution of the human species [36]. Diversity is key here, as the maternal ecosystem, in its intricate biological and cultural functions, fosters adaptability, ensuring the genetic and social variability necessary for an evolving, thriving species [43]. Without this interconnected, maternally centered foundation, the very fabric of human adaptation and survival is at risk.

8. Gender and the patriarchal colonization of knowledge

Gender, as imposed by patriarchal systems and male-default sciences [41], colonizes the societal expectations placed on women but also shapes gendered perceived roles and behaviors [44]. For example, patriarchal biopolitics has labeled dance, the Slavic Kolo, and Hora oral memory practices as cultural tourism activities. This patriarchal colonization demeans and neglects the "main functions of ritual dance in folklore culture: to convey knowledge about the structure of the world, about how to live in community, self-knowledge, knowledge about order, laws, and governance of society..." (Anna Ilieva, [12], pp. 309–10).

However, these South Slavic women war crimes and war survivors move past this colonization, illustrating how transgenerational trauma transforms and evolves through maternal epigenetic inheritance. Life experiences influence the epigenetic memory gene, highlighting the intrinsic relationships of XY and gendered identities within female biology and culture [5, 45].

For example, authors Barbra Mann and Kaarina Kailo, in their book citing the Slavic epigenome spirituality of Ancient Foremothers, consider the bear themes of birth, water, and earth goddesses as cross-cultural variants in wisdom traditions. Wisdom memory traditions are the tacit knowledge of our epigenome. The authors report that women—through female biology and gendered diversity—were highly appreciated as the first shamans and healers [46]. However, under the influence of colonialism and its interpolation of patriarchal values, this recognition of female biological and spiritual wisdom was systematically diminished [13, 46].

The women war crimes and war survivors report the Kolo, folk round dance, is the earliest origins of somatic psychology and neurobiology. What is translated is that movements that sync each other heal social communities and flourish strong social collectives. The women survivors reported the troika of breath, air, and wind. One of the largest volumes of mass on the Earth is the transparent air. The women survivors pointed to the breath work in dancing Kolos offers up a trance inducing harmony with the Moist Mother Earth so as to birth goddess Sophia—wisdom.

Then, the reverence for the bird goddess that in former Yugoslav region contains thousands of zoomorphic bird goddess artifacts [12] and the migration of birds at the equinox by ancient South Slavic shamkas (all Shamans were female in the beginning) understands the bird's ability to fan the wind, break wind so to speak, and to see what is invisible with such great trust in their leaping off into invisible without a map save for embedded instincts or cellular memory. The women war crimes and war survivors emphatically state that what matters is not the number of breaths one has in life but rather how has one inhaled and exhaled each breath of air and where it was inhaled or exhaled [34].

By fostering the women war crimes and war survivors' epigenetic memory and tacit knowledge of a stable genomic foundation, the XX chromosome contributes to both immediate survival mechanisms and long-term evolutionary advancements. This dynamic, rooted in the symbiotic relationship between XX and XY chromosomes, emphasizes the complementary roles they play in human adaptation-evolution and survival [47]. While the XX chromosome supports female longevity for the survival of the species, the XY chromosome introduces genetic mutations, inherited diseases such as sickle cell to celiac however the XY is essential for diversity, such as gendered, to eye color for evolution [48].

9. The unbroken line from mother to daughter, is sustained via epigenetics transgenerational memory infrastructure

The XX chromosome not only embodies the foundation of female biology but also sustains female indigenous ways of knowing. It is female biology when somatically interpreted refer to as female indigenous ways of knowing. Standing center in indigenous ways of knowing is the DNA mitochondria, the unbroken line from mother to daughter, is sustained via epigenetics transgenerational memory infrastructure [27].

Therefore, the XX chromosome serves as the biological foundation of female life, carrying within it an intricate system of adaptation, knowledge transmission, and survival strategies. Beyond its genetic function, it sustains female indigenous ways of knowing—embodied, somatically expressed, and preserved through transgenerational memory [38]. For example, the mitochondrial DNA, passed exclusively from mother to daughter, forms an unbroken lineage that operates as an epigenetic infrastructure, encoding the lived experiences of generations [36].

The XX chromosome is not merely a genetic sequence but an ecospheric blueprint—a dynamic map guiding adaptation, survival, and evolution in partnership with the XY chromosome [23]. This partnership, rather than a hierarchy, is an intricate process of engendering, shaping communal and biological evolution, including the full spectrum of gender diversity [27]. The existence of LGBTQIA+ identities is not an aberration but an integral part of this evolutionary process, rooted in the adaptability of human biology and cultural homeostasis [49]. Essential to female biology is a continuously evolving transgenerational memory blueprint—one that fosters adaptive responses within a living partnership with all life.

For example, the shamkas botanical knowledge in the nearby Mountains, Mt. Vlasic, the site of the 1984 Winter Olympics, the women war crimes and war survivors referred to transgenerational trauma that male perpetrators have to a plant. It is the Trava Iva- Teucrium montanum known as "sallow a Deadman alive" which grows in mountainous regions around the world used for mental and physical recovery after long illness, trauma to the body and mental exhaustion [34].

Another reference the Slavic war survivors cited often was the troika. Breath, air, wind. One of the largest volumes of mass on Earth is the transparent air. The women survivors report a shamanic breath work in dancing kolos offers up a trance inducing harmony with the Moist Mother Earth to bring us face to face with Sophia-wisdom [34]. The reverence for the bird goddess and the migration of birds at the equinox by ancient South Slavic shamkas (all Shamans were female in the beginning) understands the bird's ability to fan the wind, break wind so to speak, and to see what is invisible with such great trust in their leaping off into invisible without a map save for embedded instincts or cellular memory. This was in reference to being one of the three million women and children refugees flooding Europe during the Balkan War [50]. Often, I was asked to think of how the seasonal birds' migration know when and where to go. The women reported that what matters is not the number of breaths one has in life but rather how has one inhaled and exhaled each breath of air and where it was inhaled or exhaled.

Within, the simple but complex female biology and the tacit knowledge of the South Slavic traditions, this interconnectivity is reflected in the concept of Moist Mother Earth, a cultural and biological affirmation of the female body's role as both creator and sustainer of life, encompassing the fluid and expansive nature of gender beyond binary constraints [4, 13].

10. Female indigenous ways of knowing

Female biology fosters a partnership with the XY chromosome, ensuring adaptability through the interplay of genetic diversity and maternal ecosystems. Epigenetic mechanisms and tacit knowledge, the unspoken, innate understanding derived from life experiences—serve as a collective memory, shaping human evolution through epigenetic (transgenerational) adaptation thus evolving and transforming [51]. Again, this interconnectedness highlights the role of women as creators of culture, leveraging both biological and social knowledge to guide communities from survival to thriving.

Through the lens of Kolo-Informed Trauma (KIT), I underscore the female indigenous knowing, MCSE cultural and biological significance of oral memory practices derived from lived experiences—shaped epigenetically—and tacit knowledge, an intuitive understanding encoded genomically, in addressing transgenerational trauma [4]. Within a cultural epigenetic analysis their Slavic oral memory practices permit genomic expression to vary right down to interpersonal procedural memory tacitly [51].

KIT highlights the significance of female biology and maternal epigenetic, transgenerational inheritance, proposing that culture is created through female biology, integrating engendered roles into a woman's collective that moves from suffering to thriving within female expertise-led communities [4]. The female led expertise are grandmothers, mothers, daughters, aunties who are the major caregivers, midwives, doctors, artists, farmers, and teachers to business owners. This makes it clear that human biology is actually cultural biology, maternally centered ecosphere based on our development, how we live or have lived in socially constructed worlds [20].

I have observed many diverse ethnicities and cultures—women who, on average, were not formally educated but demonstrated exceptional intelligence in tacit knowledge rooted in female biology [52]. I define this female biological cultural process and native intelligence as a homeostatic and empowering evolutionary adaptive mechanism [9, 53]. It enables the shift from patriarchally imposed survival strategies to thriving through inclusive socially constructed collective engagement and the application of female indigenous expertise.

In my clinical work with women war survivors in regions such as Bosnia, Sub-Saharan Africa, Haiti, Afghanistan, India, and Sri Lanka demonstrate their empowerment of female-led, community-centered healing practices [34]. Their movement from survival to thriving is also detailed by Porges' polyvagal theory, which explains how our nervous system is deeply interconnected with the environment we inhabit [18, 53]. This framework aligns with the insights gained from Kolo-Informed Trauma, highlighting the importance of culturally embedded practices that integrate female biology and maternal ecosystems creating culture with safe places and spaces [54].

11. Homeostatic: Symbiosis: Oral memory

In this context, homeostasis refers to a dynamic state of balance within biological and social epigenetic memory systems [27, 55]. It emphasizes the adaptability of individuals and communities to maintain stability and coherence in response to external or internal stressors. For South Slavic women, homeostasis is achieved through cultural and the use of oral memory relational practices that shift from survival mechanisms to a thriving state within the maternal-centered ecosphere [4, 9].

Symbiosis such as pregnancy denotes a mutually beneficial relationship and is found between different systems or entities [56]. Within the maternal ecosphere, it describes the interconnectedness between individuals, their communities, and the environment, fostering healing and cultural adaptation. Symbiosis in the use of oral memory practices enables collective growth and integration of trauma experiences into communal narratives [4, 56].

Thus, oral memory encapsulates the transmission of tacit knowledge, social memory life experiences, and cultural traditions through spoken narratives and communal practices [16]. These embodied practices, such as the Slavic Kolo, the embodied circle represented in various Slavic folk dances to a sisterhood, serve as mechanisms to preserve and evolve cultural identity, facilitate healing, and foster intergenerational intensified learning [4].

Tacit knowledge refers to the unspoken, intuitive, and embodied understanding that is deeply rooted in lived experiences and passed through generations [57]. It often cannot be easily articulated but manifests through actions, traditions, and practices. In the context of South Slavic women, tacit knowledge encapsulates the collective wisdom and adaptive strategies developed in response to trauma, integrating cultural, biological, and emotional dimensions to inform intensified learning healing and survival [2, 58].

These embodied oral memory practices facilitate a homeostatic, a symbiosis shift from survival mechanisms to thriving by engaging with communal and relational healing processes [9, 56, 57]. Through the women war survivors' insights, I realized that trauma is best understood as a process of intensified learning and adaptation, contrasting sharply with the DSM's categorization of trauma and Post-Traumatic Stress as solely a mental illness [4, 34]. This perspective shifts institutionalized patriarchal survival mechanisms and trauma triggers into a process of adaptation and growth within women led-engendered collectives [18].

By examining oral memory practices, female and engendered somatic experiences, and informed trauma frameworks, KIT presents a model for addressing and healing trauma that transcends generations, demonstrating that women, as creators of culture, are central to enduring recovery and transformation- evolving and growth through change [14]. However, homeostasis dynamic regulation process is intricate as noted with female biology since it involves changing internal conditions required to survive or thrives but is ignored in the male default sciences [41, 59].

To this day humanitarian aid and governmental entities policies are not centered on homeostasis- MSCE corresponding to the culture and environment.

According to Kelvin J. Davies adaptive study homeostasis writes, "Adaptive Homeostasis, may be useful especially in studies of stress, toxicology, disease, and aging [60]. Relating the study to KIT in simpler terms adaptive homeostasis, as observed within the maternal-centered ecosphere, refers to the dynamic capacity of biological and social systems to adjust and recalibrate in response to changing environmental conditions [4, 60]. This process involves the temporary expansion or contraction of an individual's or community's adaptive range when exposed to external stressors or non-damaging stimuli such as transgenerational trauma-continual survival.

Within this framework, adaptive homeostasis embodies the interconnected nature of female biology and the maternal ecosphere, emphasizing the evolutionary capacity for intensified learning not transgenerational survival mechanisms for adaptation, and transformation [61]. It underscores how individuals and communities evolve beyond survival mechanisms, fostering a regenerative process that enables thriving amidst adversity [4].

12. Tacit knowledge, trauma, neurobiology of memory

Trauma—an event without precedent—lacks immediate vocabulary. Healing emerges through socially engaged practices that construct meaning, neuroplastic vocabulary narratives over time [25]. For instance, the neurobiology of memory, as Kandel explains, does not erase the original memory but layers it with new experiences and life lessons [62, 63]. This process is evident in the movement of women war crimes and war survivors from survival to flourishing, as they author new memories through intensified learning—manifested in oral memory rites, social engagement practices, thus, evolving cultural traditions [22, 34, 44].

Another example, the maternal bonding role, influenced by the female-specific oxytocin hormone—which is present in significantly higher amounts in females compared to males—plays a critical part in nurturing infants through to adulthood [26]. This process demonstrates how non-verbal communication, tacit knowledge, evolves into shared understanding, forming the prescience in biological and social complexity foundation for adaptive behaviors and social connections [5, 35, 64].

Communal socially engaged communities collectively recover and heal from transgenerational trauma through shared narratives and cultural rituals. KIT integrates oral memory practices and the embodied maternal ecosphere to redefine trauma as a neuroplastic portal for intensified learning [35]. The main question I ask of the female survivors of unmitigated violence to war crimes is, 'do you need to survive right now or thrive?'

Tacit knowledge, deeply embedded within female biology and cultural traditions, informs transgenerational responses to trauma [44]. South Slavic women war survivors have preserved this knowledge through oral herstories, resisting patriarchal silencing and reclaiming their maternal ecosphere narratives in the aftermath of a century of wars [34]. These herstories emphasize the interconnectedness of female biology—the maternal ecosphere—through personal stories and collective herstories in shaping healing responses for transgenerational trauma [4].

13. Preserving oral herstories

By documenting and preserving oral herstories, I accessed insights that may otherwise remain hidden and excluded in male-biased sciences [41, 59]. The women war crimes and war survivors' life experiences highlight the importance of rejecting superficial efforts to fund survival-focused skills- resiliency training and instead advocate for the integration of maternal ecospheres and female-centered cultural practices social engagement to build the homeostatic replete with a sense of safety into trauma research and interventions [5, 18].

According to Porges' study, he writes, "Basically, when humans feel safe, their nervous systems support the homeostatic functions of health, growth, and restoration, while they simultaneously become accessible to others without feeling or expressing threat and vulnerability. Several principles highlight the validity of a science of safety that when implemented in societal institutions, ranging from healthcare to education, would enhance health and sociality, and lead to greater productivity, creativity, and a sense of wellbeing. By respecting our need to feel safe as a biological imperative linked to survival, we respect our phylogenetic heritage and elevate sociality as a neuromodulator that functionally provides the scientific validation for a societal focus on promoting opportunities to experience feelings of safety and co-regulation" ([18], pp. 194–5).

In my exploration of how women war crimes and war survivors healed transgenerational trauma without access to mental health professionals, funding, or even basic necessities like food, their responses illuminated a profound truth. They often said, "When we had nothing, when we lost everything, I discovered I had everything" [34]. This statement encapsulates the depth of their tacit knowledge, rooted in an innate need for homeostasis with the wealth of the communal practices of the maternal-centered ecosphere. In doing so, rather being so, the women war crimes and war survivors are empowered to adapt and find healing even in the face of unimaginable loss [11, 50, 65]. Specific examples and references can further substantiate this shift from survival to thriving.

14. KIT case studies

I witnessed this realization firsthand in Novi Travnik, Bosnia, amidst the burned-out police station, bombed car skeletons, and bullet-ridden buildings. It was clear that sterile trauma therapy rooms failed to address the deep cultural and communal needs of the survivors in conflict, domestic violence to war afflicted regions environments. Healing in this context required culturally embedded practices that resonated with the lived experiences and collective traditions of the women to create homeostatic safe zones [4]. A sisterhood, the grandmother to women only, female expert led circles-kolos are homeostatic safe places [34]. Such spaces needed to prioritize relational and maternal ecosystems over detached clinical environments, fostering recovery through shared narratives, rituals, and community engagement [63].

For example, my Kolo: Women's Cross cultural Collaboration nonprofit through donations orchestrated the women only outings to the Bosnian coast city Neum. The women repeatedly asked to bring their families and spouses [34]. I refused their requests and demanded that the women spend more time caring for themselves and that in doing so, they were caring for their families.

Additionally, I recognized the necessity of organizing a KIT trauma-healing women-only social engagement. A retreat at a bed and breakfast accommodating over 20 women, located just a short walk from the beach, became an essential intervention. The stark contrast between the gutted and war-torn surroundings of Novi Travnik and the serene resort coastal city of Neum rejuvenated the women profoundly [4]. Many experienced deep, restorative sleep for the first time in years, though feelings of guilt surfaced over not sharing the trip with their families. We identified this as a 'green light' guilt—an indication of something desperately needed for their well-being.

The oral herstories memories shared during this time revealed just how long it had been since these women last laughed—many tracing it back to the years before the Balkan War. Yet, amidst the retreat, laughter was rediscovered. Bar jokes and songs erupted in crescendos of joy, their hilarity piercing through years of trauma, symbolizing a significant step toward healing. The elder of the Kolo Sumejja, remarked with a mix of curiosity and amusement, "You call this therapy?" I responded, "Yes, and all of it unfolded without a word from me [34]. It was your oral memory songs, shared laughter, and collective connection—all guided by the innate trauma expertise embedded within you."

The Slavic kolo archetypally symbolizes the collective and cyclical nature of healing, a symbiosis. Represented through communal socially engaged and engendered circle to folk dance, oral memory practices, and storytelling, the kolo embodies a socially engaged healing process rooted in cultural oral memory traditions [25].

This approach aligns with female indigenous practices worldwide, and the polyvagal nervous system emphasizing social engagement, to provide the interconnectedness of individual and community well-being [18]. By integrating kolo-informed trauma into research and clinical practice, professionals can better support individuals in their healing journey and empower them to draw on their cultural traditions and community networks for healing transgenerational trauma.

In Bosnia Herzegovina, the Kolo-informed trauma sessions were filled with oral memory rituals and traditions—food, music, dancing, and deeply serious laughter—all woven together with the sharing of herstorical narratives [15]. By building upon my KIT approach, I infused these sessions with female indigenous tacit knowledge, a profound understanding carried through generations.

My mother tongue, Serbo-Croatian, grounded my work, reflecting my family's identity as immigrants—displaced peoples (DPs) who endured slurs and marginalization. My mother, a survivor of the WWII Jasenovac concentration camp in former Yugoslavia, carried with her the profound weight of survival and adaptation [14, 15]. Her lived experiences became a cornerstone of my understanding of trauma and healing, deeply informing me of my approach to Kolo-informed trauma.

Incorporated lived experiences add to tacit knowledge, but often referred to as the intuitive, is the unwritten understanding encoded in life experiences [9]. It plays a crucial role in healing transgenerational trauma [66]. This knowledge is often conveyed by women war survivors as, "Every choice one makes—how they live, what they eat, what they cultivate, their movements, and behaviors—will reverberate through present and future generations" [34].

Such knowledge underscores the importance of integrating cultural traditions and oral memory practices into trauma studies and interventions. By embracing kolo-informed trauma, researchers and practitioners enhance their understanding of trauma and develop more effective, culturally sensitive interventions tailored to the needs of those most affected, women [4, 43, 59].

15. Maternal fright

A young pregnant woman from Bosnia-Herzegovina, visibly exhausted with dark circles under her eyes and trembling hands, epitomized the impact of maternal fright—a phenomenon deeply rooted in the South Slavic oral memory traditions and transgenerational trauma [34, 35]. This fear and trauma are both acute and chronic, shaped by a century of wars endured by the South Slavic peoples, including WWI, WWII, and the Balkan War.

As she rubbed her swollen belly, she spoke of her womb as a place of targeted violence, embodying what South Slavic women call maternal fright [35].

Maternal fright, as seen in this case, is not only a deeply personal experience but a transgenerational phenomenon sensitive to fear and trauma, absence of safe places and spaces for women [18]. Historically, natural disasters and life crises were primary drivers of epigenetic changes in oral memory traditions, fostering cultural thriving, evolving and adapting to the environment and life/death crisis at hand [36]. However, modern violence has exhausted these traditions, leaving them struggling under the weight of ongoing fear and trauma.

This oral herstory of a pregnant woman recounted how her husband lost 18 relatives in the 1993 Ahmica-Vitez genocide, where 150 Muslims, including children and the elderly, were slaughtered during morning prayers [8, 66]. Despite living five kilometers away, the trauma permeated their lives, influencing her pregnancy and the unborn child within her.

As she sought a way to protect her child, she instinctively created a new ritual to address this void in oral memory traditions. Using a green marker, she drew a spiral on her belly—a symbol of Slavic thaumaturgy or miracle-making—thus introducing a practice to ensure safety for her unborn child, the marriage bed into the evolving South Slavic oral memory traditions to combat maternal fright [35].

This case underscores the unique ways South Slavic women, lacking institutional support, generate responses to violence through cultural and biological frameworks [67]. Their experiences highlight the interplay of maternal fright, neurobiological trauma, and the enduring influence of oral memory traditions in shaping transgenerational healing practices.

16. Oral herstories Balkan war rape camps

The rape camps during the Balkan War were sites of systematic violence and trauma, targeting South Slavic women and other marginalized groups [50]. These camps symbolized patriarchal oppression, where women's bodies were weaponized to instill fear and dominance [68]. Despite these atrocities, women found ways to resist and move from survival to their maternal female biology ecosphere [69].

In these camps, older women—often doctors, or known lesbians- LGBTIQQ to midwives—played critical roles. They provided care, performed clandestine medical procedures, and shared knowledge about managing pregnancies resulting from rape [70]. Their oral memory efforts were acts of defiance and solidarity, rooted in the cultural ethos of the maternal ecosphere. These women not only survived but also preserved their cultural identity, ensuring the continuation of oral memory traditions and female biology and female solidarity collective that provided safe harbor in a rape camp [71].

In my clinical interviews and research with South Slavic women war crimes and war survivors, one elder from Travnik—a city nestled in the safe zone of Mount Vlašić, just five kilometers from Novi Travnik—spoke of a stream of over a thousand women refugees fleeing the rape camps. This elder, who had worked extensively with these refugees, highlighted the unspoken realities of survival in a patriarchal society deeply fractured by war [4].

When I inquired why I had never encountered a child born from the rape camps despite a decade of fieldwork, her response revealed the depths of the silence surrounding this trauma. She explained that women doctors and nurses in the camps had taken extraordinary measures, teaching women how to perform abortions under clandestine conditions [34]. For those who carried pregnancies to term, secrecy was paramount. The elder emphasized that discussing rape camp pregnancies or children was impossible in their patriarchal society, where systemic violence and the proliferation of post-war gangs and corrupt authorities made it unsafe for these women to reveal their rape camps experiences, their gender identities or children's origins [34].

17. Embodied tacit knowledge and the role of epigenetics

A critical component of the maternal ecosphere is tacit knowledge—an embodied transgenerational consciousness thus understanding that emerges from lived experience [53]. The oral herstories add to tacit knowledge and enhance the role of epigenetics.

Tacit knowledge represents a neuroplastic form of cellular memory that cannot be easily articulated but is deeply felt and intuitively understood by those within the community [21, 72]. For the South Slavic women, this knowledge is not merely intellectual; it is a visceral, bodily awareness that is transmitted through the maternal line, encoded in both biological and cultural forms [17]. Similarly, trauma lacks a vocabulary for what never happened before, while tacit knowledge does not require words.

Tacit knowledge is an unwritten but genomically written epigenetic understanding encoded in life experiences [21, 72]. I continue to observe how female biological cultural plays a crucial role in healing transgenerational trauma derived from the violence against genders and women and strategic target of rape to a century of wars for South Slavs [73]. This neuro-plastic homeostasis knowledge is often conveyed by women war survivors as cultural oral memory impacts, "We are all flesh for memory to be created replacing bad memories of my grandmother and mother before me" ([4, 34], p. 6–7).

What the women war survivors neuro-plastic homeostasis knowledge conveys describes and defines neuro-plastic homeostasis. Neuro-plastic homeostasis refers to the dynamic capacity of the nervous system to maintain balance while adapting to life experiences, whether these are rooted in trauma or growth [18, 63]. This concept intertwines the biological flexibility of neural pathways with the engendered socio-ecological framework to that of biosemiotics in which individuals and communities exist. It emphasizes the innate ability of the human brain and body to recalibrate and evolve, transforming experiences into learning processes that inform behaviors and cultural practices [72]. In the maternal ecosphere, neuro-plastic homeostasis plays a pivotal role in fostering healing and communal connection, integrating trauma into adaptive narratives that drive both individual and collective evolution.

Williams' *The Long Revolution,* expressed the creative mind, female biology of human creativity of evolved relations, tacit knowledge and deep understanding of complex systems [64]. Female biology- human epigenetic memory is enworlded and somatically embodied ([9], p. 15). It is where the environment through culture is fundamental to creative human evolutionary change [9]. According to Wendy Wheeler, "not only has inheritance of acquired characteristics been shown to be possible but such epigenetic inheritances indicates our inseparable lived relation to our environment including our cultural environment.... What we feel and experience both biologically and psychologically is capable of heritability, this has very far reaching social ethical and political implications" ([9], p. 14). What is being described is maternal ecosphere, neuro-plastic homeostasis.

Recent research in epigenetics has shed light on how life experiences, particularly traumatic ones, can influence gene expression and be inherited across generations [48]. This epigenetic transmission of trauma aligns with the South Slavic understanding of 'we are all flesh to be written upon' memory and knowledge [4, 62]. For these women, trauma and healing are not confined to the individual; they are embedded within a biological and cultural system that retains the imprints of past experiences [34].

The archetypal 'we are flesh' female biology is shown with the Balkan War landmines and ripe camps [34]. In Bosnia-Herzegovina, over a million landmines from the Balkan War continue to claim lives, disrupting traditional foraging practices such as gathering healing herbs and mushrooms [74]. Bosnian women war crimes and war survivors describe the landmines as killing fields, a haunting reminder of war's lingering destruction [34]. These killing fields still unearth grenades and bombs from WWII, further embedding trauma into the landscape. Despite surviving a century of wars, the region remains deeply connected to local food cultivation [34]. The balconies of tall apartment buildings overflow with herbs, potatoes, and flowers—acts of resistance and sustainability, embodying a thriving Moist Mother Earth practice.

The grief these women carry over the landmines extends beyond Western clinical psychological perspectives, which often view landmine clearance—despite their shelf life of over a hundred years—as the only remedy. When I asked them about their grief, nearly all referenced a traditional belief: in spring, one does not plant, dig, or strike the Moist Mother Earth until the time is ripe [34]. These symbolic inferences serve as an embodied lesson, a form of intensified learning meant to counteract transgenerational trauma and transform violence-laden memories into wisdom for survival [4, 11]. However, with the enduring presence of landmines and the legacy of rape camps, women war survivors articulate a deeper wounding: Moist Mother Earth has been violated, her womb transformed by war into a site of devastation. They express that the rape camps were not only an assault on their bodies but an assault on the land itself—the womb of Moist Mother Earth desecrated, leaving their own wombs as tombs [4, 14, 34].

The Slavic Moist Mother Earth term reflects the ecological womb [12]. As a creator of culture, women impart cultural socially learned information where the storage and transmission of knowledge in a nonliterate environment is biosemiotic in nature [9]. Women's female tacit knowledge is present in the biosemiotics research that easily translates our environment for our genome [9]. We do know that biology requires co-evolution of all life forms and their environments over vast lengths of time.

Biosemiotican Jakob von Uexküll's concept of biology presents a postmodern ecological framework that transcends patriarchal paradigms and attempts to move beyond traditional feminist discourse. However, von Uexkull inadvertently underscores the centrality of female biological processes, reinforcing the universal reality that every human is born of a woman [5, 9]. A critical aspect of von Uexküll's theory is his assertion that culture functions as the ecological womb, shaping both the environment and our genome.

Through my research, I have observed that the lack of focus on female-specific victimization is tied to a broader systemic erasure—one that extends to the destruction of culture itself [11, 75]. In our world, marked by relentless cycles of environmental devastation, climate change, and violence, the deliberate targeting of female-centered ways of life is not incidental but strategic. Culture, as a way of life, imprints itself onto the genome, shaping not only biological inheritance but also transgenerational adaptation [4, 53]. This means that laws, mandates, and policies—including those enacted through humanitarian aid and global institutions—are not merely failing women; they are actively complicit in the perpetuation of holocaustic trauma. By excluding the fundamental capacity of women to create and sustain culture, these institutions reinforce a negative transgenerational impact on the genome, further embedding trauma rather than fostering collective healing and transformation [8, 14].

Given that the uteri is only found in female bodies thus defining female biology, this transmission is especially evident in the mitochondrial DNA (mtDNA), which is exclusively matrilineal and reflects an unbroken line of inheritance from mother to child [49]. Mitochondrial DNA serves as a biological parallel to the cultural transmission of knowledge within the maternal ecosphere, supporting the continuity of shared memory and community identity [27, 40, 61].

18. Culture as homeostasis: Beyond resilience

In contrast to Western models of trauma recovery, which often emphasize female biology in generic or default to male terms Perez instead of maternal ecosystems terms, reveals the portrayal of XX chromosome-related adaptation as a coping strategy- keep building resiliency, a transgenerational survival mechanism. Continuously, surviving and building more and more resiliency skills to survive depletes the body and any sense of wellbeing. However, the South Slavic Moist Mother Earth [13] approach is the antidote via adaptive evolving cultural homeostasis [4].

Homeostasis, in this Slavic maternal ecosphere context, refers to a dynamic state of balance and neuroplastic adaptation that sustains both individual and a safe communal well-being [35]. Through practices like the Slavic embodied Moist Mother Earth oral memory such as the Kolo-embodied circle practices [12], the community maintains a stable safe environment in which trauma can be integrated rather than merely survived. This system of cultural homeostasis is not about bouncing back from adversity; it is about sustaining a life-affirming balance that allows the community to thrive even amidst disruption.

It is noted that the space and place previous to recognition, consciousness is the biological homeostasis, how the body self-regulates not just survival but more importantly to adapt thus evolving, all of which defines interception, poised on the human nervous system, the polyvagal interpreting signals [55, 76].

The Slavic Kolo-embodied socially engaged circle to round folk dances are a collective thus becomes a site of both memory and adaptation, where participants engage in a practice that reinforces social bonds and provides a framework for intensified learning transforming trauma [4]. In moving together, from the kolo folk dances to encircled, socially engaged participants create a collective rhythm that synchronizes their emotional and physiological states, fostering an environment of safety and trust [4, 18]. This collective attuned serves as a buffer against the isolating effects of trauma, allowing for the reintegration of difficult experiences into the communal narrative. By prioritizing cultural homeostasis over individual resilience, the maternal ecosphere provides a foundation for healing that is inherently social and interdependent [9, 53].

19. Female biology as a source of maternal cultural continuity

The concept of the maternal ecosphere is deeply rooted in female biology, which South Slavic women see as the source of both life and epigenetic memory knowledge. As shown in the Balkan War rape camps case study, female biological processes, such as menstruation, pregnancy, and childbirth, are not merely physical phenomena; they are also cultural events that shape the community's understanding of life, death, and continuity [23]. This focus on female biology aligns with the cultural belief that all life is born from and sustained by the female body—a perspective that echoes the Slavic Moist Mother Earth archetype. It is a concept, which venerates the Earth as a living, nurturing force [49, 66].

In this ecosphere, mitochondrial DNA—passed exclusively from mothers to their children—symbolizes an unbroken biological lineage that parallels the transmission of cultural knowledge within the community [75]. This matrilineal inheritance serves as a reminder of the continuity that exists through generations, reinforcing the importance of female biology as a stabilizing force within the community.

By acknowledging the centrality of the female body and its role in sustaining life, the South Slavic women affirm the cultural and biological foundations of their maternal ecosphere, positioning it as a vital resource for healing transgenerational trauma [77].

The term "maternal matrescence ecosphere" in this study signifies a unique female-centered social and biological environment where trauma is metabolized not solely by individuals, but within a supportive and enduring cultural framework [78]. The case study - maternal fright illustrates this ecosphere, rooted in South Slavic oral memory practices and rituals associated with the Slavic Moist Mother Earth indigenous knowledge, highlights the profound role of oral memory [12, 13, 79].

Oral memory, in this context, is defined as the epigenetic transmission of knowledge, experiences, and traditions through spoken narratives and communal practices, forming a living repository of collective history and cultural identity [35]. The female body, within this ecosphere, is framed not just as a site of biological reproduction, but as the central source of inclusive cultural continuity and social cohesion [23].

It is through this maternal ecosphere that South Slavic women war survivors anchor themselves in memory and tradition, creating a living system of knowledge that supports healing and adaptation- evolution across generations [4, 35]. Furthermore, it is not only a cultural framework since females create inclusive culture through their biology, a critical recognition.

Trauma survival mechanisms require a rhythmic, synchronized partnership that fosters collaboration and transition into the neuroplasticity of intensified learning [4, 18], This partnership, rooted in the principles of epigenetics, is inherently transgenerational—shaping, influencing, and evolving the human genome. However, what is not addressed in the male default sciences is that every single person who has ever lived, those living now, and those yet to come, are all born of a female. She is carrying forward the biological and experiential bioimprints of gynaecocracies'[3] maternal life.

The male-default sciences [41] often fail to account for the critical role of female biology in the evolution of the species, focusing instead on androcentric models that obscure the contributions of women and their biological systems. Female biology, with its capacity to drive evolutionary processes through the XX chromosome, is central to the species' survival and adaptation [43]. While technological advancements have accelerated at unprecedented rates, they have often been accompanied by a socio-modern regression that neglects the integration of cultural and biological knowledge [43].

The evolutionary processes shaping human cognition, neuroplasticity, and socio-biological development are interconnected with environmental influences and life experiences [9, 15]. Yet, the mechanistic approaches of male-default sciences fail to address the complex, nonlinear dynamics of cultural evolution and the maternal ecosystems that sustain life [41]. This neglect is evident in the reductionist portrayal of human progress, which prioritizes technological innovation over the socio-cultural systems that women have historically maintained to ensure species continuity. By reclaiming the narrative-herstories through studies of female biology and maternal-centered ecosystems, we can challenge the reductionism of androcentric paradigms and highlight the transformative role of women in shaping adaptive and evolving cultural frameworks.

Trauma is neurobiological, yet the male-biased sciences often default to the male. As Dr. Caroline Perez notes, this "habit of default male" permeates evolutionary theories, ignoring female biology, including the fact that for the first 3 months of gestation, all fetuses are female [41].

[3] Gynaecocracies' maternal life- traces back to Hellenic myths holding a biological reality that more females are born in proportion to males.

In this context, the use of South Slavic oral memory practices such as the embodied Kolo is far more than a socially engaged circle or a folk dance; it is a form of somatic maternal memory that consolidates the social bonds essential for healing. By engaging in the Kolo either in a somatic circle or folk round dances, women participate in a shared, rhythmic polyvagal somatic movement that symbolizes the cycle of life and death, continuity and change [4].

This practice allows the community to process trauma collectively, reinforcing social bonds and creating an environment of safety and support [76, 77]. Through the maternal ecosphere functions as a regenerative cultural practice, embodying the principles of connection, stability, and adaptive change.

This maternal-centered framework, which can also be termed the "Matrescence", [78] encapsulates a transformative process where female biology and cultural practices coalesce to foster transgenerational healing and cultural continuity [80].

20. Adaptive culture and transgenerational trauma healing

The South Slavic women's approach to healing transcends individual experiences of trauma and embodies an adaptive cultural system that promotes community adaptation- evolving perpetually and human flourishing- evolution [48]. Rather than focusing on individual recovery, their practices emphasize the collective process of adapting to trauma through intensified learning when facing change. By fostering social cohesion, reinforcing shared memory, and creating a space for collective reflection and growth [73]. This approach is evident in the ways the women engage in oral memory traditions and communal rituals that function as forms of cultural epigenetic continuity.

By participating in these practices, the South Slavic women create an evolving social fabric that allows for the integration of intensified learning from trauma into a larger communal narrative.

These somatic oral memory rituals, particularly the Slavic Kolo-embodied circle and/or folk round dance, are not simply remnants of tradition but are adaptive responses to both herstorical and historical and contemporary traumas [43, 45, 77]. They embody the collective strength and wisdom that comes from generations of lived experience, supporting a framework for healing that is grounded in communal solidarity rather than individualistic patriarchal coping survival mechanisms.

This collective strength fosters an environment in which trauma is not merely endured but transformed, ensuring the continuation of life-affirming values, behaviors, and social structures [25, 35, 43].

21. Epigenetic transmission of cultural memory

Epigenetic inheritance is a biological female mechanism that supports the transmission of cultural memory, allowing the inclusive experiences of one generation to influence the physiology and psychology of the next [36]. This phenomenon aligns with the South Slavic concept of inherited memory, where trauma and healing are encoded not only in oral memory stories and rituals but also in the very biology of females [30]. Through mitochondrial DNA, women inherit a biological memory for adaptation- evolving, which is then reinforced by cultural practices that echo epigenetically inherited tacit knowledge [58, 66].

In this way, the maternal ecosphere functions as a system of embodied knowledge that preserves both the memory of trauma healing and the means for healing. This epigenetic transmission of memory ensures that the knowledge of past struggles is not lost but rather transformed into a resource for future generations.

For the South Slavic women, healing transgenerational trauma involves engaging with these inherited memories through ritual, storytelling, and communal practices that activate the body's innate capacities for adaptation bypassing resilience-endless surviving. This approach to trauma recovery recognizes the profound interconnectedness of biology, culture, and memory in shaping the individual and collective experience of healing [18, 40].

22. Institutionalized violence and cultural continuity

The legacy of institutionalized violence against women, particularly in the context of the Balkan War, has created unique challenges for the South Slavic women war survivors [34, 35, 68]. These challenges include the systematic erasure of female experiences from official histories and the ongoing marginalization of women's trauma within both local and international frameworks. However, rather than accepting this marginalization, the women have leveraged their maternal ecosphere as a means of resistance, using their cultural practices to assert their agency and reclaim their herstorical narratives [4].

Through the oral memory traditions and communal gatherings, the South Slavic women have preserved their history of survival and adaptation, passing down not only stories but also the skills and wisdom needed to navigate a world shaped by patriarchal violence [21, 31]. Women's invisibility extends to their wombs and their labors, such as child-rearing and domestic life, which, despite being the cornerstone of patriarchal capitalist society, are often disregarded or marginalized.

These women have endured the strategic military targeting of their bodies in conflicts, including sexual violence and domestic violence, where their narratives are overshadowed by patriarchal systems that prioritize male perspectives and values [11, 71]. This act of cultural continuity serves as a way of switching from resistance against institutionalized erasure, to affirming the importance of women's experiences and perspectives in the broader narrative of trauma and recovery. By situating their trauma within a cultural framework that honors female biology, these women create a counter-narrative that challenges the patriarchal structures that seek to render them invisible [13, 50, 71].

23. Conclusion

This chapter calls for a paradigm shift in healthcare—one that recognizes female biology, communal healing, and cultural plurality and pliability as vital components of transgenerational trauma healing.

Integrating maternally centered social ecosphere (MCSE) principles into healthcare shifts the focus from individual pathology to collective healing. Kolo-informed trauma therapy, epigenetics, and oral memory traditions offer an all-inclusive model for mind-body health interventions, preventions healing transgenerational trauma. By embracing female-centered healthcare approaches, practitioners can develop more effective, inclusive strategies for trauma recovery and community well-being.

Female biology is the embodiment of social epigenetic memory, continuously shaping and adapting through the maternal-centered ecosphere. This ecosystem serves as an antidote to the cycles of violence, including femicide and sex trafficking, by fostering inclusive oral memory cultural practices for adaptive learning. The focus on a maternally centered ecosphere highlights the capacity of female biology to innovate, preserve, and evolve in ways that transcend survival, creating pathways for thriving amidst adversity.

This chapter emphasizes the foundational role of the maternal-centered social ecosphere in healing transgenerational trauma among South Slavic women war survivors. By intertwining biological inheritance with cultural continuity, these women have developed an adaptive framework that promotes both individual and communal well-being. Their embodied oral memory practices serve not only as mechanisms for processing trauma but as living repositories of collective memory, fostering connection, stability, and transformation.

The exploration of female biology, epigenetics, and oral memory traditions reveals the often-overlooked contributions of females to cultural evolution and species survival. By redefining trauma as intensified learning and recognizing the neuroplastic potential within communal healing practices, this chapter challenges male-default scientific perspectives that have historically marginalized the significance of female-centered ecosystems. In doing so, it calls for the integration of these frameworks into trauma research, offering a more inclusive and culturally sensitive approach to recovery and adaptation that honors the profound contributions of females as creators of life and culture.

Author details

Danica Anderson
The Kolo: Women's Cross-Cultural Collaboration, Non Profit Organization Registered in the States of Washington and Florida, USA

*Address all correspondence to: danica@kolocollaboration.org

References

[1] Do Carmo Q, Gabriela VV, Dembélé M, Ayotte-Beaudet P. Going beyond adaptation: An integrative review and ethical considerations of semi-structured interviews with elementary-aged children. Journal of Qualitative Methods. 2025. DOI: 10.1177_16094069241247474 [Accessed: January, 2025]

[2] New Study Shows Transmission of Epigenetic Memory across Multiple Generations. Santa Cruz: University of California; 2022. Available from: https://www.sciencedaily.com/releases/2022/09/220926200451.htm [Accessed January 23, 2023]

[3] Jennifer D. Female Biology. Jennifer Devers; 2025. Available from: https://books.google.com/books?id=d0zpEAAAQBAJ&lr=&source=gbs_navlinks_s [Accessed: January, 2025]

[4] Anderson D. South Slavic Women's Transgenerational Trauma Healing through Oral Memory Practices. Olympia: Lexington Books; 2023. Available from: https://rowman.com/ISBN/9781666937923/South-Slavic-Women%E2%80%99s-Transgenerational-Trauma-Healing-Through-Oral-Memory-Practices-Women-War-Crimes-and-War-Survivors [Accessed: January 7, 2024]

[5] The devastation of war extends beyond physical destruction; it **deeply alters biological and psychological health across generations**. In **post-war Bosnia and Herzegovina**, South Slavic women's **oral memory practices** and **maternal-centered healing traditions** play a crucial role in **healthcare interventions for trauma recovery**. This chapter presents a **new paradigm for mind-body healing** through the **Maternally-Centered Social Ecosphere (MCSE)**—a system that **harnesses female biology, epigenetics, and communal healing traditions** as critical components of **trauma-informed healthcare**

[6] Rikhof J. The influence of international criminal law on refugee law. Frontiers in Human Dynamics. 2023;5. DOI: 10.3389/fhumd.2023.1088033 [Accessed: December, 2024]

[7] Gillian K. State-empowered entities as sites of progress for international anti-trafficking law and policy? Frontiers in Human Dynamics. 2023;5. DOI: 10.3389/fhumd.2023.1245909 [Accessed: December, 2024]

[8] Bahtijarag R, Pim JE, Milojevic I, Grigaityte I, Anderson DB, Garic-Komnenic S, et al. Nonkilling Balkans. Honolulu: Center for Nonkilling; 2015

[9] Wheeler W. The Whole Creature, Complexity, Biosemiotics and the Evolution of Culture. London: Lawrence & Wishart; 2006

[10] Gina H. Justifying Force: A Feminist Analysis of the International Law on the Use of Force. London School of Economics and Political Science UK; 2009. Available from: https://www.proquest.com/openview/f9393b39f4331c9fc0275641ad0dfc95/1?pq-origsite=gscholar&cbl=2026366

[11] Tabaković J. Searching for Healing Amidst the Genocidal Logic: Fragmentary Exiled Bosnian (Im)Possibilities. University of Cambridge; 2024. DOI: 10.17863/CAM.113186 [Accessed: January, 2025]

[12] Marler J. From the Realm of the Ancestors; Anthology In Honor of Marija

Gimbutas. Manchester: Knowledge, Trends & Ideas; 1991

[13] Hubbs J. Mother Russia: The Feminine Myth in Russian Culture. Indiana University Press; 1993

[14] Anderson D. Blood & Honey: The Secret Herstory-Balkan Women War Crimes and War Survivors. Olympia, WA: Kolo Books; 2015. ISBN 97809-9886891-3-8

[15] Blood and Honey: Biosemiotic & Bioculinary. Kolo Press; 2012 [Accessed: January 9, 2025]

[16] Livio P. Psychobiological Footprints through Human Development: How our Experiences Shape Who we Are. Taylor & Francis; 2024. Available from: https://books.google.com/books?hl=en&lr=&id=rt0PEQAAQBAJ&oi=fnd&pg=PA1980&dq=biological+processes+and+evolutionary+adaptations+that+drive+diversity,+highlighting+the+essential+role+of+female+biology+in+shaping+human+development+and+adaptation&ots=3iKB8-aT [Accessed: January, 2025]

[17] Howard AE. Transgenerational Effects of Trauma through Epigenetic Mechanisms. Proquest; 2022. Available from: https://www.proquest.com/openview/16d640091a242177025626e37cd175ae/1?pq-origsite=gscholar&cbl=18750&diss=y [Accessed: January, 2025]

[18] Porges SW. Polyvagal theory: A science of safety. Frontiers in Neuroscience. 2022;**16**. DOI: 10.3389/fnint.2022.871227 [Accessed: January, 2025]

[19] Lehrner A, Yehuda R. Cultural trauma and epigenetic inheritance. Development and Psychopathology. 2018;**30**(5):1763-1777. DOI: 10.1017/S0954579418001153 [Accessed: January, 2025]

[20] Kirmayer LJ, Worthman CM, Kitayama S, Lemelson R, Cummings CA. Culture, Mind, and Brain: Emerging Concepts, Models, and Applications. 2020. Available from: https://books.google.com/books?id=XxH9DwAAQBAJ&dq=female+indigenous+knowing+cultural+and+biological+significance+of+oral+memory+practices+derived+from+lived+experiences%E2%80%94shaped+epigenetically%E2%80%94and+tacit+knowledge,+an+intuitive+understanding+ [Accessed: January, 2024]

[21] Mews P, Calipari ES, Day J, Lobo MK, Bredy T, Abel T. From circuits to chromatin: The emerging role of epigenetics in mental health. Journal of Neuroscience. 2021;**41**(5):873-882 [Accessed: January, 2025]. DOI: 10.1523/JNEUROSCI.1649-20.2020

[22] Womersley JS, du Plessis M, Greene MC, van den Heuwel LL, Kinyanda E, Seedat S. Advances in the molecular neurobiology of posttraumatic stress disorder from global contexts: A systematic review of longitudinal studies. Global Mental Health (Cambridge Prisms). 2023;**10**. DOI: 10.1017/gmh.2023.53 [Accessed: January, 2025]

[23] Rebecca K. Interwined: Women, Nature and Climate Justice. New Press; 2024. Available from: https://books.google.com/books?id=VUPREAAAQBAJ&dq=XX+chromosome+not+only+embodies+the+foundation+of+female+biology+but+also+sustains+female+indigenous+ways+of+knowing&lr=&source=gbs_navlinks_s [Accessed: December, 2024]

[24] Ross C. IBE-science of learning portal. In: Neuroplasticity: How the Brain Changes with Learning. 2019. Available from: https://solportal.ibe-unesco.org/articles/neuroplasticity-how-the-brain-changes-with-learning/ [Accessed: January, 2025]

[25] Michelle F. In: Falzon M, editor. Available from: https://books.google.com/books?id=5fofEQAAQBAJ&printsec=frontcover#v=onepage&q&f=falseHealing Horizons: Real Stories of Growth and Transformation from Real People. 2025 [Accessed: January, 2025]

[26] Sedwick VM. Exploring the Role of the Posterior Amygdala in the Regulation of Caregiving. ProQuest; 2024. Available from: https://www.proquest.com/openview/5d4505227b51498fe5c225a2ae1f36a0/1?pq-origsite=gscholar&cbl=18750&diss=y [Accessed: January, 2025]

[27] Rosalynn V. Mitochondrial Memory: Transgenerational Trauma, Functional Medicine, and Quantum Physics. Anthropology Faculty Publications and Presentations; 2024. Available from: https://scholarworks.utrgv.edu/anthro_fac/102/ [Accessed: December, 2024]

[28] Tuulari JJ, Bourgery M, Iversen J, Koefoed TG, Ahonen A, Ahmedani A, et al. Exposure to childhood maltreatment is associated with specific epigenetic patterns in sperm. Molecular Psychiatry. 2025. DOI: 10.1038/s41380-024-02872 [Accessed: January, 2025]

[29] Marianne G. Sperm Cells Carry Traces of Childhood Stress, Epigenetic Study Finds. 2025. Available from: https://www.livescience.com/health/fertility-pregnancy-birth/sperm-cells-carry-traces-of-childhood-stress-epigenetic-study-finds?lrh=fdeef8b60c32bd3a4826175a912b2bbddd51c2710737b0432c912e8ebcbce237 [Accessed: January, 2025]

[30] Corning Peter A, Kauffman SA, Noble D, Shapiro JA, Vane-Wright RI, editors. Evolution" on Purpose": Teleonomy in Living Systems. MIT Press; 2023. Available from: https://books.google.com/books?hl=en&lr=&id=ynOdEAAAQBAJ&oi=fnd&pg=PR7&dq=Epigenetic+mechanisms+and+tacit+knowledge%E2%80%94the+unspoken,+innate+understanding+derived+from+life+experiences%E2%80%94serve+as+a+collective+memory,+shaping+human+evolution+thro [Accessed: December, 2024]

[31] Kem G, Stewart T. Hope and Communityship: Women's Ways of Engaging in Embodied Somatic Leadership. Emerald Publishing Limited; 2024. DOI: 10.1108/978-1-83549-476-920241005 [Accessed: December, 2024]

[32] Bohleber W. Remembrance, trauma and collective memory: The battle for memory in psychoanalysis. The International Journal of Psychoanalysis. 2007;**88**(2):329-352. DOI: 10.1516/V5H5-8351-7636-7878 [Accessed: January, 2025]

[33] Margherita G, Tessitore F. Facing the traumatic field in the clinical and social work with forced migrants through a psychodynamic perspective: From "refugee trauma" to the Clinic of Social Links. 2023:379-388. DOI: 10.1007/s10615-023-00894-y [Accessed: January, 2025]

[34] Sumejja K. Women War Crimes and War Survivors, Interview by [PhD] Danica Anderson 2000-2025. Fear-Transgenerational Trauma

[35] Danica A. Maternal fright - South Slavic Oral memory Traditions; a biosemiotic epigenetic transgenerational & somatic psychobiology healing practice. Birth Psychology. 2016;**1**:34. Available from: https://www.academia.edu/24033171/Maternal_Fright_and_South_Slavic_Oral_Memory_Traditions_Biosemiotics_Epigenetics_and_Somatic_Psychobiology_Healing_Practices [Accessed: November q3, 2022]

[36] Kanherkar RR, Csoka AB. Epigenetics across the human lifespan. Frontiers in Cell and Developmental

Biology. 2014;**2**. DOI: 10.3389/fcell.2014.00049 [Accessed: December, 2024]

[37] Marler J. The Body as Sacred Metaphor. ResearchGate; 2003. Available from: file:///C:/Users/danic/Downloads/BodyofWomanasSacredMetaphor.pdf

[38] Rani K, Tambe PB, Shaikh MA, Kshirsagar S. Nutritional Epigenomics. In: Tambe PB, Shaikh MA, Kankate SKR, editors. Nutrigenomics and Nutraceuticals. Taylor Francis; 2024. p. 24. DOI: 10.1201/9781003428268-14 [Accessed: January, 2025]

[39] Haggarty P. Genetic and metabolic determinants of human epigenetic variation. Current Opinion in Clinical Nutrition and Metabolic Care. 2015. DOI: 10.1097/MCO.0000000000000194 [Accessed: January, 2025]

[40] Greiner S, Johanna S, Block R. Why are organelle genomes transmitted maternally? BioEssays. 2015;**37**(1):80-94. DOI: 10.1002/bies.201400110

[41] Criado PC. Invisible Women in a World Designed for Men. New York: Abrams Press; 2021

[42] Ann SM. The Authority Gap: Why Women Are Still Taken Less Seriously than Men, and What We Can Do About It. W.W. Norton & Company; 2022. Available from: https://books.google.com/books?id=EUM3EAAAQBAJ&lr=&source=gbs_navlinks_s [Accessed: January, 2025]

[43] Heide GA. The Way into an Egalitarian Society. 2007. Available from: https://www.goettner-abendroth.de/fileadmin/user_upload/pdf/the_way.pdf

[44] Samantha A, Simpson M, Curtis A. Men have gender and women are people: A structural approach to gender and violence. Violence against women. Violence Against Women. 2022. DOI: 10.1177/10778012221104844 [Accessed: December, 2024]

[45] Pilotto AM, Turner DC, Mazzolari R. Human skeletal muscle possesses an epigenetic memory of high intensity interval training. American Journal of Physiology-Cell Physiology. 2024. DOI: 10.1152/ajpcell.00423.2024

[46] Kaarina K. Original instructions. In: The Woman Who Married the Bear: The Spirituality of the Ancient Foremothers. 2023. p. 75

[47] Aura Z, Wapeesittipan P, Joshi A. Insights into sex and gender differences in brain and psychopathologies using big data. Life. 2023. DOI: 10.3390/life13081676 [Accessed: December, 2024]

[48] Hayley M. Molecular Biology and Genetics. Pressbooks; 2023. Available from: https://pressbooks.calstate.edu/explorationsbioanth2/chapter/3/ [Accessed: December, 2024]

[49] Peter N, Helanterä H, Kapheim KM. Research Topic: Social Evolution and the What, When, Why and How of the Major Evolutionary Transitions. 2023

[50] Julie M. War's Offensive on Women: The Humanitarian Challenge in Bosnia, Kosovo, and Afghanistan. Bloomfield: Kumarian Press, Inc; 2000

[51] Wehrs DR, Nalbantian S, Tucker DM. Cultural Memory: From the Sciences to the Humanities. Taylor & Francis; 2022. Available from: https://books.google.com/books?id=VJGZEAAAQBAJ&dq=female+indigenous+knowing+cultural+and+biological+significance+of+oral+memory+practices+derived+from+lived+experiences%E2%80%94shaped+epigenetically%E2%80%94and+tacit+knowledge,+a

n+intuitive+understanding [Accessed: January, 2025]

[52] Anne C. A Mind of her Own: The Evolutionary Psychology of Women. 2013. Available from: https://books.google.com/books?id=2FJoAgAAQBAJ&lr=&source=gbs_navlinks_s [Accessed: January, 2025]

[53] Antonio D. The Self Comes to Mind: Constructing the Conscious Brain. Pantheon; 2010

[54] Darcia N, Bradshaw GA, Fernández-Giménez ME, Ravera F, Oteros-Rozas E. Ecology and Society. 2022;**27**(2). DOI: 10.5751/ES-12794-270204

[55] Goldstein DS. How does homeostasis happen? Integrative physiological, systems biological, and evolutionary perspectives. American Journal of Physiology-Regulatory, Integrative and Comparative Physiology. 2019. DOI: R-00396-2018

[56] Lynn M. Symbiosis in Cell Evolution: Life and its Environment on the Early Earth. Freeman; 1981

[57] Milne TK. Precedented Times, Precedented Measures: Exploring the theatre-as-body's Recurrent Adaptations to. ProQuest; 2024. Available from: https://www.proquest.com/openview/3b5c97f7b58e5de7ca47f119285e3bd6/1?pq-origsite=gscholar&cbl=18750&diss=yArchive [Accessed: January, 2025]

[58] Brock R. Tacit Knowledge in Science Education. Rotterdam: Sense Publishers; 2017. DOI: 10.1007/978-94-6300-749-8_1

[59] Billman GE. Homeostasis: The underappreciated and far too often ignored central organizing principle of physiology. Frontiers in Physiology. 2020. DOI: 10.3389/fphys.2020.00200 [Accessed: January, 2025]

[60] Davies KJ. Adaptive Homeostasis. Molecular Aspects of Medicine. 2016;**49**:1-7. DOI: 10.1016/j.mam.2016.04.007 [Accessed: January 2025]

[61] Jablonka E, Lamb MJ. Evolution in Four Dimensions; Genetic, Epiengentic, Behavioral and Symbolic Variation in the History of Life. Cambridge: A Bradford Book; 2005

[62] Eric K. In Search of Memory: The Emergence of a New Science of Mind. W.W. Norton; 2007

[63] Steven R. Eric Kandel: Making memories. The Lancet. 2006:1721-1722. DOI: 10.1016/S0140-6736(06)68753-9 [Accessed: January 22, 2023]

[64] Raymond W. The Long Revolution. Columbia University Press; 1961

[65] Mertus JA, Tesanovic J, Metikos H, Boric R, West C. The Suitcase: Refugee Voices from Bosnia and Croatia. University of California Press; 1997

[66] Andrea O. Moving between Worlds: A Guide to Embodied Living and Communicating. 2022. Available from: https://books.google.com/books?id=wketEAAAQBAJ&dq=+knowledge+through+oral+memory+neuroplastic+herstories+&lr=&source=gbs_navlinks_s [Accessed: January, 2025]

[67] Delic A, Avdibegovic E. Shame and Silence in the Aftermath of War Rape in Bosnia and Hercegovina: 22 Years Later. 2015. Available from: https://www.researchgate.net/profile/Amra-Delic-2/publication/293815848_Shame_and_Silence_in_the_aftermath_of_War_Rape_in_Bosnia_and_Herzegovina_22_years_later/links/56bb97b408ae3f9793153a86/Shame-and-Silence-in-the-aftermath-of-War-Rape-in-Bosnia-and-Her [Accessed: January, 2025]

[68] McClellan DS, Knez N. Prosecuting rape, sexual enslavement, and genocide in time of war: Southeastern Europe 1991-1995. International Journal of Social Sciences. 2016;**5**(4):45-52. DOI: 10.20472/SS.2016.5.4.005 [Accessed: January, 2025]

[69] Grebo L, Ahmici T. 2023. One Day, Two Massacres: Remembering Bosnia's Ahmici and Trusina Atrocities. Available from: https://balkaninsight.com/2023/04/14/one-day-two-massacres-remembering-bosnias-ahmici-and-trusina-atrocities/ [Accessed: December 22, 2024]

[70] Annika B, Selimovic JM. Places of pain and spaces of silence Re-visiting a Bosnian rape camp. Geopolitics. 2023:1635-1658. DOI: 10.1080/14650045.2023.2265315 [Accessed: December, 2024]

[71] Stiglmayer A. Mass Rape: The War against Women in Bosnia-Herzegovina. Lincoln: University of Nebraska Press; 1994. Available from: https://books.google.com/books?id=5tJflDgysEIC&dq=Balkan+War+Rape+camps+1991-1995+Stiglmayer&lr=&source=gbs_navlinks_s [Accessed: January, 2025]

[72] Chad K-G. First-In-human experience with integration of wireless intracranial pressure monitoring device within a customized cranial implant. Congress of Neurological Surgeons. 2020. DOI: 10.1093/ons/opz431/5716909 [Accessed: January, 2025]

[73] Nicole K. She City: Designing out Women's Inequity in Cities. Bloombury Publishing; 2024. Available from: https://www.torrossa.com/en/resources/an/5681984 [Accessed: January, 2025]

[74] Ivo B, Skejic A, Zindovic B, Bender J. Geologically-driven migration of landmines and explosive remnants of war—A feature focusing on the Western Balkans. Geosciences. 2023;**13**(6):178

[75] Delic Amra M, Hasanovic E, Avdibegovic A, Dimitrijevic C, Hancheva C, Scher T, et al. Academic model of trauma healing in post-war societies. Acta Medica Academica. 2014;**43**(1):76-80. DOI: 10.5644/ama2006-124.103 [Accessed: January, 2025]

[76] Porges SW. The Polyvagal Theory: Neurophysiological Foundations of Emotions Attachment Communication Self-Regulation. New York: Norton Series on Interpersonal Neurobiology; 2011. DOI: 978-0393707007 [Accessed: December 04, 2022]

[77] Cavalli-Sforza LL. The Great Human Disa–Oras; the History of Diversity and Evolution. Milano: Perseus Books Publishing; 1993

[78] Anna R. 2024. "Matrescence," and the Transformations of Motherhood. Available from: https://www.newyorker.com/culture/persons-of-interest/matrescence-and-the-transformations-of-motherhood?utm_source=chatgpt.com [Accessed: October, 2024]

[79] Ana D, Antonijevi Z. Exploring collective memory-work in Serbia: Construction of gender and ethnicity in post-conflict context. In: Hamm R, editor. Reader Collective Memory-Work. 2021. p. 353. Available from: https://d1wqtxts1xzle7.cloudfront.net/75289260/Reader_Collective_Memory_Work_ebook_-libre.pdf?1638052353=&response-content-disposition=inline%3B+filename%3DReader_Collective_Memory_Work_ebook.pdf&Expires=1738034590&Signature=NKYIxSTp79Daah~PmixFdJYStbIy4d [Accessed: January, 2025]

[80] Hove MMJ, Steven A. Biological Psychology: 10.3: Plasticity: Experiences Can Alter the Brain. Biological Psychology. Revised ed. Available from: https://rotel.pressbooks.pub/biologicalpsychology/chapter/plasticity-experiences-can-alter-the-brain/2024 [Accessed: January, 2025]

Chapter 10

Physiological Correlates of Pain in Children during the Skin Diagnostic Testing and Prevention of Childhood Procedural Pain and Distress

Vasiliy Pyatin, Elena Borodulina, Olga Kozlova and Olga Maslova

Abstract

The chapter is devoted to procedural pain for children as the most frequent cause of anxiety and distress in children and their parents. The chapter will provide an overview of the topic and present the results of our own studies of children's psychosomatic reactions to pain during the Mantoux test and skin prick test under standard clinical conditions. The chapter will present objective data on the progressive reduction of negative emotional reactions in children from 75% in the Mantoux test to their complete absence in the skin prick test, based on the study of physiological correlates of pain during skin diagnostic testing. In the chapter, we show a ways of preventing childhood procedural pain and distress by measuring physiological correlates of pain and anxiety in children during the diagnostic skin testing.

Keywords: children procedural pain, Mantoux test, skin prick test, EMG, respiration, EDA, ECG, HRV

1. Introduction

1.1 The issue of pediatric procedural pain

Current pain therapy is in crisis [1]. This view is supported by the fact that the causes and treatment of acute pain continue to represent a major public health challenge and, on a subjective level, a profound psycho-emotional problem for children, adolescents and their parents [2].

In this chapter, we present a pilot study showing that overcoming this crisis can be achieved through the technological improvement of techniques that reduce or completely eliminate the occurrence of acute procedural pain, as the most promising way to overcome the crisis of pain therapy in pediatric medical practice. We also show that the proposed paradigm for preventing pediatric pain and distress can be effectively addressed primarily through immunization (needle prick), as the most common cause of pediatric procedural pain worldwide.

A person's response to pain and subjective experience of pain is always individualized and reflects sensory, cognitive and psychosomatic manifestations, regardless of age. The same brain structures (thalamus, anterior cingulate cortex, cerebellum, basal ganglia and periaqueductal gray) respond to pain stimuli and thus participate in pain control [3–5]. However, children are not born with innate neurophysiological mechanisms of pain control. The nociceptive regulation exhibited by the adult central nervous system develops during ontogeny [6, 7]. Children's reactions to procedural pain manifest themselves briefly during the needle prick but are known to have long-term consequences. It has been shown that children's experiences during acute painful medical procedures play an important role in the manifestation of behavioral and psychophysiological reactions that will occur during painful medical manipulations in adults later in their life [8].

Not only children's experiences of acute pain but also the behavior of parents and medical staff during a nociceptive medical procedure is recorded in the long-term memory of the child. Therefore, reducing the intensity of acute pain stimuli, parental education and involvement during the performance of acute pain stimuli, such as the Mantoux test and skin prick test, as well as high professional qualification of medical personnel are among the most important conditions for performing noxious medical procedures in children [9].

Acute pain is a severe stressor [2]. Children who have experienced repeated states of anxiety related to painful medical interventions have an increased risk of developing cognitive deficits in adulthood. It has also been shown that adults tend to avoid seeking medical care when anticipating painful medical manipulations [10]. Consequently, acute childhood pain of 'medical' genesis will be a source of pre-procedural anxiety for the adult, a cause of fear of the syringe and consequent psychosomatic tension [11, 12].

As a result, statistically, approximately 25% of adults experience fear at the sight of a syringe and needle, which they typically experience in a similar situation in childhood [13]. Moreover, negative emotional states such as fear or anxiety arising from nociceptive medical procedures increase the perception of pain [14–16]. Preventing the development of a negative emotional state in children during brief acute nociceptive medical manipulation (needle prick) through the use of antinociceptive techniques represents an effective paradigm for bringing modern pain therapy out of crisis.

1.2 Types of pain

Acute pain is pain that is directly related to a temporary injury and usually lasts for a short period of time. Procedural pain and anxiety are distress caused by medical procedures, including intravenous injections, vaccinations, administration of anesthesia and other needle-related procedures, as well as other procedures required as part of routine care, such as changing a dressing on a burn wound [17]. In medical practice, acute pain is defined as pain that lasts ≤3 months (acute postoperative pain or vaccination pain). The mechanisms of acute pain are mainly nociceptive, and it resolves after recovery. Chronic pain lasts or recurs for ≥3 months and may involve nociceptive, neuropathic and nociplastic mechanisms. Finally, in clinical cases, pain can also be described as continuous or periodic [18]. Our chapter investigates the problem of procedural pain in children and a technical option to solve the problem.

1.3 Physiological correlates of procedural pain in children and methods of study

Objective assessment of physiological correlates of acute pediatric pain, especially in conditions where subjective self-reporting cannot be performed in the context of short-term procedural manipulation (needle prick), manifestation of fear and even more so distress, seems to be relevant in clinical research. The validity of objective measurements of children's responses to acute procedural pain is extremely relevant for the development of effective antinociceptive methods to prevent childhood pain and distress [19].

In our chapter, we aimed to consider all components of the nociceptive process during childhood immunization to provide an objective multiparametric assessment of procedural childhood pain, which is based on the application of well-validated physiological signals such as electrocardiogram (ECG), electrodermal conduction, respiratory rate and depth and heart rate variability (HRV) [20] directly during procedural manipulation – Mantoux test and skin prick test.

We experimentally substantiate the informational significance of the signals of the above methods to address the working hypothesis of our clinical-physiological study. In particular, surface facial electromyography (EMG) is widely used in psychology as a non-invasive tool for assessing subtle emotional facial expressions [21] and is an objective and accessible tool for assessing physiological correlates of acute childhood pain [22]. Meanwhile, emotional facial expression during children's responses to acute pain allows us to assess the intensity of painful stimulus, regardless of gender and age of a person [23]. In addition, the direct correlation between pain stimulus strength and facial emotional expression makes the EMG method particularly informative when investigating physiological correlates of pain in children [24].

In our study, surface facial EMG was used to differentiate the strength of pain exposure in the Mantoux test and skin prick test. In acute pain in children, physiological correlates of cardiac activity are also informative in the study of childhood distress during nociceptive immunization. This is due to the fact that the neurophysiological mechanisms of interaction are based on the integrative function of stem sympathoactivating structures, in particular, multisensory neurons of the area A5 bridge, as shown in our earlier studies [25]. In the sympathoactivating area A5 bridge, we first identified multisensory neurons that receive, along with other sensory inputs, nociceptive afferent signals that stimulate sympathetic neuronal activity. The result of the integrative function of multisensory sympathoactivating neurons of the area A5 is the regulation of preganglionic sympathetic neurons [25] and, consequently, sympathetic control of cardiac activity and skin electrical activity. This is consistent with studies showing that electrical skin conductance and heart rate in acute pain and anxiety correlate with the degree of pain stimulation in school-aged children [26]. Thus, heart rate remains also the most found method for measuring pain in children [27].

It should be emphasized that under conditions of acute procedural pain in children induced by nociceptive stimuli of different intensities (Mantoux test and skin prick test), electrodermal activity has not been studied to date. In the literature, there are no publications on respiratory physiological correlates of acute procedural pain in children during immunization by the above methods. Thus, there is a report of a study about the respiratory rate which was measured for pain in healthy adults [27]. The relationship between the nociceptive sensory system and the stem mechanisms of heart rate regulation is the source of a biomarker of an integrative physiological correlate of pain in children, including HRV, which reflects the balance of influence of sympathetic and parasympathetic nervous systems on heart rate generation and according to a gender factor in children [28]. It is well known that acute pain is always associated with an increase in sympathetic influences on cardiac activity [29], but the relationship of the response with the gender and age factors of children in acute procedural pain has also not been described in the literature.

1.4 A paradigm for distracting children in pain

Despite its ubiquity, pain is a major unresolved problem for people, families, healthcare providers and society as a whole [18]. Among the many techniques to reduce pain in children, distraction techniques are widely used. These interventions are based on cognitive, behavioral or cognitive-behavioral techniques. These include hypnosis or pain coping skills training. Most known distraction techniques are used to reduce pain or distress in children and adolescents during needle procedures [30]. Methods aimed at changing emotions and behavior during medical procedures that cause acute pain can be a combination of cognitive-behavioral interventions [30, 31] for children and parents [9]. The authors note that clinicians and parents should carefully consider the use of distraction as a pain reduction strategy for children and adolescents during painful medical procedures, such as needle pricks [32]. In doing so, the choice of distraction should be determined by context, the child's preferences and accessibility.

Other traditional means of distracting children during nociceptive stimulation in pediatric practice include books or toys and the presence of parents during nociceptive procedures. That said, the role of parents, as well as behavioral training for children prior to nociceptive medical interventions, is not unequivocally positive and remains an unresolved issue in reducing childhood pain [9, 30, 33–36]. The list of distraction techniques for children during nociceptive medical procedures can be supplemented with techniques such as listening to music, animation, watching videos, interacting with clowns, animals, telling stories or talking about another topic to reduce anxiety, distress and pain in children [26, 30, 37–45]. It has been shown that the anti-pain effect of distraction techniques in children is correlated with the age factor: for example, music as a distraction causes a reduction in pain. However, the antinociceptive effect of music is absent in adolescents under similar experimental conditions [46].

An innovative method of distraction in pediatric practice is virtual reality (VR) [47, 48]. The use of immersive VR technologies has emerged as a potential tool in medicine to distract patients and change their perception of pain. However, according to researchers, the use of VR in clinical practice remains limited [49]. In pediatric practice, the effectiveness of VR to reduce pain and distress has been shown in studies in intravenous needle drips, as well as other diagnostic and medical procedures involving needles [50]. For example, when performing the pediatric skin prick-test, distraction in VR reduces anxiety both before and during this procedure [51]. Overall, the benefit of digital distraction for reducing pain and distress in children over non-digital distraction requires further research [32]. The authors believe that optimal clinical conditions for use should be created to confirm the effectiveness of VR in pediatrics, and such studies should be conducted according to the established guidelines [47].

In our opinion, the numerous variations of distraction for procedural pain in children [31] are likely indicative of the low efficacy of this technique. According to our working hypothesis, a reduction of procedural pain, for example, in the most massively diagnostic Mantoux test, can be achieved using a technique with minimal nociceptive stimulation. Our comparative study was conducted during the performance of the Mantoux test and skin prick test. The Mantoux test is associated with intense nociceptive irritation, but the skin prick test, on the other hand, should be associated with minimal nociceptive irritation of skin receptors in children. The technique of the painful Mantoux test is known to involve intradermal injection of allergen using a syringe [52], while the skin prick test is performed using a tuberculin injection lancet [51, 53, 54]. Therefore, in our study, we assumed a priori that the skin prick test elicits minimal nociceptive stimulus in children during a medical procedure [55–59].

This chapter analyses for the first time the physiological correlates of the Mantoux test and skin prick-test pain in children and presents a paradigm for dealing with acute procedural pediatric pain and distress, which we propose should be based on a method of minimal nociceptive exposure. We have previously highlighted that immunization is the most widely used medical nociceptive intervention worldwide and is among the most common sources of acute pain and distress in children [31]. The development and use of micro-needles or the administration of needle-free substances, such as through sprays into the nasal passages, has been aimed at reducing pain irritation [13]. However, the use of psychological techniques to reduce distress in children during immunization has not been successful [31]. Parental presence during painful medical procedures, including immunization, reduces fear but not pain in children [9]. Therefore, the key aim of our study is to prove the efficacy of using minimal nociceptive stimulation to prevent pediatric procedural pain and distress.

2. Methods

The study of the physiological correlates of pain in children is a complex problem and has ethical and methodological considerations [60, 61]. Seventy-five children (from 3 to 15 years old) participated in our study on the basis of informed parental consent. The study was approved by the Bioethics Committee of Samara State Medical University. A summary of the groups of children is presented in **Table 1**. Children with severe chronic diseases and children registered with a neuropsychologist were excluded. The study of physiological correlates of pain in children was conducted in the course of routine tuberculin diagnostic activities in the medical facility with the participation of qualified medical personnel using the Mantoux test method in a standard dilution of purified tuberculin (2 TE of PPD-L) and the skin prick-test method [53, 54].

Physiological research methods	Boys	Girls	Total	Age
Surface facial EMG	22	23	45	7,57 ± 0,54
Electrodermal activity				
Respiratory rate and amplitude				
ECG				
HRV	14	16	30	
Total	36	39	75	

Table 1.
The physiological research methods and subject groups.

Instrumental support of the study and research procedure. The electrophysiological complex BIOPAC System (USA) was used for data recording in children using surface facial EMG, skin electrical activity, respiratory rate and depth and ECG. The data were analyzed offline, starting with successive transformations of the original signal. HRV was recorded with the device 'ELOX-01 m' (Russia). The study protocol included physiological recordings immediately before and during the children's Mantoux test and skin prick test.

Surface electromyography of facial muscles (EMG). Active electrodes were fixed on the skin in the projection of m.levator labii superioris and the indifferent electrode was fixed on the earlobe. The average power of the integrated EMG and the difference between the maximum and minimum amplitude of the integrated EMG signal were analyzed.

Electrodermal activity (EDA). Electrodes were fixed at the base of the last phalanx of the index and middle fingers of the hand. EDA was measured in delta microsiemens (ΔμS).

Investigation of respiratory rate and depth. The sensor of the device was fixed in the upper zone of the chest by a belt.

Heart rate study. Electrodes for ECG recording were fixed in the second standard lead.

Heart rate variability (HRV) study. The sensor of the device was placed on the distal phalanx of the index finger of the left hand. When registering using this method, the structural unit of the heart rate is the time interval between the highest points of the pulse waves – the NN (NN) interval, an analog of the RR interval of the electrocardiogram. Primary data processing in the ELOGRAPH 3.0 program made it possible to determine the values of 18 heart rate parameters using standard methods [62]. Measured parameters are follows: heart rate; NN mode; the amplitude of the NN mode; standard deviation NN; the square root of the mean squares of the difference of consecutive NN; percentage of consecutive NN pairs differing by more than 50 ms; variation range NN; HRV index; triangular interpolation index of the histogram NN; parameters of the spectrum of NN oscillations (by the method of Fourier transforms) in the range of very low (VLF), low (LF) and high (HF) frequencies, spectrum power (total), parameters of the ratio LF and HF (pLF, pHF and LF/HF); the index of activity of the sympathetic (SYM) and parasympathetic (PAR) divisions of the autonomic nervous system, the index of tension of regulatory systems according to Baevsky (Baevsky index).

Statistical processing of the results. The study data were processed statistically using the SPSS 13.0 software package by parametric and non-parametric methods with a preliminary test of normality using the Kolmogorov-Smirnov test. All results are presented in the form of mean values (M) and their standard error (m), as well as in the form of relative data (deviations in percent from baseline values). Changes in parameters were considered reliable at $p \leq 0.05$.

3. Results

Objectivities of physiological correlates of procedural pain in the Mantoux test and skin prick test were carried out on the basis of analysis of surface facial EMG, EDA, respiratory activity and ECG signals in 45 children (22 boys and 23 girls). During routine diagnostic activities, the Mantoux test and skin prick test were conducted to investigate physiological correlates of procedural pain by the HRV method in 30 children. Overall, the study revealed significant differences in physiological correlates of procedural pain between groups of boys and girls, as well as between methods of execution of noxious tests (**Table 2**).

Measured parameters	Tests	Parameter increase during test execution
Δ power EMG (mV)	Mantoux test	0,045 ± 0,01 ($p < 0.01$)
	Skin prick-test	0,015 ± 0,005 ($p < 0.05$)
Δ EDA (ΔμS)	Mantoux test	1705 ± 0,45 ($p < 0.01$)
	Skin prick-test	1093 ± 0,467 ($p < 0.05$)
Δ Respiratory rate/min-1	Mantoux test	11,12 ± 0,74 ($p < 0.01$)
	Skin prick-test	2,0 ± 0,66 ($p < 0.05$)
Δ Heart rate/min-1	Mantoux test	14,2 ± 3,4, $p < 0.01$)
	Skin prick-test	9,85 ± 3,28 ($p < 0.01$)

Table 2.
Changes in physiological correlates of procedural pain in children during execution diagnostic tests.

3.1 Surface facial EMG

During the Mantoux test, the value of mean EMG power increased relative to the baseline in all children (**Table 2**). In girls, the increase in this parameter was 0.076 ± 0.01 mV ($p < 0.01$) by 76% (0.058 ± 0.01, $p < 0.001$) more than in boys mV (**Figure 1A**). Under the same conditions, the skin prick test in all children was accompanied by an increase in mean EMG power by 0.015 ± 0.005 mV ($p < 0.05$), which was by 67% (0.03 ± 0.007 mV, $p < 0.01$) less than in the Mantoux test. Under these conditions, the increase in this parameter in girls was by 63% (0.014 ± 0.006 mV, $p < 0.01$) more than in boys. Overall, the EMG power gain during the skin prick test in boys and girls was 55% (0.010 ± 0.004 mV, $p < 0.01$) and 71% (0.054 ± 0.019 mV, $p < 0.001$) less than during the Mantoux test, respectively.

3.2 Electrodermal activity

During the Mantoux test in children, the mean signal power of electrodermal activity (EDA) increased relative to baseline (**Table 2**). The increase in this parameter in girls was 2.058 ± 0.52 ΔμS ($p < 0.01$) by 51% (1.057 ± 0.68 ΔμS, $p < 0.001$) more than in boys (**Figure 1B**). During the skin prick test in children, the mean EDA signal power increased by 1.093 ± 0.467 ΔμS ($p < 0.05$) and was by 36% (0.612 ± 0.459 ΔμS, $p < 0.01$) less than during the Mantoux test. At the same time, the boy's group showed no difference in EDA signal power for both types of acute pain exposure. However, the increase in EDA signal power during the skin prick test in girls was 46% (0.944 ± 0.51 ΔμS, $p < 0.01$) less than during the Mantoux test.

The amplitude of the EDA signal was also an informative indicator of the response to acute procedural pain. In all children, the Mantoux test increased this parameter by 8.389 ± 1.78 ΔμS ($p < 0.001$) above baseline. In girls, the increase of this parameter was 8.906 ± 1.78 ΔμS ($p < 0.001$) that was by 17% (1.55 ± 1.56 ΔμS, $p < 0.01$) more than in boys. During the skin prick test, EDA amplitude increased by 3.472 ± 0.85 ΔμS ($p < 0.01$) and was by 59% (4.917 ± 1.32 ΔμS, $p < 0.01$) less than during the Mantoux test. Overall, in boys and girls, the increase in EDA signal amplitude in the skin prick test was by 88% (6.505 ± 2.74 ΔμS, $p < 0.001$) and by 46% (4.123 ± 1.41 ΔμS, $p < 0.01$) less than during the Mantoux test.

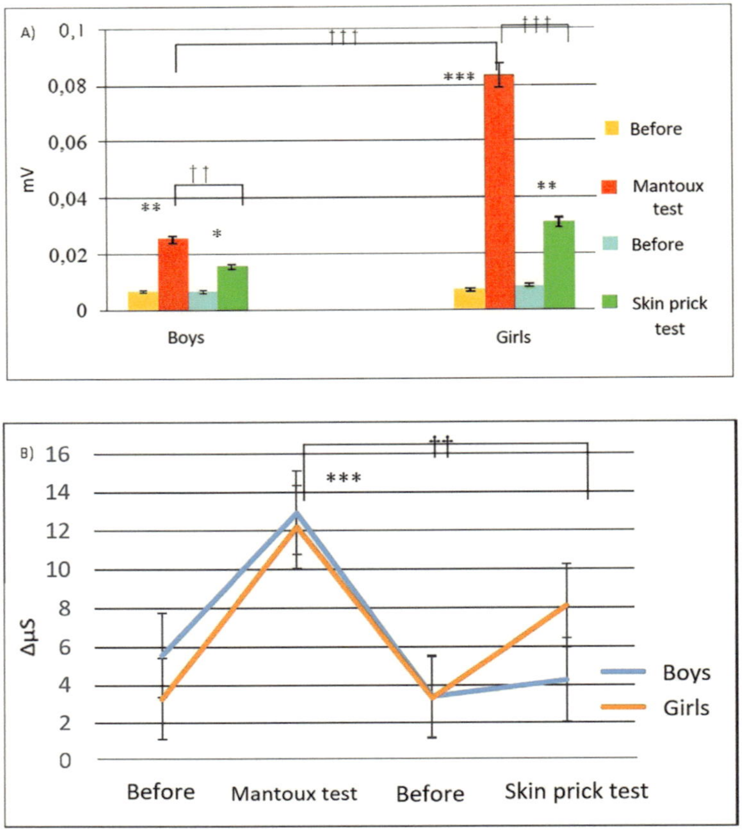

Figure 1.
*Physiological correlates of procedural pain in children during performance of the Mantoux test and skin prick test. A) EMG signal power, B) Skin-galvanic response signal power. Note: Reliability of the change of parameters relative to the background level: *- p <0.05; ** - p <0.01; *** - p <0.001. Reliability of parameter changes between groups and methods of tests accordingly: †† - p <0,01; ††† - p <0,001.*

3.3 Respiratory rate and amplitude

During the Mantoux test, the respiratory rate increased in all children by 44% (11.12 ± 0.74 $мин^{-1}$, $p < 0.01$) relative to the baseline (**Figure 2A**). The response of this parameter was associated with the gender factor. Respiratory rate in girls increased by 43% (11.56 ± 0.80 $мин^{-1}$, $p < 0.001$) and was by 61% (7.0507 ± 0.96 $мин^{-1}$, $p < 0.001$) more than in boys. The respiratory rate increased by 19% (4.5093 ± 1.44 $мин^{-1}$, $p < 0.01$) in boys. During the skin prick test, respiratory rate increased in all children by 8% (2.0 ± 0.66 $мин^{-1}$, $p < 0.05$) relative to baseline, which was by 82% (9.12 ± 0.70 $мин^{-1}$, $p < 0.001$) less than during the Mantoux test. In both boys and girls, respiratory rate increased by 3.01 ± 1.69 $мин^{-1}$ ($p < 0.001$) and 9.78 ± 0.69 $мин^{-1}$ ($p < 0.01$), which was less than during the Mantoux test.

The amplitude of respiratory movements during the Mantoux test increased in all children by 141% ($p < 0.001$) relative to the baseline. At the same time, the increase in respiratory amplitude in boys was 79% ($p < 0.01$), and in girls – 178% ($p < 0,001$). When performing the skin prick test, the increase in respiratory depth relative to baseline in all children was 59% ($p < 0.01$) and 82% ($p < 0.01$) less than in the Mantoux test.

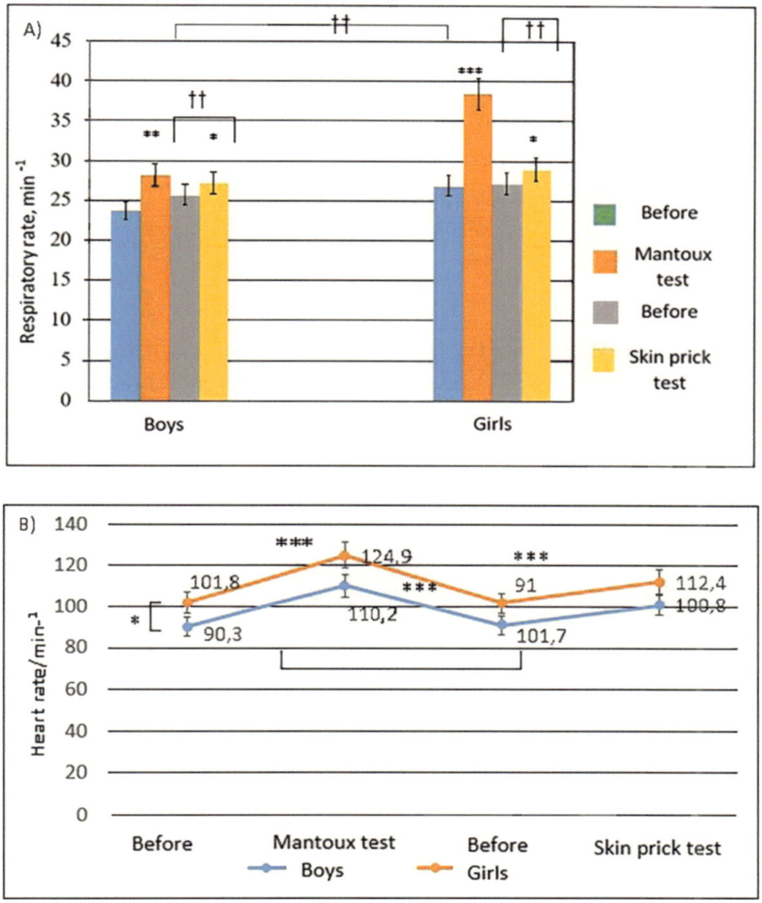

Figure 2.
*Physiological correlates of procedural pain in children during performance of the Mantoux test and skin prick test. A) Respiratory rate, B) Heart rate. Note: Fragment B shows the absolute value of the heart rate. Reliability of the change of parameters relative to the background level: *- p <0.05; ** - p <0.01; *** - p <0.001. Reliability of parameter changes between groups and methods of tests accordingly: †† - p <0,01.*

3.4 Heart rate variability

In our work, heart rate variability in children during the Mantoux test and skin prick test was investigated for the first time. Thirty boys (n = 14) and girls (n = 16) participated in the study (**Table 1**). In this series of studies, the Mantoux test (2TE) and skin prick test were also performed according to the standardized methodology [53, 54].

3.4.1 Mantoux test

HRV in boys and girls increased by 22% (21.7 ± 3.41 beats/min, $p < 0.001$) relative to baseline. Moreover, HRV increased in boys by 19.9 ± 6.13 beats/min ($p < 0.001$) and in girls by 23.2 ± 2.86 beats/min ($p < 0.001$) (**Figure 2B**). Under these conditions, NN50, which shows the number of CI pairs differing from neighboring ones by more than 50 ms and reflects the overall HRV, decreased in all children by 72% (29.5 ± 7.76 c.u., $p < 0.001$) relative to baseline. NN50 decreases in boys and girls by

63% (35.78 ± 14.22 c.u., $p < 0.001$) and 88% (24.0 ± 5.49 c.u, $p < 0.001$) relative to baseline, respectively. Triangular index as a geometric method of HRV estimation decreased in two groups of children by 27% (0.021 ± 0.004 c.u., $p < 0.01$) relative to baseline. Moreover, in boys and girls, the value of the RRti parameter decreases relative to baseline by 31% (0.027 ± 0.007 c.u., $p < 0.01$) and 21% (0.015 ± 0.005 c.u., $p < 0.01$), respectively, and reflects the characteristic tendency of increased sympathetic activity under the conditions of acute procedural pain. The PAR index increases by 29% (3.53 ± 1.12 c.u, $p < 0.01$) under these conditions.

3.4.2 Skin prick test

During the skin prick test in all children, the duration of cardiointerval decreased by 9% (0.058 ± 0.022 s, $p < 0.001$) relative to baseline without statistically significant differences between groups of boys and girls. Under these conditions, the increase in HRV in the skin prick test averaged 10.3 ± 3.06 beats/min ($p < 0.001$) with similar dynamics of the parameter in boys and girls. The parameter NN50 decreases in two groups of children by 66% (19.3 ± 4,46 c.u., $p < 0,001$), also with approximately equal dynamics in boys and girls ($p < 0,001$) relative to baseline. RRti decreased in boys and girls by 11% (0.008 ± 0.003 c.u., $p < 0.001$) and 18% (0.012 ± 0.004 c.u., $p < 0.001$) compared to baseline. HRV allows a multiparametric evaluation of noxious stimulation during the Mantoux test (2TE) and skin prick test (**Table 3**).

Parameter	Gender	Baseline	Mantoux test	Baseline	Skin prick-test
NN50 (ms)	♂	0,701± 0,039	0,578 ± 0,038***	0,691 ± 0,039	0,631± 0,039 ***†††
	♀	0,600± 0,019‡	0,488 ± 0,012***	0,599 ± 0,016	0,543± 0,013 ***†††
SDNN (ms)	♂	0,056± 0,005	0,043 ± 0,006	0,053 ± 0,008	0,051± 0,007
	♀	0,041± 0,004‡	0,045 ± 0,007	0,040 ± 0,003	0,038± 0,004
RRti (units)	♂	0,087± 0,008	0,059 ± 0,006**	0,074 ± 0,009	0,066± 0,005*
	♀	0,069± 0,006	0,055 ± 0,003**	0,066 ± 0,004	0,054± 0,004*
SYM (units)	♂	2,86± 0,62	4,86 ± 1,60	4,14± 0,93	3,14± 0,73††
	♀	4,56± 0,63‡	4,94 ± 0,73	3,88± 0,42	3,50± 0,45

*Note: data are presented in the form of the mean value of the parameter and its standard error (M ± m). ♂- group of boys, ♀- group of girls. NN (ms) – cardiointerval duration; STDNN (ms) – standard deviation of cardiointervals; RRti (c.u.) – triangular index; SYM (c.u.) – sympathetic system activity index; change of parameter relative to baseline: * - p < .05, ** - p < .01, *** - p < .001; between Mantoux test and skin prick-test: † – p < .05, †† – p < .01, ††† – p < .001; between groups - ‡ – p < .05.*

Table 3.
Indicator parameters of HRV response in boys and girls during Mantoux test and skin prick-test.

Investigated feature	Mantoux test Abs. (%)	Skin prick-test Abs. (%)	p ≤ 0,05
Behavioral responses of children	91 (75,8%)	0	p < 0,001
Difficulties for medical personnel	96 (80%)	0	p < 0,001
Execution defects	42 (35%)	0	p < 0,001

Table 4.
Assessment of behavioral reactions of children and medical personnel during the execution the Mantoux test and skin prick-test in a group of children.

Along with the physiological correlates of procedural pain in children during the Mantoux test and skin prick test, the behavioral response of children and medical personnel was assessed (**Table 4**), which showed that the greatest issues occur during the Mantoux test, which also influences on certain number of defects in execution and diagnostic of this test (**Table 4**).

4. Discussion

Pain is subjective and individualized. However, physiological tests make it possible to measure pain [63]. Injections (needle pricks) are the most common cause of procedural pain in children and are distressing for both children and their parents. This is a difficult emotional situation for medical personnel [13]. Anxious behavior of parents during injections significantly affects the psychophysiological state of children and increases the manifestations of distress during nociceptive stimulation [64, 65].

Many techniques for identifying children's pain have been proposed including techniques for assessing pain perception from children's behavior [66]. However, no optimal unified scale has been created for use with all types of pain or a universal scale for children of different ages [19, 67–69].

Our study, given the above, was primarily aimed at identifying several objective physiological correlates (EMG, EDA, respiration, ECG and HRV) of procedural acute pain in children, as this paradigm dominates in the assessment of children's response to acute pain [68]. In the working hypothesis paradigm, we first analyzed the physiological correlates of procedural pain during the Mantoux test and skin prick test. In addition, we have shown in our work that objective resolution of acute procedural pain is related to nociceptive acute medical manipulation in children. Especially since the elimination of acute pain and distress in children remains an urgent problem of pediatrics and phthisiatrics [1, 54, 61, 70],

Second, the analysis of the results shows that the manifestation of the studied physiological correlates of procedural pain in children depends on the intensity of the nociceptive stimulus. Thus, we believe that reducing the intensity of painful stimuli (skin prick test) opens the way for preventing the manifestations of procedural pain and distress in children. Moreover, such a solution to the paradigm of pediatric procedural pain is supported by the diagnostic accuracy of skin prick test results relative to the diagnostic accuracy of Mantoux test results [54].

Third, in our work, we established the dependence of the studied physiological correlates of procedural pain on the factor of children's gender. Although the relationship between the gender factor and the intensity of nociceptive stimulation is described in the literature [71], we established a real trend of decreasing dependence between these factors using the diagnostic skin prick test as an example.

Finally, the study of integrative physiological correlates of pain in children during the Mantoux test and skin prick test is also well illustrated by HRV and actualizes the solution of the working hypothesis of preventing procedural pain in children by minimal and potentially non-painful acute manipulations. HRV is known to reflect the complex balance of regulatory influences of the sympathetic and parasympathetic nervous system on heart rate generation and reliably reflects the relationship between the intensity of nociceptive stimulus, on the one hand, and the factors of gender and age in HRV responses in children on the other [28, 72]. In the paradigm of sympathetic activation during maximal (Mantoux test) and minimal (skin prick test) nociceptive acute procedural medical manipulations, the significant informative potential of HRV in objectifying and addressing pediatric procedural pain has been shown.

5. Conclusion

The chapter presents data on the analysis of multiparametric physiological correlates of procedural pain in children during routine Mantoux test and skin prick testing. On this basis, the authors formulated a paradigm for solving the problem of acute procedural pain and distress in children through the application (development) of methods and techniques with minimal nociceptive effects on the nociceptive system of children. The chapter describes the informative value of the objective assessment of physiological correlates (surface facial EMG, electordermal activity, ECG, respiration and HRV) to measure the intensity of nociceptive exposure and the objective possibility to establish a relationship between nociceptive irritation during the Mantoux test and skin prick-test, on the one hand, and the physiological correlates of procedural pain, a factor of children's gender and age, on the other hand. The study actualizes the development, implementation and validation of antinociceptive manipulations that do not cause acute procedural pain in children, to solve the problem of therapy of children's pain and distress.

Conflict of interest

The authors declare that the research was conducted in the absence of any commercial or financial relationships that could be construed as a potential conflict of interest.

Author details

Vasiliy Pyatin[1*], Elena Borodulina[2], Olga Kozlova[3] and Olga Maslova[4]

1 Neurointerfaces and Neurotechnologies Laboratory of Research Institute of Neurosciences, Samara State Medical University, Samara, Russia

2 Department of Phthisiology and Pulmonology, Samara State Medical University, Samara, Russia

3 Medical University "Reaviz", Samara, Russia

4 Department of Science, Eurasian Technological University, Almaty, Kazakhstan

*Address all correspondence to: pyatin.vf@gmail.com

References

[1] Manion J, Waller MA, Clark T, Massingham JN, Neely GG. Developing modern pain therapies. Frontiers in Neuroscience. 2019;**13**:1370. DOI: 10.3389/fnins.2019.01370

[2] Di Nora A, Sciuto L, Finocchiaro MC, Trobia G, Minardi C, Di Stefano A, et al. Acute pain in children: A reappraisal on the modalities of grade evaluation and on treatment strategies (review). World Academy of Sciences Journal. 2025;**7**:10. DOI: 10.3892/wasj.2024.298

[3] Vogt BA. Pain and emotion interactions in subregions of the cingulate gyrus. Nature Reviews Neuroscience. 2005;**6**(7):533-544. DOI: 10.1038/nrn1704

[4] Tracey I, Mantyh PW. The cerebral signature for pain perception and its modulation Affiliations Expand. Neuron. 2007;**55**(3):377-391. DOI: 10.1016/j.neuron.2007.07.012

[5] Borsook D, Sava S, Becerra L. The pain imaging revolution: Advancing pain into the 21st century. The Neuroscientist. 2010;**16**(2):171-185. DOI: 10.1177/1073858409349902

[6] Fitzgerald M. The development of nociceptive circuits. Nature Reviews. Neuroscience. 2005;**6**:507-520. DOI: 10.1038/nrn1701

[7] Kohut SA, Riddell RP. Does the neonatal facial coding system differentiate between infants experiencing pain-related and non-pain-related distress? The Journal of Pain. 2009;**10**(2):214-220. DOI: 10.1016/j.jpain.2008.08.010

[8] Young KD. Pediatric procedural pain. Annals of Emergency Medicine. 2005;**45**(2):160-171. DOI: 10.1016/j.annemergmed.2004.09.019

[9] McCarthy AM, Kleiber C, Hanrahan K, Zimmerman BM, Westhus N, Allen S. Factors explaining children's responses to intravenous needle insertions. Nursing Research. 2010;**59**(6):407-416. DOI: 10.1097/NNR.0b013e3181f80ed5

[10] Pate JT, Blount RL, Cohen LL, Smith AJ. Childhood medical experience and temperament as predictors of adult functioning in medical situations. Children's Health Care. 1996;**25**(4):281-298. DOI: 10.1207/s15326888chc2504_4

[11] Badali MA, Pillai RR, Craig KD, Giesbrecht K, Chambers CT. Accuracy of children's memory for a novel painful procedureю. Pain Research and Management. 2000;**4**(2):161-168. DOI: 10.1155/2000/705436

[12] Hohmeister J, Kroll A, Wollgarten-Hadamek I, Zohsel K, Demirakça S, Flor H, et al. Cerebral processing of pain in school-aged children with neonatal nociceptive input: An exploratory fMRI study. Pain. 2010;**150**(2):257-267. DOI: 10.1016/j.pain.2010.04.004

[13] Taddio A, Chambers CT, Halperin SA, Ipp M, Lockett D, Rieder MJ, et al. Inadequate pain management during childhood immunizations: The nerve of it. Clinical Therapeutics. 2009;**31**(2):S152-S167. DOI: 1 0.1 016/J.c1lnthera.2009.07.022

[14] Rhudy JL, Meagher MW. Fear and anxiety: Divergent effects on human pain thresholds. Pain. 2000;**84**(1):65-75. DOI: 10.1016/S0304-3959(99)00183-9

[15] Rhudy JL, Meagher MW. Negative affect: Effects on an evaluative

measure of human pain. Pain. 2003;**104**(3):617-626. DOI: 10.1016/S0304-3959(03)00119-2

[16] Keogh E, Cochrane M. Anxiety sensitivity, cognitive biases, and the experience of pain. The Journal of Pain. 2002;**3**(4):320-329. DOI: 10.1054/jpai.2002.125182

[17] Won AS, Bailey J, Bailenson J, Tataru C, Yoon IA, Golianu B. Immersive virtual reality for pediatric pain. Children. 2017;**4**:52. DOI: 10.3390/children4070052

[18] Eccleston C, Fisher E, Howard RF, Slater R, Forgeron P, Palermo TM, et al. Delivering transformative action in paediatric pain: A Lancet Child & Adolescent Health Commission. Lancet Child Adolesc Health. 2020;**5**(1):47-87. DOI: 10.1016/S2352-4642(20)30277-7

[19] Hatfield LA, Ely EA. Measurement of acute pain in infants. Biological Research for Nursing. 2015;**17**(1):100-111. DOI: 10.1177/1099800414531448

[20] Subramaniam SD, Doss B, Chanderasekar LD, Madhavan A, Rosary AM. Scope of physiological and behavioural pain assessment techniques in children—A review. Healthcare Technology Letters. 2018;**5**(4):124-129. DOI: 10.1049/htl.2017.0108

[21] Rutkowska JM, Ghilardi T, Vacaru SV, van Schaik JE, Meyer M, Hunnius S, et al. Optimal processing of surface facial EMG to identify emotional expressions: A data driven approach. Behavior Research Methods. 2024;**56**:7331-7344. DOI: 10.3758/s13428-024-02421-4

[22] Ma C, Wang C, Zhu D, Chen M, Zhang M, He J. The investigation of the relationship between individual pain perception, brain electrical activity, and facial expression based on combined EEG and facial EMG analysis. Journal of Pain Research. 2025;**18**:21-32. DOI: 10.2147/JPR.S477658

[23] Ashraf AB, Lucey S, Cohn JF, Chen T, Ambadar Z, Prkachin KM, et al. The painful face – Pain expression recognition using active appearance models. Image and Vision Computing. 2009;**27**(12):1788-1796. DOI: 10.1016/j.imavis.2009.05.007

[24] Kunz M, Chatelle C, Lautenbacher S, Rainville P. The relation between catastrophizing and facial responsiveness to pain. The Journal of Pain. 2008;**140**(1): 127-134. DOI: 10.1016/j.pain.2008.07.019

[25] Pyatin VF, Tatarnikov VS, Glazkova EN. Activation of neurons of zone A5 of the rat brain upon hypoxic and thermonociceptive stimulation and switching off of the central respiratory generator. Neurophysiology. 2006;**38**(4):253-260. DOI: 10.1007/s11062-006-0054-6

[26] Cohen LL, MacLaren JE, Fortson BL, Friedman A, DeMore M, Lim CS, et al. Randomized clinical trial of distraction for infant immunization pain. Pain. 2006;**125**:165-171. DOI: 10.1016/j.pain.2006.05.01

[27] Korving H, Sterkenburg PS, Barakova EI, Feijs LMG. Physiological measures of acute and chronic pain within different subject groups: A systematic review. Pain Research and Management. 2020;**2020**:9249465. DOI: 10.1155/2020/9249465

[28] Lu Q, Zeltzer LK, Tsao JC, Kim SC, Turk N, Naliboff BD. Heart rate mediation of sex differences in pain tolerance in children. The Journal of Pain. 2005;**118**(1-2):185-193. DOI: 10.1016/j.pain.2005.08.008

[29] Haas K, Lu Q, Evans S, Tsao JCI, Zeltzer LK. Relationship between resting

blood pressure and laboratory-induced pain among healthy children. Gender Medicine. 2011;**8**(6):388-398. DOI: 10.1016/j.genm.2011.07.002

[30] Uman LS, Birnie KA, Noel M, Parker JA, Chambers CT, McGrath PJ, et al. Psychological interventions for needle-related procedural pain and distress in children and adolescents. Cochrane Database of Systematic Reviews. 2013;**10**:CD005179. DOI: 10.1002/14651858.CD005179.pub3

[31] Chambers CT, Taddio A, Uman LS, McMurtry CM, HELPinKIDS Team. Psychological interventions for reducing pain and distress during routine childhood immunizations: A systematic review. Clinical Therapeutics. 2009;**31**(2):S77-S103. DOI: 10.1016/j.clinthera.2009.07.023

[32] Gates M, Hartling L, Shulhan-Kilroy J, MacGregor T, Guitard S, Wingert A, et al. Digital technology distraction for acute pain in children: A meta-analysis. Pediatrics. 2020;**145**(2):e20191139. DOI: 10.1542/peds.2019-1139

[33] Chambers CT, Craig KD, Bennett SM. The impact of maternal behavior on children's pain experiences: An experimental analysis. Journal of Pedtatric Psychology. 2002;**27**(3):293-301. DOI: 10.1093/jpepsy/27.3.293

[34] Taddio A, McMurtry CM, Shah V, Riddell RP, Chambers CT, Noel M. Reducing pain during vaccine injections: Clinical practice guideline. Canadian Medical Association Journal. 2015;**187**(13):975-982. DOI: 10.1503/cmaj.150391

[35] Hyland EJ, D'Cruz R, Harvey JG, Moir J, Parkinson C, Holland AJA. An assessment of early child life therapy pain and anxiety management: A prospective randomized controlled trial. Burns. 2015;**41**(8):1642-1652. DOI: 10.1016/j.burns.2015.05.017

[36] Matziou V, Chrysostomo A, Vlahioti E, Perdikaris P. Parental presence and distraction during painful childhood procedures. British Journal of Nursing. 2013;**22**(8):470-475. DOI: 10.12968/bjon.2013.22.8.470

[37] Yoo H, Kim S, Hur H-K, Kim H-S. The effects of an animation distraction intervention on pain response of preschool children during venipuncture. Applied Nursing Research. 2011;**24**(2):94-100. DOI: 10.1016/j.apnr.2009.03.005

[38] Felluga M, Rabach I, Minute M, Montico M, Giorgi R, Lonciari I, et al. A quasi randomized-controlled trial to evaluate the effectiveness of clown therapy on children's anxiety and pain levels in emergency department. European Journal of Pediatrics. 2016;**175**(5):645-650. DOI: 10.1007/s00431-015-2688-0

[39] Sahiner NC, Bal MD. The effects of three different distraction methods on pain and anxiety in children. Journal of Child Health Care. 2016;**20**(3):277-285. DOI: 10.1016/j.jopan.2014.05.011

[40] Rezai MS, Goudarzian AH, Jafari-Koulaee A, Bagheri-Nesami M. The effect of distraction techniques on the pain of venipuncture in children: A systematic review. Journal of Pediatric Review. 2016;**5**(1):1-11. DOI: 10.17795/jpr-9459

[41] Vagnoli L, Caprilli S, Vernucci C, Zagni S, Mugnai F, Messeri A. Can presence of a dog reduce pain and distress in children during venipuncture? Pain Management Nursing. 2015;**16**(2):89-95. DOI: 10.1016/j.pmn.2014.04.004

[42] Wolyniez I, Rimon A, Scolnik D, Gruber A, Tavor O, Havir E, et al. The effect of a medical clown on pain during intravenous access in the pediatric emergency department: A randomized prospective pilot study. Clinical Pediatrics. 2013;**52**(12):1168-1172. DOI: 10.1177/0009922813502257

[43] Trottier ED, Doré-Bergeron M-J, Chauvin-Kimoff L, Baerg K, Ali S. Managing pain and distress in children undergoing brief diagnostic and therapeutic procedures. Paediatrics and Child Health. 2019;**24**(8):509-521. DOI: 10.1093/pch/pxz026

[44] Goldberg A, Stauber T, Peleg O, Hanuka P, Eshayek L, Confino-Cohen R. Medical clowns ease anxiety and pain perceived by children undergoing allergy prick skin tests. Allergy. 2014;**69**(10):1372-1379. DOI: 10.1111/all.12463

[45] Yinger OS, Gooding LF. A systematic review of music-based interventions for procedural support. Journal of Music Therapy. 2015;**52**(1):1-77. DOI: 10.1093/jmt/thv004

[46] Birnie KA, Chambers CT, Taddi A, McMurtr CM, Noel M, Riddell R, et al. Psychological interventions for vaccine injections in children and adolescents: Systematic review of randomized and quasi-randomized controlled trials. The Clinical Journal of Pain. 2015;**31**(10):S72-S89. DOI: 10.1097/AJP.0000000000000265

[47] Chan E, Foster S, Sambell R, Leong P. Clinical efficacy of virtual reality for acute procedural pain management: A systematic review and meta-analysis. PLoS One. 2018;**13**(7):e0200987. DOI: 10.1371/journal.pone.0200987

[48] Ang SP, Montuori M, Trimba YMN, Patel D, Chen QC. Recent applications of virtual reality for the Management of Pain in burn and pediatric patients. Current Pain and Headache Reports. 2021;**25**:4. DOI: 10.1007/s11916-020-00917-0

[49] Teh JJ, Pascoe DJ, Hafeji S, Parchure R, Koczoski A, Rimmer MP, et al. Efficacy of virtual reality for pain relief in medical procedures: A systematic review and meta-analysis. BMC Medicine. 2024;**22**:64. DOI: 10.1186/s12916-024-03266-6

[50] Gold JI, Kim SH, Kant AJ, Joseph MH, Rizzo AS. Effectiveness of virtual reality for pediatric pain distraction during IV placement. Cyberpsychology & Behavior. 2006;**9**:207-212. DOI: 10.1089/cpb.2006.9.207

[51] Stassart C, Giebels K. Effectiveness of virtual reality for pediatric pain and anxiety management during skin prick testing. Open Journal of Medical Psychology. 2022;**11**:89-102. DOI: 10.4236/ojmp.2022.113007

[52] Zhuang L, Yang L, Li L, Ye Z, Gong W. Mycobacterium tuberculosis: Immune response, biomarkers, and therapeutic intervention. MedComm. 2024;**5**(e419):1-33. DOI: 10.1002/mco2.41

[53] Aksenova VA, Baryshnikova LA. Efficacy of the recombinant tuberculosis allergen for early identification of latent tuberculosis in children and adolescents in general healthcare settings. Voprosy sovremennoi pediatrii—Current Pediatrics. 2015;**14**(3):358-362. DOI: 10.15690/vsp.v14i3.1371

[54] Borodulina EA. Screening for TB infection. State of the problem. Epidemiology and Vaccinal Prevention. 2016;**15**(1):28-33. DOI: 10.31631/2073-3046-2016-15-1-28-33

[55] Carr WW, Martin B, Howard RS, Cox L, Borish L. Comparison of test devices for skin prick testing. The Journal of Allergy and Clinical Immunology. 2005;**116**:341-346. DOI: 10.1016/j.jaci.2005.03.035

[56] Heinzerling L, Mari A, Bergmann K-C, Bresciani M, Burbach G, Darsow U, et al. The skin prick test – European standards. Clinical and Translational Allergy. 2013;**3**(1):3. DOI: 10.1186/2045-7022-3-3

[57] Coop CA, Forester JP. Comparison of pain during skin-prick testing, immunizations, and phlebotomy. Allergy and Asthma Proceedings. 2016;**37**(5):93-97. DOI: 10.2500/aap.2016.37.3961

[58] Svelto C, Matteucci M, Pniov A, Pedotti L. Skin prick test digital imaging system with manual, semiautomatic, and automatic wheal edge detection and area measurement. Multimedia Tools and Applications. 2018;**77**(8):9779-9797. DOI: 10.1007/s11042-018-5823-x

[59] Karaatmaca B, Sahiner UM, Soyer O, Sekerel BE. The impact of skin prick testing on pain perception and anxiety in children and parents. Allergol Immunopathol (Madr). 2021;**49**(2):72-79. DOI: 10.15586/aei.v49i2.68

[60] Kankkunen P, Vehviläinen-Julkunen K, Pietilä AM. Ethical issues in paediatric nontherapeutic pain research. Nursing Ethics. 2002;**9**(1):80-91. DOI: 10.1191/0969733002ne483oa

[61] Van Dijk M, Ceelie I, Tibboel D. Endpoints in pediatric pain studies. European Journal of Clinical Pharmacology. 2011;**67**(1):S61-S66. DOI: 10.1007/s00228-010-0947-6

[62] Baevsky RM, Chernikova AG. Heart rate variability analysis: Physiological foundations and main methods. Cardiometry. 2017;**10**:66-76. DOI: 10.12710/cardiometry.2017.10.6676

[63] Cetinkaya S. Pain Management in Pediatric Nursing. Open Journal of Pediatrics. 2023;**13**:379-393. DOI: 10.4236/ojped.2023.133043

[64] Nader R, Korol C, Craig K. Parental judgments of pain in infants 2, 4, 6 and 12-months exposed to routine immunization injections. Journal of Pain. 2005;**6**(3):S67

[65] Williams AE, Rhudy JL. The influence of conditioned fear on human pain thresholds: Does preparedness play a role? The Journal of Pain. 2007;**8**(7):598-606. DOI: 10.1016/j.jpain.2007.03.004

[66] Cohen LL, Lemanek K, Blount RL, Dahlquist LM, Lim CS, Palermo TM, et al. Evidence-based assessment of pediatric pain. Journal of Pediatric Psychology. 2008;**33**(9):939-955. DOI: 10.1093/jpepsy/jsm103

[67] Stinson JN, Kavanagh T, Yamada J, Gill N, Stevens B. Systematic review of the psychometric properties, interpretability and feasibility of self-report pain intensity measures for use in clinical trials in children and adolescents. Pain. 2006;**125**(1-2):143-157. DOI: 10.1016/j.pain.2006.05.006

[68] Tomlinson D, von Baeyer CL, Stinson JN, Sung L. A systematic review of faces scales for the self-report of pain intensity in children. Pediatrics. 2010;**126**(5):e1168-e1198. DOI: 10.1542/peds.2010-1609

[69] Dufton LM, Dunn M, Slosky LS, Compas BE. Compas self-reported and laboratory-based responses to stress in children with recurrent pain and anxiety. Journal of Pediatric Psychology. 2011;**36**(1):95-105. DOI: 10.1093/jpepsy/jsq070

[70] Twycross A. Managing pain in children: Where to from here? Journal of Clinical Nursing. 2010;**19**(15-16):2090-2099. DOI: 10.1111/j.1365-2702.2010.03271.x

[71] Kunz M, Gruber A, Lautenbacher S. Sex differences in facial encoding of pain. The Journal of Pain. 2006;**7**(12):915-928. DOI: 10.1016/j.jpain.2006.04.012

[72] Tousignant-Laflamme Y, Rainville P, Marchand S. Establishing a link between heart rate and pain in healthy subjects: A gender effect. The Journal of Pain. 2005;**6**(6):341-347. DOI: 10.1016/j.jpain.2005.01.351

Chapter 11

Acceptance and Self-Compassion: Mind-Body Approaches to Psychosomatic Disorders

Engin Büyüköksüz

Abstract

Psychosomatic disorders involve a complex interplay between psychological distress and physical symptoms, often exacerbated by maladaptive cognitive and emotional responses. This chapter explores the role of Acceptance and Commitment Therapy (ACT) and self-compassion as effective mind-body interventions for managing these conditions. ACT fosters psychological flexibility, enabling individuals to accept distressing thoughts and bodily sensations without avoidance while engaging in values-based actions. Self-compassion, on the other hand, helps reduce self-criticism, emotional distress, and maladaptive coping mechanisms by promoting self-kindness, mindfulness, and a sense of shared humanity. Empirical research highlights the efficacy of ACT and self-compassion interventions in reducing symptom distress, anxiety, depression, and functional impairment in individuals with chronic pain and psychosomatic disorders. Clinical applications, including group therapy models, online interventions, and assessment tools, demonstrate their adaptability across different therapeutic settings. By integrating mindfulness, acceptance, and compassion-based strategies, these interventions not only alleviate psychological suffering but also enhance overall well-being. This chapter synthesizes current research, clinical methodologies, and intervention strategies, offering a comprehensive framework for incorporating ACT and self-compassion into treatment approaches for psychosomatic disorders. The findings emphasize the importance of shifting from symptom elimination to values-driven living, providing a holistic and sustainable approach to mental and physical health.

Keywords: acceptance and commitment therapy, self-compassion, psychosomatic disorders, psychological flexibility, mindfulness, chronic pain

1. Introduction

Acceptance and commitment therapy (ACT) reformulates and synthesizes the cognitive-behavioral therapy (CBT) tradition, offering a novel understanding of previously explored therapeutic questions, themes, and areas. It adopts an experimental, principle-based approach, emphasizing sensitivity not only to form but also

IntechOpen

to the context and function of psychological phenomena. Since ACT is grounded in the pragmatic variant of functional contextualism, known as contextual behavioral science, it integrates both direct and didactic strategies alongside experiential and contextual change methodologies [1, 2]. From a broader perspective, ACT is a functional contextual intervention approach rooted in relational frame theory (RFT).

The foundation of functional contextualism lies in "behavior in context." Its fundamental components include focusing on the entirety of an event, sensitivity to the role of context in understanding the nature and function of an event, emphasis on pragmatic truth criteria, and the application of scientific foundations to these pragmatic measures [3, 4]. ACT conceptualizes psychological events as ongoing interactions between the organism and its historically and situationally defined context. When a therapist removes a client's problematic behaviors from their respective contexts, they risk overlooking the nature of the problem and potential solutions [3, 5].

ACT enables individuals to behave flexibly according to present contingencies and opportunities, regardless of whether internal events are desirable, undesirable, or neutral. This emphasis on *psychological flexibility* serves as the underlying model of ACT [6, 7]. Psychological flexibility is defined as the ability to remain fully engaged with the present moment, without unnecessary defense, while persistently pursuing valued goals or modifying behavior based on situational demands (**Figure 1**) [8, 9].

1.1 Psychological inflexibility in ACT

ACT models psychological distress as *psychological inflexibility*, which consists of six dimensions: experiential avoidance, cognitive fusion, lack of present-moment awareness, attachment to a conceptualized self, weakened contact with values, and impulsive or dysfunctional behaviors [6]. The *Hexaflex Model of Psychological Inflexibility* illustrates these dimensions (**Figure 2**).

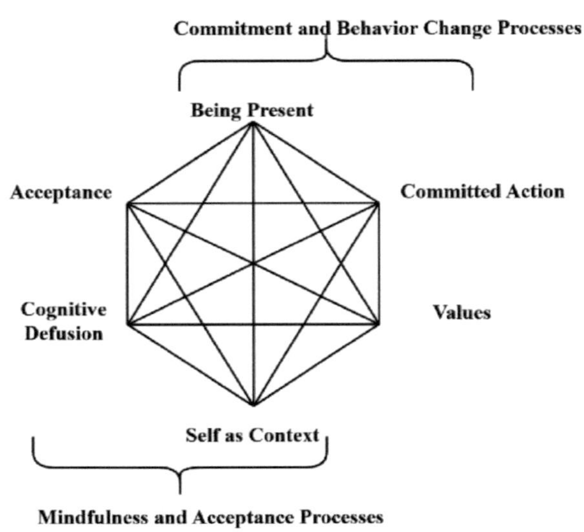

Figure 1.
Psychological flexibility [8].

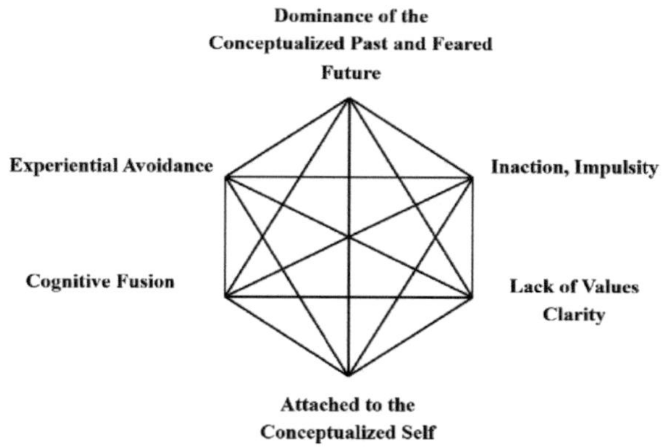

Figure 2.
Psychological inflexibility [8].

Psychological inflexibility arises when inflexibility of psychological reactions dictates actions rather than chosen values and possibilities. This occurs when individuals engage in *cognitive fusion*—the process by which thoughts dominate behavior as if they were literal truths—while simultaneously engaging in *experiential avoidance*—the attempt to suppress or control unwanted internal experiences [3, 10]. From the ACT perspective, these two processes are central to the development and maintenance of psychological distress [11].

1.1.1 Acceptance as an alternative to experiential avoidance

Experiential avoidance occurs when an individual seeks to modify the form, frequency, or context of an aversive psychological experience, despite such attempts leading to actions that contradict personal values and goals [10, 12]. This process has been widely recognized as a pathological mechanism in various therapeutic approaches [3]. Research has linked experiential avoidance to a range of mental health issues, including depression [13, 14], post-traumatic stress disorder [15], anxiety disorders [16, 17], and personality disorders [18, 19].

In contrast, ACT promotes *acceptance*, defined as *a willing, open, and nonjudgmental engagement with one's present experiences, including distressing thoughts, emotions, and bodily sensations* [6, 20]. Acceptance in ACT is not a passive resignation but an active and flexible stance that facilitates goal-directed behavior. This is essential for psychological well-being, as resisting or suppressing emotions often exacerbates distress, while mindful engagement enhances resilience [21].

1.1.2 Cognitive fusion vs. cognitive defusion

ACT distinguishes between *cognitive fusion*—where individuals are entangled with their thoughts—and *cognitive defusion*, which allows individuals to step back and observe their thoughts without becoming dominated by them [6, 22]. Cognitive defusion techniques, such as verbal distancing strategies and mindfulness practices, help individuals see thoughts as transient mental events rather than absolute truths [23]. This shift enables greater psychological flexibility, allowing individuals to behave in ways aligned with their values rather than being dictated by distressing thoughts or emotions [24].

1.1.3 The role of values and committed action

A core component of ACT is *values clarification*, which involves helping individuals identify meaningful life directions and commit to behaviors that align with those values [25]. Unlike traditional cognitive-behavioral models that emphasize symptom reduction, ACT focuses on *building a fulfilling and values-based life*, even in the presence of psychological distress.

2. Self-compassion: Conceptualization, dimensions, and psychological processes

At the beginning of the twenty-first century, Neff [26] introduced the concept of *self-compassion* into psychological science, a notion that has existed for thousands of years within Buddhist philosophy "given that self-compassion is considered analogous to compassion toward others [27]." In her self-compassion model, Neff [26] demonstrated that self-compassion follows a hierarchical structure, ranging from high to low, and consists of three dimensions, each with an opposing pole: *self-kindness vs. self-judgment, common humanity vs. isolation, and mindfulness vs. over-identification*.

Self-compassion is cultivated through *expressing kindness toward oneself, recognizing shared human experiences, and enhancing mindfulness*, which concurrently reduces *self-criticism, isolation, and over-identification with distressing thoughts and emotions* [26]. Neff and Dahm [28] further explicate the dimensions of self-compassion: *Self-kindness* refers to one's ability to respond to personal suffering with warmth and a willingness to alleviate it; *common humanity* reflects the understanding that painful thoughts and emotions are universal rather than uniquely personal; and *mindfulness* involves maintaining a balanced awareness of experiences without becoming engulfed in them, allowing for psychological distance and reflection.

According to Neff [26, 29], the *dimensions of self-compassion* are as follows:

a. *Self-kindness*: Instead of engaging in harsh self-criticism, individuals treat themselves with understanding and care in the face of suffering or failure.

b. *Common humanity*: Contrary to feelings of isolation, individuals recognize that suffering and negative experiences are fundamental aspects of the human condition.

c. *Mindfulness*: A balanced awareness that prevents over-identification with distressing thoughts and emotions, facilitating their acceptance rather than suppression.

Self-compassion is intricately linked to *the degree to which individuals identify with their suffering. Over-identification* occurs when individuals become so absorbed in their emotional responses that they struggle to engage with alternative cognitive appraisals or emotional perspectives. This excessive self-judgment, particularly during experiences of failure or perceived inadequacy, intensifies feelings of isolation and distress. However, as one's *self-concept expands to acknowledge the universality of suffering and disappointment*, distress is mitigated.

2.1 Empirical findings on self-compassion and psychological processes

Over the past two decades, substantial research has explored the relationship between self-compassion and psychological well-being through both *descriptive* [30, 31] and *interventional* [32, 33] studies. Klimecki et al. [34] found a *positive association between self-compassion, mental health, and emotional regulation*, whereas MacBeth and Gumley [35] reported a *negative relationship between self-compassion and psychological distress, with a significant effect size*. Additionally, constructs such as *self-criticism, isolation, and over-identification* have been identified as significant *predictors of psychological distress* [36, 37].

In response to these findings, various *compassion-based interventions* have been developed with the specific aim of fostering self-compassion [38]. Increasingly, self-compassion is recognized as a *key explanatory variable in understanding mental health and psychological resilience*.

A meta-analysis conducted by Zessin et al. [39] identified a *strong positive relationship between self-compassion and well-being*. Notably, *cognitive and psychological well-being exhibited a stronger correlation with self-compassion than emotional well-being*, suggesting that self-compassion has a *causal impact on well-being*. Furthermore, *self-esteem was examined as a potential mediating variable* in this relationship.

Similarly, Marsh et al. [40] explored the relationship between self-compassion and psychological well-being in *adolescents*, analyzing existing literature to estimate the effect size. Their findings indicate *a significant negative association between self-compassion and anxiety, depression, and stress*, demonstrating *a large effect size*.

In another meta-analysis, Ferrari et al. [31] examined the *psychosocial outcomes of self-compassion interventions*, analyzing pretest-posttest and follow-up data from both experimental and control groups. Among 27 studies, *11 reported significant improvements in psychosocial outcomes following self-compassion interventions*. Notably, the impact was most pronounced in *eating behaviors and rumination measures*, while moderate effect sizes were found for *stress, depression, mindfulness, self-criticism, and anxiety*. These findings further support the *efficacy of self-compassion-based interventions across diverse psychological processes and populations*.

3. Clinical implications of ACT

ACT has shown significant efficacy in treating various psychological disorders, including anxiety, depression, chronic pain, substance use disorders, and post-traumatic stress disorder. By targeting psychological inflexibility, ACT helps individuals engage in meaningful activities despite experiencing distressing thoughts and emotions.

ACT is particularly effective in treating anxiety and depression by addressing cognitive fusion and experiential avoidance—two key processes that contribute to emotional distress. In anxiety disorders, ACT helps individuals defuse from catastrophic thoughts and reduce avoidance behaviors, thereby fostering adaptive coping mechanisms. For depression, ACT interventions emphasize values clarification and committed action, helping individuals re-engage in life activities despite persistent low mood and negative thoughts. Studies have shown that ACT produces long-term benefits by enhancing resilience and reducing relapse rates.

One of the most significant clinical applications of ACT is in the management of chronic pain. Traditional pain management approaches focus on symptom reduction, which can reinforce avoidance behaviors and exacerbate suffering. In contrast, ACT encourages individuals to accept pain as a part of life while redirecting their focus toward values-based activities. By fostering psychological flexibility, ACT reduces the emotional distress associated with pain and improves overall functioning. Research indicates that ACT-based interventions can significantly enhance the quality of life for individuals suffering from chronic pain conditions.

ACT has profound implications for psychosomatic disorders, where emotional distress manifests as physical symptoms. Conditions such as irritable bowel syndrome (IBS), fibromyalgia, and tension headaches often have a strong psychological component, exacerbated by stress, emotional suppression, and avoidance behaviors. ACT helps individuals develop acceptance of their bodily sensations without excessive reactivity, reducing the psychological reinforcement of symptoms. By addressing cognitive fusion and increasing mindfulness, ACT enables patients to break the cycle of symptom amplification caused by maladaptive thought patterns.

In psychosomatic conditions, ACT interventions focus on reducing stress-related physiological responses by enhancing present-moment awareness and cognitive defusion. Studies have shown that ACT-based treatments improve pain tolerance, decrease symptom severity, and enhance emotional resilience. By shifting the focus from symptom elimination to values-based living, ACT empowers individuals to regain control over their lives despite ongoing physical discomfort.

ACT promotes psychological flexibility, which is a key determinant of mental well-being. The six core processes of ACT—acceptance, cognitive defusion, present-moment awareness, self-as-context, values, and committed action—help individuals navigate life's challenges more effectively. By fostering mindfulness and reducing the impact of distressing thoughts, ACT enables individuals to respond to difficulties in a way that aligns with their values and long-term goals. This makes ACT a valuable therapeutic approach across diverse clinical settings.

3.1 Clinical assessment tools of ACT

ACT employs various clinical assessment tools to measure key processes such as psychological flexibility, experiential avoidance, cognitive fusion, and values-based action. These tools are integral in both research and clinical practices to assess client progress and treatment efficacy.

Over the past 20 years, researchers have developed measurement scales designed to assess psychological inflexibility in adults, particularly in the wake of the creation of the Acceptance and Action Questionnaire [41]. In parallel with the development and application of ACT, self-report scales interrelate experiential avoidance, cognitive fusion, and mindfulness. For example, the Acceptance and Action Questionnaire-II [12], the Cognitive Fusion Questionnaire [24], the Committed Action Questionnaire [42], the Comprehensive Assessment of Acceptance and Commitment Therapy Processes [43], the Difficulties in Emotion Regulation Scale [44], the Drexel Defusion Scale [23], the Five Facet Mindfulness Questionnaire [45], the Multidimensional Experiential Avoidance Questionnaire [46], the Multidimensional Psychological Flexibility Inventory [47], and the Valuing Questionnaire [48] (see [49], respectively alphabetically).

3.2 The contents of ACT treatment: An 8-session group therapy plan for somatic symptom management

3.2.1 Session 1: Introduction to ACT and psychological flexibility in somatic symptom management

Objectives

- Introduce participants to the principles of ACT in the context of somatic symptom disorders.
- Establish group norms and expectations.
- Define psychological flexibility and its role in coping with physical symptoms.

Key activities:

- Icebreaker activity to build rapport among group members.
- Psychoeducation on ACT: The Hexaflex Model [50] with a focus on bodily distress.
- Experiential exercise: "Passengers on the Bus" metaphor to illustrate cognitive fusion related to somatic symptoms.
- Mindfulness practice: Observing bodily sensations without resistance.

  Homework: Participants track moments of psychological inflexibility related to physical discomfort and its impact on daily life.

Research insights:
ACT has been demonstrated as effective for chronic pain and functional somatic syndromes, such as fibromyalgia and vestibulodynia [51, 52].

3.2.2 Session 2: Understanding cognitive fusion and Defusion for somatic symptoms

Objectives:

- Teach participants about cognitive fusion and its impact on somatic symptom distress.
- Introduce defusion techniques to create psychological distance from distressing bodily sensations.

Key activities:

- Mindfulness practice: Observing bodily sensations without resistance.
- Group discussion on common health-related anxious thoughts and bodily focus.

- Experiential exercise: "Leaves on a Stream" meditation for cognitive defusion from bodily discomfort.
- Role-playing exercise: Practicing defusion techniques when experiencing distressing physical sensations.
- Homework: Apply at least one defusion technique daily and journal its effects.

Research insights:
Studies show ACT can reduce somatic symptom severity by addressing cognitive fusion [53].

3.2.3 Session 3: Exploring acceptance and willingness in the presence of physical discomfort

Objectives

- Differentiate between experiential avoidance and acceptance in relation to somatic symptoms.
- Encourage participants to embrace discomfort without unnecessary struggle.

Key activities:

- Mindfulness practice: Observing bodily sensations without resistance.
- Identifying personal avoidance strategies related to bodily discomfort.
- Experiential exercise: "Struggling in Quicksand" metaphor applied to chronic physical symptoms.
- Homework: Monitor and challenge avoidance behaviors related to pain and discomfort.

Research insights:
ACT interventions improve acceptance and reduce avoidance behaviors in chronic somatic conditions [54].

3.2.4 Session 4: Values clarification and commitment to well-being despite symptoms

Objectives:

- Help participants identify core personal values that are not dictated by symptom reduction.
- Guide them in making values-based commitments despite somatic distress.

Key activities:

- Mindfulness practice: Observing bodily sensations with warmth and self-care.
- Group exercise: Values card sort related to health and well-being.

- Experiential exercise: "The Funeral Speech" to reflect on life priorities beyond symptom focus.
- Homework: Identify three small actions aligned with personal values, independent of physical discomfort.

Research insights:
Engagement in values-based action improves coping with somatic symptoms [50].

3.2.5 Session 5: Committed action - Engaging in life despite symptoms

Objectives:

- Teach strategies for engaging in meaningful activities despite somatic symptoms.
- Psychoeducation: Overview of ACT (Hexaflex Model) and self-compassion (Kristin Neff's model: self-kindness, common humanity, mindfulness).
- Address barriers to committed action.

Key activities:

- Mindfulness practice: Observing bodily sensations with self-kindness.
- Identifying internal and external barriers to action due to physical discomfort.
- Behavioral activation exercise: "Taking Small Steps Toward Change" despite symptoms.
- Homework: Create a weekly action plan incorporating self-compassion in goal-setting.

Research insights:
ACT promotes valued living despite somatic distress [50].

3.2.6 Session 6: Self-as-context and perspective-taking in health narratives

Objectives:

- Explore the concept of self-as-context beyond illness identity.
- Encourage flexible perspective-taking about somatic symptoms.
- Develop a long-term self-compassionate ACT practice for symptom management.

Key activities:

- Mindfulness exercise: Viewing health narratives with a self-compassionate lens.
- Experiential exercise: "The Chessboard Metaphor" applied to somatic experiences.

- Rewriting one's health story with a compassionate and empowering narrative.
- Homework: Practice flexible perspective-taking in daily interactions.

Research insights:
Self-as-context exercises enhance psychological flexibility and reduce distress [55].

3.2.7 Session 7: Psychological flexibility in managing symptoms in relationships

Objectives:

- Apply ACT principles to interpersonal relationships affected by somatic symptoms.
- Address communication barriers through mindfulness and acceptance.

Key activities:

- Self-compassion meditation: Loving-kindness meditation for self and others.
- Role-playing exercise: Communicating symptom-related needs effectively.
- Group discussion on maintaining valued relationships despite health challenges.
- Homework: Apply mindfulness to a challenging relationship.

Research insights:
ACT-based interpersonal flexibility improves emotional regulation and social support [56].

3.2.8 Session 8: Review, integration, and long-term ACT strategies

Objectives:

- Reflect on progress and lessons learned.
- Develop a long-term plan for continued ACT practice in somatic symptom management.
- Address barriers to action with self-kindness.

Key activities:

- Mindfulness exercise: Observing thoughts as external events with self-compassion.
- Group reflection: Sharing key takeaways from the program.

- Goal-setting exercise: Creating a personal ACT commitment plan.
- Experiential exercise: "Looking Back, Looking Forward."

Research insights:
ACT principles maintain long-term well-being in somatic symptom management [51].

3.3 Clinical applications and outcomes of ACT and self-compassion for somatic symptoms

ACT and self-compassion interventions have been increasingly investigated for their efficacy in managing somatic symptoms and chronic pain conditions. The uploaded documents provide extensive empirical support for the effectiveness of ACT and self-compassion in improving psychological flexibility, reducing symptom distress, and enhancing quality of life in individuals with functional somatic syndromes (FSS). Below is a comprehensive synthesis based on the reviewed studies.

3.3.1 Efficacy of ACT for somatic symptoms and chronic pain

Numerous studies have indicated that ACT represents a promising intervention for the management of chronic pain, functional somatic syndromes (FSS), and the psychological distress that often accompanies these conditions. Research has shown that ACT can effectively diminish pain-related interference and emotional distress in individuals suffering from fibromyalgia. A feasibility study focusing on a brief ACT intervention for fibromyalgia revealed moderate enhancements in physical functioning, sleep quality, and emotional well-being [52]. Furthermore, a meta-analysis established that ACT interventions significantly improve pain acceptance, quality of life, and psychological flexibility, yielding long-term advantages for patients with fibromyalgia [56]. Group-based ACT programs, such as AHEAD, designed for adolescents experiencing multiple functional somatic syndromes, have demonstrated notable improvements in illness perceptions, psychological inflexibility, and symptom-related distress [57]. Additionally, internet-based ACT interventions have proven to be a viable and effective alternative to traditional face-to-face therapy, particularly in alleviating pain interference and psychological distress. A systematic review reported moderate-to-large effects in enhancing pain acceptance, emotional regulation, and psychological flexibility [53]. In a randomized controlled trial involving provoked vestibulodynia, online ACT significantly enhanced sexual functioning, pain acceptance, and quality of life when compared to a waitlist control group [51]. Women with vulvodynia who engaged in an ACT-based online intervention experienced increased pain acceptance, decreased distress, and improved sexual satisfaction [54]. Overall, ACT-based interventions have shown effectiveness in alleviating chronic fatigue, depression, and functional impairment among individuals with fibromyalgia and related disorders [58]. The effectiveness of ACT in mitigating repetitive negative thinking (RNT) among individuals with fibromyalgia was substantiated by research that demonstrated notable decreases in symptoms of depression, anxiety, and cognitive fusion [59].

3.3.2 Role of self-compassion in ACT for somatic symptoms

Self-compassion has garnered increasing attention as a vital component in enhancing psychological well-being and managing symptoms in individuals suffering from chronic pain and somatic disorders. It plays a mediating role in the relationship between ACT and the alleviation of distress, anxiety, and depression. Furthermore, self-compassion acts as a protective mechanism against self-criticism and ineffective coping strategies [55]. Research on ACT interventions that emphasize self-compassion has shown improvements in resilience, a decrease in avoidance behaviors, and better emotional regulation among patients with chronic pain [54]. ACT approaches that integrate mindfulness-based self-compassion techniques have yielded significant benefits in lowering emotional distress and enhancing functional adaptation in populations with chronic illnesses [51]. Additionally, Mindfulness-Based Stress Reduction programs that incorporate self-compassion have proven particularly effective in alleviating pain-related disability and anxiety [55].

3.3.3 Key clinical outcomes of ACT and self-compassion interventions

3.3.3.1 Decrease in psychological distress and depression

ACT interventions have been shown to produce notable reductions in depression, anxiety, and psychological distress among individuals suffering from chronic pain and functional somatic syndromes [58]. The incorporation of self-compassion exercises within ACT frameworks has been found to improve emotional regulation and mitigate catastrophizing tendencies [59].

3.3.3.2 Enhancement of pain ACT and functional outcomes

There is a correlation between increased psychological flexibility and pain acceptance with diminished disability and enhanced participation in daily activities [52]. ACT interventions have resulted in fewer medical consultations, better social functioning, and an overall improvement in quality of life [55].

3.3.3.3 Efficacy in adolescents with functional somatic syndromes

Group-based ACT initiatives targeting adolescents with various functional somatic syndromes, such as the AHEAD program, have demonstrated significant advancements in physical health, a reduction in symptom burden, and improved emotional well-being (**Table 1**) [57].

Integrating *ACT* with *self-compassion* techniques offers a promising approach to managing somatic symptom disorders. Research indicates that patients with SSDs often exhibit lower levels of self-compassion compared to the general population, which correlates with increased physical symptoms and reduced quality of life [60]. Studies have demonstrated the effectiveness of ACT in improving psychosomatic symptoms and enhancing mindfulness in patients with psychosomatic disorders [61]. Additionally, self-compassion has been identified as a resilience factor, potentially buffering against mental disorders and aiding in symptom management [60]. Incorporating self-compassion into ACT interventions can address the unique challenges faced by individuals with SSDs. For instance, a study exploring the mediating effects of self-compassion and alexithymia found that enhancing self-compassion through mindfulness-based cognitive therapy significantly reduced psychosomatic distress in SSD patients [62]. By fostering a kinder, more accepting relationship with

Articles	n	Gender	Assessment	Treatment	Control group	Time post-assault
Buhrman et al. [51]	278	Mostly female	Pain acceptance, functional disability, quality of Life	Guided internet-based ACT	Waitlist, treatment as usual	Post-treatment, follow-up (3–12 months)
Eastwood and Godfrey [56]	384	Mostly female	CPAQ, FIQ, depression, anxiety, pain intensity	ACT (online, group, one-to-one)	Waiting list, TAU, active therapy	Post-intervention, follow-up (3–6 months)
Trindade et al. [53]	312	Mixed	Psychological flexibility, values-based action, pain intensity	Online ACT	Waitlist, TAU	Post-treatment, follow-up (3–6 months)

Table 1.
The summary of the meta-analysis studies.

oneself, patients can develop greater psychological flexibility and resilience, leading to improved management of somatic symptoms.

4. Conclusion

This chapter explored the integration of ACT and self-compassion as effective mind-body approaches for managing psychosomatic disorders. ACT, with its emphasis on psychological flexibility, provides individuals with tools to navigate distressing thoughts and physical symptoms without avoidance or excessive control. By fostering acceptance, cognitive defusion, values-based action, and mindfulness, ACT empowers individuals to engage in meaningful life activities despite ongoing challenges.

Similarly, self-compassion plays a crucial role in mitigating distress, reducing self-criticism, and enhancing emotional resilience. By cultivating self-kindness, recognizing shared humanity, and maintaining mindfulness, individuals with chronic pain and somatic symptoms can develop a more adaptive and compassionate relationship with their experiences. Research indicates that self-compassion interventions, particularly when integrated with ACT, contribute to improved psychological well-being, reduced symptom distress, and enhanced overall functioning.

The clinical applications of ACT and self-compassion highlight their efficacy in treating conditions such as fibromyalgia, chronic pain, functional somatic syndromes, and stress-related disorders. Empirical findings suggest that these approaches not only alleviate psychological distress but also promote sustainable well-being by shifting the focus from symptom elimination to valued living. The structured intervention plans and clinical assessment tools reviewed in this chapter further demonstrate the practical applicability of these therapeutic modalities.

In conclusion, ACT and self-compassion provide a robust framework for addressing the complex interplay between psychological and physiological symptoms in psychosomatic disorders. Their integration offers a holistic approach to enhancing mental and physical health, making them valuable components of modern therapeutic interventions. Future research should continue to explore their long-term efficacy and potential for adaptation in diverse clinical settings.

Conflict of interest

The authors declare no conflict of interest.

Author details

Engin Büyüköksüz
Psychological Counseling and Guidance Center, Istanbul Technical University, Istanbul, Turkey

*Address all correspondence to: buyukoksuz@itu.edu.tr

References

[1] Biglan A, Hayes SC. Should the behavioral sciences become more pragmatic? The case for functional contextualism in research on human behavior. Applied and Preventive Psychology. 1996;**5**(1):47-57. DOI: 10.1016/S0962-1849(96)80026-6

[2] Ming S, Gould E, Fiebig JH. Understanding and Applying Relational Frame Theory: Mastering the Foundations of Complex Language in our Work and Lives as Behavior Analysts. Oakland, CA: New Harbinger Publications; 2023

[3] Hayes SC, Wilson KG, Gifford EV, Follette VM, Strosahl K. Experiential avoidance and behavioral disorders: A functional dimensional approach to diagnosis and treatment. Journal of Consulting and Clinical Psychology. 1996;**64**(6):1152-1168. DOI: 10.1037/0022-006X.64.6.1152

[4] Zettle RD, Wilson KG. Progression of ACT. In: Twohig MP, Levin ME, Petersen JM, editors. The Oxford Handbook of Acceptance and Commitment Therapy. New York, NY: Oxford University Press; 2023. pp. 3-24. DOI: 10.1093/oxfordhb/9780197550076.001.0001

[5] Staubitz JL, Staubitz JE, Pollack MS, Haws RA, Hopton M. Effects of an enhanced choice model of skill-based treatment for students with emotional/behavioral disorders. Journal of Applied Behavior Analysis. 2022;**55**(4):1306-1341. DOI: 10.1002/jaba.952

[6] Hayes SC, Strosahl KD, Wilson KG. Acceptance and Commitment Therapy: The Process and Practice of Mindful Change. 2nd ed. New York: Guilford Press; 2012

[7] Ong CW, Ciarrochi J, Hofmann SG, Karekla M, Hayes SC. Through the extended evolutionary meta-model, and what ACT found there: ACT as a process-based therapy. Journal of Contextual Behavioral Science. 2024;**32**:100734. DOI: 10.1016/j.jcbs.2024.100734

[8] Hayes SC, Luoma JB, Bond FW, Masuda A, Lillis J. Acceptance and commitment therapy: Model, processes and outcomes. Behaviour Research and Therapy. 2006;**44**(1):1-25. DOI: 10.1016/j.brat.2005.06.006

[9] Ciarrochi J, Hernández C, Hill D, Ong C, Gloster AT, Levin ME, et al. Process-based therapy: A common ground for understanding and utilizing therapeutic practices. Journal of Psychotherapy Integration. 2024;**34**(3):265-290. DOI: 10.1037/int0000348

[10] Russell LH, Bardeen JR, Clayson KA, Dolan SL, Fergus TA. The closed response style and posttraumatic stress: Examining the interaction between experiential avoidance and cognitive fusion among women experiencing sexual trauma. Psychological Trauma. 2020;**12**(6):627-634. DOI: 10.1037/tra0000580

[11] Hayes SC, Strosahl KD, Bunting K, Twohig M, Wilson KG. What is Acceptance and Commitment Therapy? In: Hayes SC, Strosahl KD, editors. A practical guide to acceptance and commitment therapy. New York: Springer Science & Business Media; 2004. pp. 3-29

[12] Bond FW, Hayes SC, Baer RA, Carpenter KC, Guenole N, Orcutt HK, et al. Preliminary psychometric properties of the acceptance and action questionnaire-II: A revised measure of

psychological flexibility and acceptance. Behavior Therapy. 2011;**42**(4):676-688. DOI: 10.1016/j.beth.2011.03.007

[13] Cribb G, Moulds ML, Carter S. Rumination and experiential avoidance in depression. Behavior Change. 2006;**23**(3):165-176. DOI: 10.1375/bech.23.3.165

[14] Moroz M, Dunkley DM. Self-critical perfectionism, experiential avoidance, and depressive and anxious symptoms over two years: A three-wave longitudinal study. Behaviour Research and Therapy. 2019;**112**:18-27. DOI: 10.1016/j.brat.2018.11.006

[15] Barlow MR, Turow REG, Gerhart J. Trauma appraisals, emotion regulation difficulties, and self-compassion predict posttraumatic stress symptoms following childhood abuse. Child Abuse and Neglect. 2017;**65**:37-47. DOI: 10.1016/j.chiabu.2017.01.006

[16] Bardeen JR, Fergus TA. The interactive effect of cognitive fusion and experiential avoidance on anxiety, depression, stress and posttraumatic stress symptoms. Journal of Contextual Behavioral Science. 2016;**5**(1):1-6. DOI: 10.1016/j.jcbs.2016.02.002

[17] Berman NC, Wheaton MG, McGrath P, Abramowitz JS. Predicting anxiety: The role of experiential avoidance and anxiety sensitivity. Journal of Anxiety Disorders. 2010;**24**(1):109-113. DOI: 10.1016/j.janxdis.2009.09.005

[18] Chapman AL, Specht MW, Cellucci T. Borderline personality disorder and deliberate self-harm: Does experiential avoidance play a role? Suicide and Life-Threatening Behavior. 2005;**35**(4):388-399. DOI: 10.1521/suli.2005.35.4.388

[19] Iverson KM, Follette VM, Pistorello J, Fruzzetti AE. An investigation of experiential avoidance, emotion dysregulation, and distress tolerance in young adult outpatients with borderline personality disorder symptoms. Personality Disorder. 2012;**3**(4):415-422. DOI: 10.1037/a0023703

[20] Chambers R, Stoliker D, Simonsson O. Psychedelic-assisted psychotherapy and mindfulness-based cognitive therapy: Potential synergies. Mindfulness. 2023;**14**(9):2111-2123. DOI: 10.1007/s12671-023-02206-4

[21] Cook D, Hayes SC. Acceptance-based coping and the psychological adjustment of Asian and Caucasian Americans. International Journal of Behavioral Consultation and Therapy. 2010;**6**(3):186-197. DOI: 10.1037/h0100907

[22] Savarimuthu VDP, Joseph DAM, Irulandi M. Emotion regulation through cognitive strategies. In: Ibrahim M, editor. Emotional Regulation - Theory and Application across Clinical Settings. 2024. pp. 1-24. DOI: 10.5772/intechopen.1003516

[23] Forman EM, Herbert JD, Juarascio AS, Yeomans PD, Zebell JA, Goetter EM, et al. The Drexel defusion scale: A new measure of experiential distancing. Journal of Contextual Behavioral Science. 2012;**1**(1-2):55-65. DOI: 10.1016/j.jcbs.2012.09.001

[24] Gillanders DT, Bolderston H, Bond FW, Dempster M, Flaxman PE, Campbell L, et al. The development and initial validation of the cognitive fusion questionnaire. Behavior Therapy. 2014;**45**(1):83-101. DOI: 10.1016/j.beth.2013.09.001

[25] Moran DJ, Bach PA, Batten SV. Committed Action in Practice: A clinician's Guide to Assessing, Planning, and Supporting Change in your

Client. Oakland, CA: New Harbinger Publications; 2018

[26] Neff KD. The development and validation of a scale to measure self-compassion. Self and Identity. 2003;**2**(3):223-250. DOI: 10.1080/15298860309027

[27] Neff KD. Self-compassion and psychological well-being. Constructivism Human Science. 2004;**9**(2):27-37

[28] Neff KD, Dahm KA. Self-compassion: What it is, what it does, and how it relates to mindfulness. In: Ostafin B, Robinson M, Meier B, editors. Handbook of Mindfulness and Self-Regulation. New York: Springer; 2015. pp. 121-137. DOI: 10.1007/978-1-4939-2263-5_10

[29] Neff KD. Self-compassion: An alternative conceptualization of a healthy attitude toward oneself. Self and Identity. 2003;**2**(2):85-101. DOI: 10.1080/15298860309032

[30] Duarte J, Pinto-Gouveia J, Cruz B. Relationships between nurses' empathy, self-compassion and dimensions of professional quality of life: A cross-sectional study. International Journal of Nursing Studies. 2016;**60**:1-11. DOI: 10.1016/j.ijnurstu.2016.02.015

[31] Ferrari M, Hunt C, Harrysunker A, Abbott MJ, Beath AP, Einstein DA. Self-compassion interventions and psychosocial outcomes: A meta-analysis of RCTs. Mindfulness. 2019;**10**(8):1455-1473. DOI: 10.1007/s12671-019-01134-6

[32] Kirschner H, Kuyken W, Wright K, Roberts H, Brejcha C, Karl A. Soothing your heart and feeling connected: A new experimental paradigm to study the benefits of self-compassion. Clinical Psychological Science: A Journal of the Association for Psychological Science. 2019;**7**(3):545-565. DOI: 10.1177/2167702618812438

[33] Mantzios M, Wilson JC. Mindfulness, eating behaviours, and obesity: A review and reflection on current findings. Current Obesity Reports. 2015;**4**(1):141-146. DOI: 10.1007/s13679-014-0131-x

[34] Klimecki OM, Leiberg S, Ricard M, Singer T. Differential pattern of functional brain plasticity after compassion and empathy training. Social Cognitive and Affective Neuroscience. 2014;**9**(6):873-879. DOI: 10.1093/scan/nst060

[35] MacBeth A, Gumley A. Exploring compassion: A meta-analysis of the association between self-compassion and psychopathology. Clinical Psychology Review. 2012;**32**(6):545-552. DOI: 10.1016/j.cpr.2012.06.003

[36] Körner A, Coroiu A, Copeland L, Gomez-Garibello C, Albani C, Zenger M, et al. The role of self-compassion in buffering symptoms of depression in the general population. PLoS One. 2015;**10**(10):e0136598. DOI: 10.1371/journal.pone.0136598

[37] Neff KD. The self-compassion scale is a valid and theoretically coherent measure of self-compassion. Mindfulness. 2016;**7**(1):264-274. DOI: 10.1007/s12671-015-0479-3

[38] Neff KD, Germer CK. A pilot study and randomized controlled trial of the mindful self-compassion program. Journal of Clinical Psychology. 2013;**69**(1):28-44. DOI: 10.1002/jclp.21923

[39] Zessin U, Dickhäuser O, Garbade S. The relationship between self-compassion and well-being: A meta-analysis. Applied Psychology. Health

and Well-Being. 2015;**7**(3):340-364. DOI: 10.1111/aphw.12051

[40] Marsh IC, Chan SW, MacBeth A. Self-compassion and psychological distress in adolescents—A meta-analysis. Mindfulness. 2018;**9**(4):1011-1027. DOI: 10.1007/s12671-017-0850-7

[41] Hayes SC, Strosahl KD, Wilson KG, Bissett RT, Pistorello J, Toarmino D, et al. Measuring experiential avoidance: A preliminary test of a working model. Psychological Record. 2004;**54**:553-578. DOI: 10.1007/BF03395492

[42] McCracken LM. Committed action: An application of the psychological flexibility model to activity patterns in chronic pain. The Journal of Pain. 2013;**14**(8):828-835. DOI: 10.1016/j.jpain.2013.02.009

[43] Francis AW, Dawson DL, Golijani-Moghaddam N. The development and validation of the comprehensive assessment of acceptance and commitment therapy processes (CompACT). Journal of Contextual Behavioral Science. 2016;**5**(3):134-145. DOI: 10.1016/j.jcbs.2016.05.003

[44] Gratz KL, Roemer L. Multidimensional assessment of emotion regulation and dysregulation: Development, factor structure, and initial validation of the difficulties in emotion regulation scale. Journal of Psychopathology and Behavioral Assessment. 2004;**26**:41-54. DOI: 10.1023/B:JOBA.0000007455.08539.94

[45] Baer RA, Smith GT, Hopkins J, Krietemeyer J, Toney L. Using self-report assessment methods to explore facets of mindfulness. Assessment. 2006;**13**(1):27-45. DOI: 10.1177/1073191105283504

[46] Gámez W, Chmielewski M, Kotov R, Ruggero C, Watson D. Development of a measure of experiential avoidance: The multidimensional experiential avoidance questionnaire. Psychological Assessment. 2011;**23**:692-713. DOI: 10.1037/a003447310.1037/a0023242

[47] Rolffs JL, Rogge RD, Wilson KG. Disentangling components of flexibility via the hexaflex model: Development and validation of the multidimensional psychological flexibility inventory (MPFI). Assessment. 2018;**25**(4):458-482. DOI: 10.1177/1073191116645905

[48] Smout M, Davies M, Burns N, Christie A. Development of the valuing questionnaire (VQ). Journal of Contextual Behavioral Science. 2014;**3**(3):164-172. DOI: 10.1016/j.jcbs.2014.06.001

[49] Büyüköksüz E. The Turkish validation of the short form of the avoidance and fusion questionnaire (AFQ-Y8): Factor structure, measurement invariance, and incremental validity. Journal of Contextual Behavioral Science. 2025;**35**:100864. DOI: 10.1016/j.jcbs.2024.100864

[50] Hofmann SG, Asmundson GJ, Hayes SC. The efficacy of acceptance and commitment therapy in emotion regulation: A meta-analytic review. Journal of Contextual Behavioral Science. 2023;**30**:45-56. DOI: 10.1016/j.jcbs.2023.01.005

[51] Buhrman M, Hällström H, Fridén A, Kettis Moden E, Grahn G, Carlfjord M, et al. Guided internet-based acceptance and commitment therapy for provoked vestibulodynia: A randomized controlled trial. European Journal of Pain. 2024;**28**(7):1185-1201. DOI: 10.1002/ejp.2253

[52] Gómez-Pérez MC, García-Palacios A, Castilla D, Zaragozá I, Suso-Ribera C.

Brief acceptance and commitment therapy for fibromyalgia: Feasibility and effectiveness of a replicated single-case design. Pain Research & Management. 2020;**2020**(1):7897268. DOI: 10.1155/2020/7897268

[53] Trindade IA, Guiomar R, Carvalho SA, Duarte J, Lapa T, Menezes P, et al. Efficacy of online-based acceptance and commitment therapy for chronic pain: A systematic review and meta-analysis. The Journal of Pain. 2021;**22**(11):1328-1342. DOI: 10.1016/j.jpain.2021.04.003

[54] Chisari C, McCracken LM, Cruciani F, Moss-Morris R, Scott W. Acceptance and commitment therapy for women living with vulvodynia: A single-case experimental design study of a treatment delivered online. Journal of Contextual Behavioral Science. 2022;**23**:15-30. DOI: 10.1016/j.jcbs.2021.11.003

[55] Villatte JL, Vilardaga R, Villatte M, Vilardaga JCP, Atkins DC, Hayes SC. Acceptance and commitment therapy modules: Differential impact on treatment processes and outcomes. Behaviour Research and Therapy. 2016;**77**:52-61. DOI: 10.1016/j.brat.2015.12.001

[56] Eastwood F, Godfrey E. The efficacy, acceptability and safety of acceptance and commitment therapy for fibromyalgia–a systematic review and meta-analysis. British Journal of Pain. 2024;**18**(3):243-256. DOI: 10.1177/20494637231221451

[57] Akbarian M, Mohammadi Shirmahleh F, Borjali A, Hasanabadi H, Abolghasemi S. Effect of acceptance and commitment therapy on depression, chronic fatigue, and pain intensity in patients with fibromyalgia syndrome: A study with expectancy effect. Internal Medicine Today. 2021;**28**(1):70-85. DOI: 10.32598/hms.28.1.3599.1

[58] Kallesøe KH, Schröder A, Wicksell RK, Preuss T, Jensen JS, Rask CU. Feasibility of group-based acceptance and commitment therapy for adolescents (AHEAD) with multiple functional somatic syndromes: A pilot study. BMC Psychiatry. 2020;**20**:457. DOI: 10.1186/s12888-020-02862-z

[59] López-Palomo LE, Vargas-Nieto JC, Ruiz FJ. Efficacy of acceptance and commitment therapy focused on repetitive negative thinking in fibromyalgia: A randomized multiple-baseline design. Revista de Psicoterapia. 2022;**33**(122):85-104. DOI: 10.33898/rdp.v33i122.1150

[60] Dewsaran-van der Ven C, van Broeckhuysen-Kloth S, Thorsell S, Scholten R, De Gucht V, Geenen R. Self-compassion in somatoform disorder. Psychiatry Research. 2018;**262**:34-39. DOI: 10.1016/j.psychres.2017.12.013

[61] Sayyar Khesmakhi S, Goli F, Omidi A, Scheidt CE, Givehki R. Effectiveness of acceptance and commitment therapy on psychosomatic symptoms and mindfulness in patients with psychosomatic disorders. Practice in Clinical Psychology. 2019;**7**(2):79-86. DOI: 10.32598/jpcp.7.2.79

[62] Xu L, Shi J, Li C. Addressing psychosomatic symptom distress with mindfulness-based cognitive therapy in somatic symptom disorder: Mediating effects of self-compassion and alexithymia. Frontiers in Psychiatry. 2024;**15**:1289872. DOI: 10.3389/fpsyt.2024.1289872

Chapter 12

Neuropsychological Assessments and Neurodegenerative Disorders

Ines Tchienga and Brittany Heavens

Abstract

Neuropsychological assessments are essential for choosing mindfulness-based interventions (MBIs) and clinical treatments for neurodegenerative disorders. These assessments detect cognitive impairment, emotional and behavioral difficulties, and motor impairments, enabling the development of individualized interventions that promote cognitive resilience and emotional regulation. The integration of mindfulness practices, movement-based therapies, biofeedback, manualized psychotherapy, and standard treatment can slow disease progression and enhance the quality of life. In all, this chapter will provide a comprehensive, evidence-based framework for integrating neuropsychological assessments into mind-body interventions and clinical treatments for neurodegenerative disorders, to bridge the gap between neuroscience, psychology, and holistic health. Lastly, the limitations (e.g., lack of standardized protocols, limited large-scale studies, and treatment feasibility) and future directions will also be discussed.

Keywords: neurodegenerative disorder, neuropsychological assessments, dementia, treatment recommendations, holistic health

1. Introduction to neurodegenerative disorders

Neurodegenerative disorders (NDDs) are characterized as chronic, progressive diseases that cause decline over time due to degradation in the structure and function of neurons, consequently leading to death. These disorders primarily affect the brain, spinal cord, and peripheral nerves, resulting in a range of cognitive, motor, and behavioral deficits. Common examples include Alzheimer's disease (AD), Parkinson's disease (PD), Amyotrophic Lateral Sclerosis (ALS), and Multiple Sclerosis (MS). Although they exhibit different clinical features, these disorders frequently share common underlying factors, including abnormal protein accumulation, mitochondrial dysfunction, oxidative stress, inflammation, and synaptic loss. Major contributing elements include genetic predispositions, environmental influences, and aging. With the global life expectancy increasing, the incidence of neurodegenerative disorders is rising, presenting significant challenges for healthcare systems and caregivers. In 2020, over 55 million people worldwide were reported to be living with dementia, and this number is expected to double every 20 years, reaching 82 million in 2030 and

IntechOpen

152 million in 2050 (Alzheimer's Disease International). In the coming years, the most significant increase in dementia prevalence is expected in low and middle-income countries, which shows patterns of increasing cardiovascular disease, hypertension, and diabetes [1]. The distribution of dementia worldwide varies according to cultural and socioeconomic differences among nations. As these conditions are often irreversible and currently lack a cure, early diagnosis, supportive care, and innovative research are essential for enhancing patient outcomes.

2. What characterizes neurodegenerative disorders?

As with most branches of science, root words are used in compounds to express complex processes. Thus, to define neurodegenerative disorders (NDD), it might help to break the term down. "Neuro" is a root word relating to nerves or the nervous system as a whole. For example, the root word neuro combined with the word science (meaning, in short, the systematic study of the world [2] produces the compound word neuroscience (meaning, the systematic study of the nervous system [3]. The next most important term to define would be degeneration. Degeneration is defined as an impairment or decline of physical structure or function [4]. Combined, it follows that neurodegenerative disorders involve a decline in the functioning of the neurons in the central or peripheral nervous systems. More specifically, the term encompasses a group of neurological diseases that are mostly heterogeneous in nature [5]. The principal hallmark of these disorders is that they are "characterized" by neuron loss [6, 7]. Nerve cells progressively lose their function and subsequently die. Eventually, this cell death leads to loss of neural networks that is deleterious to "communicative circuitry" and thus significantly impairing our cognition and behavior [5]. Another shared characteristic is that age is a primary risk factor in developing an NDD [8]. Of the NDDs to be discussed in this chapter, age as the primary risk factor is true for all but one – Huntington's disease. Still, age remains a major factor regarding its progression. That being said, while age is a well-established and empirically supported risk factor for NDD, recent research has suggested that genetics and environmental factors may have comparable influences [6]. This development is instrumental to further understanding these types of disorders since up to 20 years ago the pathogenesis of many NDDs was unknown [9]. Armstrong [10] proposed a hypothesis suggesting that NDDs are associated with multiple risk factors with age being the most important [10]. He further emphasized that NDs are characterized by numerous pathologies and, as Wilson et al. [5] suggested, heterogeneity [5, 10]. Specifically, pathogenic proteins, phenotypes, and neuroanatomical pathways interact differentially for each of these diseases [10]. Despite a general lack of pathogenic understanding, the notion of underlying proteins as a categorization for NDDs has long been in mind as evidenced by research done by [7]. This research suggested a link between NDD and abnormal protein behaviors. To further the argument on pathogenesis, Wilson et al. [5] posited other potential hallmarks, including but not limited to inflammation [11], defects in Deoxyribonucleic acid (DNA) and Ribonucleic acid (RNA), defects in synaptic and neuronal networks, etc. [5]. Wilson et al. [5] also argued that this same pathogenesis underlines the need for multi-targeted treatment of NDD, given that there are currently no cures [5]. The current authors believe that multitargeted therapies, which are only attuned to internal influences, may also prove limited. While the literature for the contribution of environmental factors to NDDs needs further development, recent research suggests facets like environmental pollutants affecting hormones, temperature, lifestyle [11], as well as the environment's role in mental health [12] Moreover, given the lack of cures, current treatments plans that intertwine psychological interventions have proven beneficial [13]. Thus, targeting environmental aspects such as the ones discussed above in addition to pathogenic protein defects, neuro inflammation etc., may provide the best chance of developing a cure down the road.

2.1 Types of neurodegenerative disorders

In the following section, we will cover some of the most common NDDs, their global and national prevalence rates, and their associated cognitive and behavioral manifestations. Globally, according to the World Health Organization, approximately 50 million people are affected by NDDs [14]. In the United States alone, almost 6.5 million of this number have been identified as having an NDD. To date, the most common NDs are Alzheimer's Disease and Parkinson's disease both globally and nationally.

2.1.1 Alzheimer's disease

Alzheimer's Disease (AD) is the most common form of dementia [15] and the most common cause of dementia in people over 65 years old [16]. It is a progressive disease that "results in generalized cerebrocortical dysfunction and dementia" with subsequent deficits in cognitive domains such as executive function, attention, processing speed, and visuospatial skills [17]. In AD, lesions observed in imaging or via autopsy are due to neuron loss associated with neurotic plaques (amyloid) and neurofibrillary tangles (tau) [17].

Outside of age, other potential risk factors include increased cardiovascular risk, diabetes, traumatic brain injuries (TBI), history of major depression, and lower education [17]. That being said, its incidence in the African American populace is twice that of caucasians. Research suggests that this may be highly related to two of the aforementioned risk factors (cardiovascular risk and lower quality education) as well as diminished access to healthcare [17]. Overall, the prevalence in the United is estimated to be approximately 5.7 million [17]. AD is currently the 5th and the 6th leading cause of death in individuals of its incidental age group [17]. It is estimated that most of this is due to complications related to having AD.

2.1.2 Parkinson's disease

Parkinson's Disease (PD) is the second most common neurodegenerative disease [18, 19], affecting approximately 10 million people globally [20]. The Parkinson's Foundation listed nearly one million people in the United States as living with PD [21]. Similar to other NDs, age is the most prominent risk factor [18] as PD mostly affects adults ages 60 and over [20]. Moreover, men are 1.5 times more likely than women to be diagnosed with it due to increased susceptibility among other epidemiological factors [17, 19]. PD is a chronic disease with increasing prevalence and mortality rates. Ben-Slomo et al. [19] proposes that this might be because individuals with PD are "more likely to live with their disease," and then subsequently "die of disease related complications" as the disease progresses [19]. Additionally, contributions such as variations in epidemiological factors across countries of different socioeconomic status (SES) and inevitable interactions with demographic factors should be considered. While research supporting the incidence of PD due to ethnicity is limited, the literature points to industrialization in urbanized countries as creating environmental conditions that increase or at least significantly contribute to susceptibility [20].

The neuron loss associated in PD is observed in substantia nigra [17] which is a part of the basal ganglia. The combination of dopaminergic and GABAergic neurons located there significantly contributes to our ability to control our actions [22]. Thus, PD is primarily known as a movement disorder. Diagnostically, features such as bradykinesia (slowness of movement), rigidity (stiffness and velocity), and rest tremor ("in a limb that is at rest and is suppressed with movement initiation" [17]) are main criteria of PD. Other aspects include the presence of Lewy bodies, depleted dopamine in the striatum, patient response to dopaminergic treatment, and frontal subcortical circuitry dysfunction [17]. However, reliance on these hallmarks alone have been speculated to contribute to late diagnoses of PD indicating the possibility of other symptoms that might predate the average age of presentation. Recent research has pointed to the possibility of non-motor symptoms [18]. These non-motor symptoms *may* predate motor symptoms and are harder to pick up on as diagnostic criteria of PD. In most patients, non-motor symptoms such as "hyposmia, constipation, urinary dysfunction, orthostatic hypotension, memory loss, depression, pain, and sleep disturbances" [18]. Cognition is also a major issue for those diagnosed with PD. "Longitudinal studies have found that 75% or more [of individuals diagnosed with PD] will develop PD overtime [17].

Both cognitive and behavioral symptomatology should be carefully reviewed when entertaining the possibility of someone having PD. Additionally, though age is a significant risk factor, there have been cases of young-onset (prior to 50) as well as juvenile (prior to age 21) [18, 21]. Juvenile PD is thought to be more likely to have a genetic basis [23]. While on the topic of genetics, another neuropathological feature of PD is its sporadicity. Namely, approximately 90% of cases are sporadic while around 10% of cases are found to have had a positive family history [17]. Taken together, it seems as though PD symptomatology is widely heterogeneous in nature. This heterogeneous presentation supports the need for continued exploration of PDs development and progression as well as individualized multitargeted treatments based on that research.

3. Role of neuropsychological assessment in neurodegenerative disorders

Clinical neuropsychology examines the relationship between the brain, cognitive processes, and behavior by investigating how injuries and disorders affect brain function. This field encompasses neurocognitive, neurological, psychiatric, and neurodevelopmental elements [24]. Neuropsychological assessments are essential for evaluating various cognitive areas, as well as behavioral and emotional functioning, aiding in diagnosing and treating neurodegenerative diseases and psychiatric disorders. Additionally, these assessments are often employed for the early detection of cognitive impairments, which helps slow disease progression. Neuropsychological evaluations also play a key role in distinguishing normal age-related changes from different forms of dementia. Studies have shown that Alzheimer's Disease often overlaps with cerebrovascular disease [25]. Furthermore, various types of dementia exhibit specific neuropsychological impairments; thus, understanding these characteristics can facilitate accurate diagnosis and support the customization of approaches for individual patients. As mentioned, clinically sound assessments are necessary to differentiate dementia types, which rely heavily on clinical judgment and experience, given the limitations of neuropsychological assessments, which do not demonstrate strong psychometric properties (e.g., poor sensitivity and specificity).

Mood disorders, such as depression and anxiety, are commonly comorbid with neurodegenerative diseases. Notably, standard psychometric tools may not align precisely with the comprehensive cognitive neuropsychological analysis of deficits. However, understanding the patterns of impairment can serve as a foundation for further investigations into individual patients and for enhancing management and rehabilitation strategies [26–28]. Moreover, greater complexities can also arise if a demented patient presents with a psychiatric condition that also causes cognitive symptoms; a neuropsychological evaluation should be used to clarify overlapping symptoms between the psychiatric condition and neurodegenerative diseases.

A comprehensive neuropsychological battery should examine all cognitive domains as well as emotional and behavioral functioning to accurately identify affected regions due to the neurodegenerative disorder. However, the extensive time requirement makes this process often cumbersome and mentally taxing (e.g., cognitive fatigue, emotional distress, and physical strain) for both the patient and their caregiver. Researchers and clinicians maintain mixed beliefs about using a shorter versus an extensive battery to establish a patient's specific impairment profile [29–32]. Nevertheless, strategies have been suggested to minimize the cognitive and emotional burden caused by prolonged testing. These recommendations include implementing shortened batteries, conducting multiple short testing sessions, employing ecologically valid measures, and incorporating caregiver input to enhance direct testing [33–36]. While these suggestions seem sound, some limitations should also be considered regarding the adaptation, such as accessibility to clinically and culturally appropriate neuropsychological measures. We do not have reliable protocols and tools for assessing dementia in resource-scarce regions. Consequently, this complicates comparisons of results across studies in different centers, hindering research progress, particularly regarding contributions to a common data set for each country worldwide [37]. While our grasp of prevalent neurodegenerative disorders has advanced via neuropsychological assessments and neuroimaging, we must not forget the existing gaps in the literature concerning the relevance of our current measurement tools.

4. Understanding the mind: Body connection - Neurodegenerative disorders

The mind-body connection involves the intricate interplay between our thoughts, emotions, actions, and physical health. This connection is enabled by complex systems, such as the nervous, endocrine, immune systems, and the gut-brain axis. It is vital for sustaining overall health and influences the development and progression of chronic illnesses, including neurodegenerative disorders. As the prevalence of NDD increases, exploring the links between psychological and physiological factors opens new avenues for prevention, treatment, and healing.

4.1 Stress and inflammation

A substantial and expanding body of research has elucidated several mechanisms involved in cellular responses to psychosocial stress and emotional factors [38].

Indeed, Selye was successful in his career-long efforts to promote the importance of stress in physiology and medicine, so that many contemporary theories relating to the etiology of chronic diseases include stress as a precipitating variable [39, 40]. Moreover, stress has recently been shown to play an essential role in the onset of cardiovascular diseases, immunological disorders, and the pathophysiological consequences of normal aging [41, 42]. Furthermore, a body of research has demonstrated that neurodegeneration and stress are connected. For example, recent evidence suggests a linkage between the intensity of the stress response, the rate of age-dependent neurodegeneration, and the individual's life expectancy [43]. Additionally, it has been proposed that an inherent hyperactivity to stressors is linked to a shorter life span and to accelerated age-dependent neurodegeneration [43]. This hyperactive or 'excessive' stress response may be genetically determined or (behaviorally) acquired in early life [44]. Nevertheless, the pathophysiological effects of stress on the nervous system are closely connected with the functions of the hippocampus [45]. The formation of the central nervous system (CNS) is profoundly related to memory performance and is essential in inhibiting fear conditioning in the amygdala. Thus, stress has an impact upon these areas of biological integrity: Stress can contribute to neuronal degeneration in the brain, especially in the hippocampus formation, and here, the release of corticotropin-releasing hormone (CRH) and/or corticosterone (e.g., as part of the stress response) represents a critical precondition [46]. Moreover, it is well documented that prolonged and high stress, fear, and arousal levels commonly induce learning deficits and memory loss [45, 47].

4.2 Immune system dysregulation

The immune system plays a crucial role in protecting the body from infections, injuries, and diseases. Nonetheless, when it is dysregulated, either overactive or underactive, it can lead to chronic inflammation and autoimmunity. There is growing evidence that such dysregulation significantly contributes to the development of NDD. Neurodegenerative disorders are associated with age-dependent deposition of aggregated and misfolded proteins, cognitive disturbances, locomotive dysfunction, and neuronal loss [48]. The amyloid cascade hypothesis in AD cases posits that the primary etiopathological event is beta-amyloid (Aβ) aggregation and deposition, followed by downstream neurotoxicity [49]. A fragment found in senile plaques is generated from the sequential endoproteolytic cleavage of the type I transmembrane glycoprotein, β-amyloid precursor protein (β-APP), by β- and γ-secretases [50]. In other words, accumulating A plaques trigger a dysregulated microglial response, causing chronic inflammatory agents that exacerbate neuronal damage [51]. Inflammation has also been reported in PD, which is the second-most common NDD after Alzheimer's Disease. The histopathological hallmarks of PD are as follows: 1) age-related neurodegeneration of extrapyramidal motor neurons, particularly the loss of dopaminergic neurons of the basal ganglia from the substantia nigra pars compacta (SNpc) to the striatum (caudate and putamen), 2) Lewy bodies formed of intracellular proteinaceous inclusions containing α-synuclein (AS), and 3) chronic neuroinflammation. The third feature is characterized by the presence of activated microglia in the putamen, hippocampus, transentorhinal cortex, cingulate cortex, and temporal cortices of patients, associated with mild astrogliosis and increased numbers of infiltrating lymphocytes [52–54]. For years, the brain was believed to be protected from immune response. However, recent studies have shown that dysregulation in the immune system affects the microglia, the glymphatic systems, and peripheral CNS communication, which are essential factors in NDD. Consequently, this causes compromised immune pathways that can increase the rate of disease progression. As the boundaries between neurology and immunology fade, developing a more cohesive understanding of the neuro-immune axis will be crucial for future research and therapies.

4.3 Microbiome-gut-brain axis

The brain-gut axis refers to the two-way communication pathway between the "big brain" in the skull and the "little brain" (the enteric nervous system) located in the abdomen. For some time, infections of various types have been linked to neurodegenerative disorders. Mention has already been made of the link between Helicobacter pylori and PD [55]; infection with Helicobacter pylori has been associated with impaired levodopa absorption [56] as well as disease severity and progression [57, 58]. Furthermore, although the data are somewhat limited, eradicating H. pylori has resulted in clinical improvement [59, 60]. Given the high prevalence of gastrointestinal dysfunction in PD [61] and the more recent suggestion that the disease process in PD may originate in the gut [62], the microbiota of PD subjects has attracted considerable attention. Not surprisingly, given its high prevalence of gut dysmotility, PD has also been linked to small intestinal bacterial overgrowth [63]. Utilizing molecular techniques to identify bacterial virulence or recognition factors, prior exposure to bacterial infections has also been associated with AD and PD [64, 65]. The emergence of high-throughput sequencing, metagenomics, metabolomics, and similar techniques has transformed research on gut microbiota and its metabolism, with numerous studies already conducted on individuals with PD and AD. Studies in PD have consistently demonstrated a microbial composition that deviates significantly from that of appropriate controls; however, the nature of that deviation has been less consistent. These studies have variably shown a suppression of Prevotellaceae [66, 67] and anti-inflammatory genera such as Blautia, Coprococcus, Roseburia, and Fecalibacterium, alongside an increase of pro-inflammatory Proteobacteria [68], Enterococcaceae, and Enterobacteriaceae, the latter of which is correlated with postural instability and difficulty with gait [69].

Although these human studies typically support the microbiota-gut-brain axis's role in PD and AD, it is essential to recognize their limitations. The sample sizes are usually small, and the study population does not always represent the general disease population. All but one [69] relied on fecal sampling alone, and all were prey to the many factors that may confound any study of the human microbiome in health or disease: diet, medications, and co-morbidity, to mention but a few [70, 71]. In one of the larger studies, Hill-Burns and colleagues attempted to correct for several confounders and were able to define a microbial signature in PD independent of the observed effects of diet, age, and region of residence, gender, and medication [72]. Depression is a common co-morbidity in AD and PD; given the pro-inflammatory phenotype and the altered microbiota signatures associated with depression, per se, it may prove difficult to differentiate the relative contributions of depression and either AD or PD to a given microbial pattern [73, 74]. The interaction between disease mechanisms and the microbiome can be bidirectional; it's important to consider that the disease might influence changes in the microbiota, rather than the reverse [75].

5. Integrating neuropsychological assessment with mind: Body interventions

5.1 Neuropsychological assessment

NP assessments are used to measure an individual's current cognitive and/or academic abilities [76]. They are performance-based and usually administered via a battery in order to capture a range of potential cognitive deficits. The subsequent scoring of the results are based on demographically informed normative data in relation to performance as expected in a given population. A battery guides the collection of data and a person's skills in some or all of the following domains: achievement, attention/concentration, processing speed, visuospatial perception, learning and memory function, language functioning, executive functioning, motor functioning, premorbid functioning, and behavioral/emotional functioning. Interpretively, these results, as dictated by norms, are used to compare the individual to themselves (intraindividual strengths and weaknesses) as well as to the performance of a demographically matched group (interindividual). The individual's current functioning may also be compared against the individual's premorbid functioning and/or prior NP assessment, especially considering the referral question and symptom profile. This information can be used for things like "diagnosis, differential diagnosis, prediction of functional potential, measuring treatment response, and clinical correlation with imaging findings" [76].

5.2 Mind: Body interventions

Mind-body interventions target the relationship and interactions between the brain, body, mind, and behavior [77]. Given NDD's cognitive and behavioral manifestations, these interventions include meditation, yoga, relaxation, biofeedback, tai chi, and qigong, breathing techniques, and hypnosis. Meditation and hypnosis promote health by increasing one's focused attention. Similarly, breathing techniques reduce physiologic responses to stress while improving focused attention. Yoga, biofeedback, tai chi, and qigong help regulate breathing, gentle movement, and balance. One small pilot program found that six out of eight people with PD reported perceiving a physical benefit attributed to tai chi practice, with improved balance being the most frequently reported benefit [78]. Another small uncontrolled study with 17 community-dwelling adults with PD who completed a 5-day, 90-minute/day tai chi class showed a significant pretest-posttest change in three physical performance measures [79]. These preliminary pilot studies warrant larger controlled trials to study the effect of tai chi in people with PD. In a 6-month yoga RCT (n = 69) by Oken and colleagues, participants in the yoga intervention showed significant improvement in measures of fatigue compared to a wait-list control, and this improvement was comparable to that of an exercise control, using a stationary bicycle [80]. MBIs improve memory, attention, and mood in early AD and MCI. Studies have shown that meditation and yoga can increase brain-derived neurotrophic factor levels and reduce hippocampal volume loss [81].

5.3 Integration

Regarding the assessment of the course of degenerative disorders, findings can provide insight into current levels of global cognitive impairments, as is expected with ND. Moreover, these findings can enable the individual, their family, and the medical care team to begin planning for both short-term and long-term care. These plans can and should be highly individualized, based on the individual's current level of functioning, to provide supportive care where necessary while utilizing adaptations and compensatory strategies to maximize their autonomy. Interventions tailored to current areas of deficit can help the individual adapt to the inevitable cognitive and lifestyle changes. Proactivity in this way may also help individuals track their emotional functioning and mitigate some of the more challenging aspects of ND that negatively impact quality of life (QoL). Given our prior discussion on the mind-body connection and its contribution to the development or exacerbation of NDDs, it makes sense that practices that mitigate precipitating factors should be highly integrated into the treatment process. While assessment can measure the extent to which these disorders are worsening, we can use that information to bolster or improve current function through supportive care combined with mind-body interventions.

6. Limitations

Comprehensive neuropsychological assessments require broad measures with appropriate psychometric properties that adequately evaluate cognitive, emotional, and behavioral functioning for patients with NDs. However, some limitations are worth noting. First, NA may not fully capture the cognitive demands of specific cultures, potentially leading to inaccurate assessments. Furthermore, the current measures lack cultural sensitivity due to inherent biases in their content and formats. Second, the cost and availability of NA can pose barriers, especially in resource-limited settings (e.g., rural or underserved areas). Third, some tests lack sufficient normative data, particularly for older adults, making accurate comparisons of individual scores difficult. A greater challenge arises when clinical samples include older adults, a population that receives inadequate research attention. Fourth, some tests have limited sensitivity and specificity, which can affect diagnostic accuracy and lead to inappropriate interventions that may worsen disease progression. Moreover, discrepancies can exist between test scores and an individual's actual functional abilities in daily life. In individuals with severe dementia, some argue that neuropsychological assessments may be ineffective, as these individuals may be unable to participate or provide meaningful information. Additionally, evaluating the severity of cognitive impairment in severe cases to assess functional recovery can be challenging. Although MBIs are beneficial, their applicability also presents some challenges, making it difficult to draw strong conclusions. For example, most studies have smaller sample sizes with less diversity in the population, fewer randomized trials, and less variability in intervention protocols.

7. Conclusions

NP assessment provides sensitive measures of cognitive decline related to ND. The ability to compare an individual's premorbid functioning and current functioning, as well as anticipate functional potential or decline based on both normative data and the specific individual's strengths and weaknesses, is a powerful tool that should be wielded with care and in a manner that prioritizes the patient through a medical team approach. NP can be used to inform research through its use of longitudinal studies of these disorders. It can also be used to psychoeducate through clinical findings the families or the teams providing supportive care to individuals diagnosed with NDDs. Given the wide range of heterogeneity in the neuropathogenesis of NDs, as well as the various cognitive and behavioral manifestations, treatment should be individualized and draw from a range of research-backed interventions. The connection between mind and body allows space for mind-body interventions to be a helpful tool in groups diagnosed with NDs, as well as their caregivers. MBI can help improve the overall QoL, thereby mitigating confounding domains in assessment, such as sleep, stress, and pain. Providing caregivers and patients with activities that are easy, accessible, and sometimes immediately effective in alleviating some of their day-to-day symptoms may lead to better treatment adherence. Nonetheless, more research is required to expand the body of literature on MBI and their effectiveness in groups with NDD.

Author details

Ines Tchienga* and Brittany Heavens
Nova Southeastern University, Fort Lauderdale, Florida, United States

*Address all correspondence to: it212@mynsu.nova.edu

References

[1] Alshahrani M, Sabatini S, Mohan D, Brain J, Pakpahan E, Tang EYH, et al. Dementia risk prediction modelling in low- and middle-income countries: Current state of evidence. Frontiers in Epidemiology. 2024;**4**:1397754. DOI: 10.3389/fepid.2024.1397754

[2] Heintz M. Have you ever wondered what the definition of science is? Materials Today. 2009;**12**:1. DOI: 10.1016/S1369-7021(09)70097-5

[3] About Neuroscience. 2018. Available from: https://www.nichd.nih.gov/health/topics/neuro/conditioninfo [Accessed: March 29, 2025]

[4] Degeneration. n.d. Available from: https://www.merriam-webster.com/dictionary/degeneration [Accessed: March 29, 2025]

[5] Wilson MD, Cookson RM, Van Den Bosch L, Zetterberg H, Holztman MD, Dewatcher I. Hallmarks of neurodegenerative diseases. Cell Press. 2023;**186**:693-714. DOI: 10.1016/j.cell.2022.12.032

[6] Lamptey NLR, Chaulagain B, Trivedi R, Gothwal A, Layek B, Singh J. A review of the common neurodegenerative disorders: Current therapeutic approaches and the potential role of nanotherapeutics. International Journal of Molecular Sciences. 2022;**23**:1-18. DOI: 10.3390/ijms23031851

[7] Jellinger K. Recent advances in our understanding of neurodegeneration. Journal of Neural Transmission. 2009;**116**:1111-1162. DOI: 10.1007/s00702-009-0240-y

[8] Hou Y, Dan X, Babbar M, Wei Y, Hasselbalch GS, Croteau LD, et al. Ageing as a risk factor for neurodegenerative disease. Nature Reviews Neurology. 2019;**15**:565-581. DOI: 10.1038/s41582-019-0244-7

[9] Brown CR, Lockwood HA, Sonawane RB. Neurodegenerative diseases: An overview of environmental risk factors. Environmental Health Perspectives. 2005;**113**(9):1250-1256. DOI: 10.1289/ehp.756

[10] Armstrong R. What causes neurodegenerative disease? Folia Neuropathologica. 2020;**58**(2):93-112. DOI: 10.5114/fn.2020.96707

[11] Giri MP, Banerjee A, Ghosal A, Layek B. Neuroinflammation in neurodegenerative disorders: Current knowledge and therapeutic implications. International Journal of Molecular Sciences. 2024;**25**:1-29. DOI: 10.3390/ijms25073995

[12] Ayeni AE, Aldossary MA, Ayejoto AD, Gbadegesion AL, Alshehri AA, Alfassam AH, et al. Neurodegenerative diseases: Implications of environmental and climatic influences on neurotransmitters and neuronal hormones activities. International Journal of Environmental Research and Public Health. 2022;**19**:1-24. DOI: 10.3390/ijerph191912495

[13] Pinto C, Geraghty AW, McLoughlin C, Pagnini F, Yardley L, Dennison L. Experiences of psychological interventions in neurodegenerative diseases: A systematic review and thematic synthesis. Health Psychology Review. 2022;**17**(3):416-438. DOI: 10.1080/17437199.2022.2073901

[14] Uncovering the Culprits of Neurodegenerative Disorders. 2024.

Available from: https://news.feinberg.northwestern.edu/2024/04/11/uncovering-the-culprits-of-neurodegenerative-disorders/ [Accessed: March 29, 2025]

[15] Wareham KL, Liddlelow AS, Temple S, Benowitz IL, Di Polo A, Wllington C, et al. Solving neurodegeneration: Common mechanisms and strategies for new treatments. Molecular Neurodegeneration. 2022;**17**(23):1-29. DOI: 10.1186/s13024-022-00524-0

[16] Weintraub S. Neuropsychological assessment in dementia diagnosis. Continuum. 2022;**28**(3):781-799. DOI: 10.1212/CON.0000000000001135

[17] Stucky JK, Kirkwood WSM, Donders J, editors. Clinical Neuropsychology Study Guide and Board Review. 2nd ed. New York: Oxford University Press; 2020

[18] Tolosa E, Garrido A, Scholz WS, Poewe W. Challenges in the diagnosis of Parkinson's disease. Lancet Neurology. 2021;**20**(5):385-397. DOI: 10.1016/S1474-4422(21)00030-2

[19] Ben-Slomo Y, Darweeh S, Llibr-Guerra J, Marras C, San Luciano M, Tanner C. The epidemiology of Parkinson's disease. Lancet. 2024;**403**(10423):283-292. DOI: 10.1016/S0140-6736(23)01419-8

[20] Ball N, Teo W, Chandra S, Chapman J. Parkinson's disease and the environment. Frontiers in Neurology. 2019;**218**(10):1-8. DOI: 10.3389/fneur.2019.00218

[21] Statistics: Get Informed about Parkinson's Disease with These Key Numbers. 2025. Available from: https://www.parkinson.org/understanding-parkinsons/statistics [Accessed: April 22, 2025]

[22] Halliday G. Substantia Nigra and Locus Coeruleus. In: Paxinos G, Mai KJ, editors. The Human Nervous System. 2nd ed. Elsevier Inc: Academic Press; 2004. pp. 1349-1366. DOI: 10.1016/B978-0-12-547626-3.X5000-5

[23] Anwar A, Saleem S, Akhtar A, Ashraf S, Ahmed FM. Juvenile Parkinson disease. Cureus. 2019;**11**(8):1-4. DOI: 10.7759/cureus.5409

[24] Benton AL, Sivan AB. Clinical neuropsychology: A brief history. Disease-a-Month. 2007;**53**(3):142-147

[25] Morris RG. The neuropsychology of dementia: Alzheimer's disease and other neurodegenerative disorders. Handbook of the Clinical Psychology of Ageing. 2008;**2**:161-184

[26] Gracey DJ, Morris RG. Neuropsychological assessment of dementia. Psychiatry. 2004;**3**(12):18-22

[27] Morris RG, McKiernan F. Neuropsychological approaches to the assessment of dementia. In: Burns A, Levy R, editors. Dementia. London: Chapman & Hall; 1994. pp. 327-354

[28] Morris RG, Worsley CL, Matthews D. Neuropsychological assessment in older people: Old principles and new directions. Advances in Psychiatric Treatment. 2000;**6**:362-372

[29] Randolph C, Tierney MC, Mohr E, Chase TN. The repeatable battery for the assessment of neuropsychological status (RBANS): A preliminary clinical validation. Journal of Clinical and Experimental Neuropsychology. 2015;**20**(3):310-319. DOI: 10.1076/jcen.20.3.310.823

[30] Jefferson AL, Byerly LK, Vanderhill S, Lambe S. Characterizing functional abilities in individuals with

mild cognitive impairment. Alzheimer's & Dementia. 2011;**7**(5):568-574. DOI: 10.1016/j.jalz.2010.12.004

[31] Ready RE, Ott BR, Grace J. Patient versus informant perspectives of quality of life in mild cognitive impairment and Alzheimer's disease. International Journal of Geriatric Psychiatry. 2001;**19**(3):256-265. DOI: 10.1002/gps.1134

[32] Gomersall SR, Astell AJ, Nygård L. The use of technology in dementia care: Current practice and future directions. Aging & Mental Health. 2015;**19**(3):235-240. DOI: 10.1080/13607863.2014.962004

[33] Lezak MD, Howieson DB, Bigler ED, Tranel D. *Neuropsychological Assessment*. 5th ed. New York: Oxford University Press; 2012

[34] Silverberg ND, Panenka W, Iverson GL. The ecological validity of neuropsychological assessment and functional outcomes in dementia. Archives of Clinical Neuropsychology. 2020;**35**(2):215-227. DOI: 10.1093/arclin/acz058

[35] Schulz R, Martire LM. Family caregiving of persons with dementia: Prevalence, health effects, and support strategies. American Journal of Geriatric Psychiatry. 2004;**12**(3):240-249. DOI: 10.1176/appi.ajgp.12.3.240

[36] Mittelman MS, Haley WE, Clay OJ, Roth DL. Improving caregiver well-being delays nursing home placement of patients with Alzheimer disease. Neurology. 2006;**67**(9):1592-1599. DOI: 10.1212/01.wnl.0000242727.81172.91

[37] Costa A, Bak T, Caffarra P, Caltagirone C, Ceccaldi M, Collette F, et al. The need for harmonisation and innovation of neuropsychological assessment in neurodegenerative dementias in Europe: Consensus document of the joint program for neurodegenerative diseases working group. Alzheimer's Research & Therapy. 2017;*9*:1-15

[38] Muehsam D, Lutgendorf S, Mills PJ, Rickhi B, Chevalier G, Bat N, et al. The embodied mind: A review on functional genomic and neurological correlates of mind-body therapies. Neuroscience & Biobehavioral Reviews. 2017;*73*:165-181

[39] Esch T. Health in stress: Change in the stress concept and its significance for prevention, health and lifestyle. Gesundheitswesen (Bundesverband der Arzte des Offentlichen Gesundheitsdienstes (Germany)). 2002;*64*(2):73-81

[40] Jones F, Bright J, Clow A. Stress: Myth, Theory and Research. New York: Prentice Hall; 2001

[41] Esch T, Stefano GB, Fricchione GL, Benson H. An overview of stress and its impact in immunological diseases. Modern Aspects of Immunobiology. 2002a;*2*(4):187-192

[42] Esch T, Stefano GB, Fricchione GL, Benson H. Stress in cardiovascular diseases. Signature. 2002b;*8*(5):101

[43] Gilad GM, Gilad VH. Strain, stress, neurodegeneration and longevity. Mechanisms of Ageing and Development. 1995;*78*(2):75-83

[44] Habib KE, Gold PW, Chrousos GP. Neuroendocrinology of stress. Endocrinology and Metabolism Clinics. 2001;*30*(3):695-728

[45] Mizoguchi K, Kunishita T, Chui DH, Tabira T. Stress induces neuronal death in the hippocampus of castrated rats. Neuroscience Letters. 1992;*138*(1):157-160

[46] Esch T, Stefano GB, Fricchione GL, Benson H. The role of stress in neurodegenerative diseases and mental disorders. Neuroendocrinology Letters. 2002c;*23*(3):199-208

[47] Joseph R. The neurology of traumatic "dissociative" amnesia: Commentary and literature review. Child Abuse & Neglect. 1999;*23*(8):715-727

[48] Forman MS, Trojanowski JQ, Lee VM. Neurodegenerative diseases: A decade of discoveries paves the way for therapeutic breakthroughs. Nature Medicine. 2004;*10*(10):1055-1063

[49] Hardy J, Allsop D. Amyloid deposition as the central event in the aetiology of Alzheimer's disease. Trends in Pharmacological Sciences. 1991;*12*:383-388

[50] Hardy J, Selkoe DJ. The amyloid hypothesis of Alzheimer's disease: Progress and problems on the road to therapeutics. Science. 2002;*297*(5580):353-356

[51] Heneka MT, Carson MJ, El Khoury J, Landreth GE, Brosseron F, Feinstein DL, et al. Neuroinflammation in Alzheimer's disease. The Lancet Neurology. 2015;*14*(4):388-405

[52] Brochard V, Combadière B, Prigent A, Laouar Y, Perrin A, Beray-Berthat V, et al. Infiltration of CD4+ lymphocytes into the brain contributes to neurodegeneration in a mouse model of Parkinson disease. The Journal of Clinical Investigation. 2009;**119**:182-192

[53] Hirsch EC, Hunot S. Neuroinflammation in Parkinson's disease: A target for neuroprotection? Lancet Neurology. 2009;**8**:382-397

[54] Miklossy J, Doudet DD, Schwab C, Yu S, McGeer EG, McGeer PL. Role of ICAM-1 in persisting inflammation in Parkinson disease and MPTP monkeys. Experimental Neurology. 2006;**197**:275-283

[55] Shen X, Yang H, Wu Y, Zhang D, Jiang H. Meta-analysis: Association of Helicobacter pylori infection with Parkinson's diseases. Helicobacter. 2017;*22*(5):e12398

[56] Pierantozzi M, Pietroiusti A, Sancesario G, Lunardi G, Fedele E, Giacomini P, et al. Reduced L-dopa absorption and increased clinical fluctuations in helicobacter pylori-infected Parkinson's disease patients. Neurological Sciences. 2001;*22*:89-91

[57] Dobbs SM, Dobbs RJ, Weller C, Charlett A, Bjarnason IT, Lawson AJ, et al. Differential effect of *Helicobacter pylori* eradication on time-trends in brady/hypokinesia and rigidity in idiopathic parkinsonism: Report on completion of a randomized, double-blind, placebo-controlled efficacy study. Helicobacter. 2010;*15*(4):279-294

[58] Tan AH, Mahadeva S, Marras C, Thalha AM, Kiew CK, Yeat CM, et al. Helicobacter pylori infection is associated with worse severity of Parkinson's disease. Parkinsonism & Related Disorders. 2015;*21*(3):221-225

[59] Dobbs SM, Dobbs RJ, Weller C, Charlett A, Augustin A, Taylor D, et al. Peripheral aetiopathogenic drivers and mediators of Parkinson's disease and co-morbidities: Role of gastrointestinal microbiota. Journal of Neurovirology. 2016;*22*:22-32

[60] Hashim H, Azmin S, Razlan H, Yahya NW, Tan HJ, Manaf MRA, et al. Eradication of helicobacter pylori infection improves levodopa action, clinical symptoms and quality of life in

patients with Parkinson's disease. PLoS One. 2014;*9*(11):e112330

[61] Mukherjee A, Biswas A, Das SK. Gut dysfunction in Parkinson's disease. World Journal of Gastroenterology. 2016;*22*(25):5742

[62] Perez-Pardo P, Kliest T, Dodiya HB, Broersen LM, Garssen J, Keshavarzian A, et al. The gut-brain axis in Parkinson's disease: Possibilities for food-based therapies. European Journal of Pharmacology. 2017;*817*:86-95

[63] Cassani E, Barichella M, Cancello R, Cavanna F, Iorio L, Cereda E, et al. Increased urinary indoxyl sulfate (indican): New insights into gut dysbiosis in Parkinson's disease. Parkinsonism & Related Disorders. 2015;*21*(4):389-393

[64] Andreadou E, Pantazaki AA, Daniilidou M, Tsolaki M. Rhamnolipids, microbial virulence factors, in Alzheimer's disease. *Journal of Alzheimer's Disease*. 2017;*59*(1):209-222

[65] Goldman SM, Kamel F, Ross GW, Jewell SA, Marras C, Hoppin JA, et al. Peptidoglycan recognition protein genes and risk of Parkinson's disease. Movement Disorders. 2014;*29*(9):1171-1180

[66] Scheperjans F, Aho V, Pereira PA, Koskinen K, Paulin L, Pekkonen E, et al. Gut microbiota are related to Parkinson's disease and clinical phenotype. Movement Disorders. 2015;*30*(3):350-358

[67] Bedarf JR, Hildebrand F, Coelho LP, Sunagawa S, Bahram M, Goeser F, et al. Functional implications of microbial and viral gut metagenome changes in early-stage L-DOPA-naïve Parkinson's disease patients. Genome Medicine. 2017;*9*:1-13

[68] Keshavarzian A, Green SJ, Engen PA, Voigt RM, Naqib A, Forsyth CB, et al. Colonic bacterial composition in Parkinson's disease. Movement Disorders. 2015;*30*(10):1351-1360

[69] Hopfner F, Künstner A, Müller SH, Künzel S, Zeuner KE, Margraf NG, et al. Gut microbiota in Parkinson disease in a northern German cohort. Brain Research. 2017;*1667*:41-45

[70] Quigley EM. Gut microbiome as a clinical tool in gastrointestinal disease management: Are we there yet? Nature Reviews Gastroenterology & Hepatology. 2017a;*14*(5):315-320

[71] Wu GD, Compher C, Chen EZ, Smith SA, Shah RD, Bittinger K, et al. Comparative metabolomics in vegans and omnivores reveal constraints on diet-dependent gut microbiota metabolite production. Gut. 2016;*65*(1):63-72

[72] Hill-Burns EM, Debelius JW, Morton JT, Wissemann WT, Lewis MR, Wallen ZD, et al. Parkinson's disease and Parkinson's disease medications have distinct signatures of the gut microbiome. Movement Disorders. 2017;*32*(5):739-749

[73] Sherwin E, Sandhu KV, Dinan TG, Cryan JF. May the force be with you: The light and dark sides of the microbiota–gut–brain axis in neuropsychiatry. CNS Drugs. 2016;*30*(11):1019-1041

[74] Yu M, Jia H, Zhou C, Yang Y, Zhao Y, Yang M, et al. Variations in gut microbiota and fecal metabolic phenotype associated with depression by 16S rRNA gene sequencing and LC/MS-based metabolomics. Journal of Pharmaceutical and Biomedical Analysis. 2017;*138*:231-239

[75] Quigley EM. Microbiota-brain-gut axis and neurodegenerative diseases. Current Neurology and Neuroscience Reports. 2017b;*17*:1-9

[76] Harvey P. Clinical applications of neuropsychological assessment. Dialogues in Clinical Neuroscience. 2012;**14**(1):91-99. DOI: 10.31887/DCNS.2012.14.1/pharvey

[77] Bo A, Mao W, Lindsey AM. Effects of mind–body interventions on depressive symptoms among older Chinese adults: A systematic review and meta-analysis. International Journal of Geriatric Psychiatry. 2017;**32**(5):509-521. DOI: 10.1002/gps.4688

[78] Li F, Harmer P, McAuley E, Fisher KJ, Duncan TE, Duncan SC. Tai Chi, self-efficacy, and physical function in the elderly. Prevention Science. 2001;*2*:229-239

[79] Wahbeh H, Elsas SM, Oken BS. Mind–body interventions: Applications in neurology. Neurology. 2008;**70**(24):2321-2328

[80] Oken BS, Kishiyama S, Zajdel D, Bourdette D, Carlsen J, Haas M, et al. Randomized controlled trial of yoga and exercise in multiple sclerosis. Neurology. 2004;*62*(11):2058-2064

[81] Lavretsky H et al. A pilot study of yogic meditation for family dementia caregivers with depressive symptoms. International Journal of Geriatric Psychiatry. 2013;**28**(1):57-65